Children and Exercise XI

Proceedings of the Eleventh International Congress
on Pediatric Work Physiology
held in Papendal, The Netherlands
September 1983

International Series on Sport Sciences

Volume 15

Series Editor

Chauncey A. Morehouse, PhD
The Pennsylvania State University
University Park, Pennsylvania, USA

CHILDREN AND EXERCISE XI

Edited by:

Rob A. Binkhorst, PhD
Department of Physiology
University of Nijmengen
Geert Grooteplein Noord 21 a
6525 EZ Nijmegen
The Netherlands

Han C.G. Kemper, PhD
Coronel Laboratory for Occupational and
Environmental Health
University of Amsterdam
Jan Swammerdam Institute
1e Constantijn Huygensstraat 20
1054 BW Amsterdam
The Netherlands

Wim H.M. Saris, MD
Department of Human Biology
University of Limburg
Beeldsnijdersdreef 101
6200 MD Maastricht
The Netherlands

Human Kinetics Publishers, Inc.
Champaign, Illinois 61820

Production Director
Sara Chilton

Copy Editor
John Sauget

Managing Editor
Sue Wilmoth

Typesetters
Aurora Garcia
Sandra Meier
Yvonne Sergent
Angela Snyder

Text Layout
Janet Davenport

Cover Design
Jack Davis

Printed by
Edwards Brothers, Inc.

ISBN
0-87322-019-6

ISSN
0160-0559

Copyright © 1985 by Human Kinetics Publishers, Inc.

All rights reserved. Except for use in a review, the reproduction or utilization of this work in any form or by any electronic, mechanical, or other means, now known or hereafter invented, including xerography, photocopying, and recording, and in any information storage and retrieval system is forbidden without the written permission of the publisher.

Printed in the United States of America.

Human Kinetics Publishers, Inc.
Box 5076, Champaign, Illinois 61820

Contents

Preface   xiii

INTRODUCTORY PAPERS

Exercise in Youth: Investing in a Healthier Future
   Egbart Dekker   1

Risk Indicators for Cardiovascular Disease in Relation
to Physical Activity in Youth
   Henry J. Montoye   3

CIRCULATION

Children With Cardiac Disease and Exercise
   Rolf Mocellin   26

Ventilatory Anaerobic Threshold in Children With Atrial or
Ventricular Septal Defects
   Tony Reybrouck, Maria Weymans, Hugo Stijns,
   and Luc Van der Hauwaert   42

Dynamic Exercise in Children With Sickle Cell Anemia and
Sickle Cell Trait
   Ian C. Balfour, William B. Strong, Wesley Covitz,
   and Bruce S. Alpert   50

Comparison of Nine Exercise Tests Used in Pediatric Cardiology
   Gordon R. Cumming and Steve Langford   58

The Effects of Sprint Running on Cardiac Function During Recovery
in 6- to 11-Year-Old Boys and Girls
   Katsumi Asano and Naka Nakamura   69

RESPIRATION

Children with Lung Disease and Exercise
   Herman J. Neijens   81

Exercise in Postoperative Tricuspid Atresia
Hans U. Wessel, Ronald L. Stout, and Milton H. Paul   93

Spiroergometric Criteria of Patients With Idiopathic Scoliosis:
A Long-Term Study
Hans Stoboy and Bärbel Speierer-Kharazi   100

ANAEROBIC THRESHOLD AND AEROBIC POWER

Anaerobic Threshold in Children
Milos Mácek and Jan Vávra   110

Influence of Age and Sex on the Ventilatory Anaerobic Threshold
in Children
Maria Weymans, Tony Reybrouck, Hugo Stijns, and Jacqueline Knops   114

Development of Anaerobic Capacity in Early and Late Maturing Boys
Donald H. Paterson and David A. Cunningham   119

The Optimization of Endurance Training in Adolescent
Middle-Distance Runners
Georgine Gaisl and Hubert König   129

Effects of Supplemental Physical Activity on Body Composition,
Aerobic and Anaerobic Power in 13-Year-Old Boys
Anthony J. Sargeant, Patricia Dolan, and Adrian Thorne   135

Treadmill Endurance Times, Blood Lactate, and Exercise
Blood Pressures in Normal Children
Gordon R. Cumming, Laverne Hastman, and Joy McCort   140

Reference Values for Aerobic Power of Healthy 4- to 18-Year-Old
Dutch Children: Preliminary Results
*Wim H.M. Saris, Annemieke M. Noordeloos, Bini E.M. Ringnalda,
Martin A. Van't Hof, and Rob A. Binkhorst*   151

Is a Leveling-Off Criterion in Oxygen Uptake a Prerequisite for a
Maximal Performance in Teenagers?
Jan Willem Ritmeester, Han C.G. Kemper, and Robbert Verschuur   161

Max-O_2 Reference Values for Children in Relation to Body Mass
*Rob A. Binkhorst, Martin A. Van 't Hof, Wim H.M. Saris,
and Annemieke Noordeloos*   170

PHYSICAL ACTIVITY, ENERGY EXPENDITURE, AND TRAINING

Spontaneous Physical Activity in Preschool Children
   Miroslav Kucera   175

The Relation Between Physical Activity and Energy Intake of
8- and 13-Year-Old Children in Sweden
   Jan Sunnegardh, Lars-Eric Bratteby, Stig Sjölin, Ulla Hagman, and Anna Hoffstedt   183

Habitual Physical Activity in Dutch Teenagers Measured by
Heart Rate
   Robbert Verschuur and Han C.G. Kemper   194

Physical and Psychological Effects of Physical Training on
Handicapped Children
   Monique H.W. Dresen   203

Work Efficiency of Children During Submaximal Bicycle Exercise
   Klaus Klausen, Birger Rasmussen, Lone K. Glensgaard, and Ole V. Jensen   210

Energy Intake and Energy Expenditure in Top Female Gymnasts
   Marie-Agnes van Erp-Baart, Lilly W.H.M. Fredrix, Rob A. Binkhorst, Tresi C.L. Lavaleye, Peter C.J. Vergouwen, and Wim H.M. Saris   218

LONGITUDINAL STUDIES: EXERCISE AND HABITUAL ACTIVITY

The Organization of Developmental Studies
   Martin A. van 't Hof   224

The Problems of Analyzing Longitudinal Data From the Study
"Growth and Health of Teenagers"
   Han C.G. Kemper, Hans Dekker, Gré Ootjers, Bertheke Post, Jan Willem Ritmeester, Jan Snel, Paul Splinter, Lucienne Storm-van Essen, and Robbert Verschuur   233

Long-Term Studies of Physical Activity in Children—
The Trois Rivières Experience
   Roy J. Shephard   252

Changes in Lung Function, Ball-Handling Skills, and Performance
Measures During Adolescence in Normal School Boys
   David A. Brodie   260

MOTOR PERFORMANCE AND MOTOR LEARNING

Organization and Learning of Movements
Jan J. Denier van der Gon and Marianne H. Vincken — *269*

Motor Performance as Related to Somatotype in Adolescent Boys
Gaston Beunen, Albrecht Claessens, Michel Ostyn, Roland Renson, Jan Simons, and Dirk Van Gerven — *279*

Physical Performance Capacity and Specific Skills in
Young Soccer Players
Jacques Vrijens and Christiaan Van Cauter — *285*

Body Composition, Strength, and Motor Performance
in Undernourished Boys
Robert M. Malina and Bertis B. Little — *293*

Somatotype and Motor Function Changes in Children
Ivan Szmodis, Tamas Szabo, Zsuzsa Temesi, and Maria Rendi — *301*

LOCOMOTOR APPARATUS AND MUSCLE

The Influence of Exercise and Training on the Locomotor System
of Children: A Longitudinal Study of Adolescent Tennis Players
Hans M. Sommer — *308*

A Longitudinal Study of the Locomotor System in Trained Children
Jirina Mácková, Jan Javurek, Milos Mácek, and Jan Vávra — *319*

The Composition of Muscle Fibers in a Group of Adolescents
Mornay P. du Plessis, Paul J. Smit, Louresns A.S. du Plessis, Hennie J. Geyer, Glenda Mathews, and Hennie N.J. Louw — *323*

MISCELLANEOUS

Passive versus Active Exposures to Dry Heat as Methods
of Heat Acclimatization in Young Children
Omri Inbar, Rafi Dotan, Oded Bar-Or, and Bernard Gutin — *329*

Assessment of Biological Development by Anthropometric Variables
Mészáros Janos, Mohácsi Janos, Szasbó Tamas, and Szmodis Ivan — *341*

CHILDREN, EXERCISE, AND TRAINING: POSSIBILITIES AND LIMITATIONS

Some Notes on Physiological and Medical Considerations
for Exercise and Training of Children
Oded Bar-Or   *346*

Long-Term Effects of Excessive Training Procedures
on Young Athletes
Joseph Rutenfranz   *354*

CONGRESS ORGANIZATION

This volume represents the Proceedings of the XIth International Congress on Pediatric Work Physiology, held in Papendal, The Netherlands, in September 1983.

Scientific and Organizing Committee

R.A. Binkhorst, Chairman
H.C.G. Kemper
W.H.M. Saris

Administrative Staff

Miss L. Brouwer
Miss A. Minke
Miss A.M. Noordeloos
Mr. W.J.H. Ijsenbrandt

Sponsors

The Ministry of Welfare, Health and Cultural Affairs	Rijswijk
The Netherlands Asthma Foundation	Leusden
The Netherlands Heart Foundation	's-Gravenhage
The Dutch Dairy Bureau	Rijswijk
Depex B.V.	De Bilt
D.M.V.-Campina	Veghel
Fisons B.V.	Leusden
I.C.I.-Farma B.V.	De Bilt
Medical Fitness Equipment	Maarn
Mijnhardt B.V.	Odijk
Servier B.V.	Zoetermeer
De Vrieseborch	Haarlem
Sportieve protokost - Wander B.V.	Uden

The organizers wish to thank the sponsors who made the symposium financially possible. Our host, the staff of the National Sportscentre, Papendal, contributed very much to the excellent atmosphere of the symposium.

Preface

The subject "Children and Exercise" could be approached with the idea that it is natural for children to exercise, for if they don't, they might experience health problems. In that situation, one should determine what condition the child might contract and how it might be cured. Surely, this diagnostic and curative way of looking at the subject is valuable. There is, however, another possible approach, which is the study of children and exercise from the point of view that physical activity in youth should be optimized so that when the child grows up, activity will be an integral part of life and might contribute to a healthy way of living. This applies not only to the healthy child but also to those children with congenital or acquired physical or mental defects. A study of different aspects of children and exercise is necessary in order to be able to optimize physical activity for different groups of children or the individual child. Several of those aspects were covered in previous symposia on pediatric work physiology. Topics during this symposium were, for example, the cardiorespiratory system, maximal aerobic and anaerobic performance, learning of movements, motor performance, daily physical activity and the locomotor system. Special sessions were dedicated to the design, analysis, and results of longitudinal studies on the effects of exercise and training and to the possibilities and limitations for children who train and exercise strenuously at an early age. The discussion papers for this last session are also included in the Proceedings as they were presented. The editors are convinced that these papers will contribute to valuable discussions in groups that are concerned with children, exercise, training, and sport. These include but are not limited to the children themselves, the parents, pediatricians, teachers of physical education, trainers and coaches, sport physicians, and so forth. These discussions might contribute to an approach to exercise and sports by children that will improve their health, both now and in the future.

R.A. Binkhorst
H.C.G. Kemper
W.H.M. Saris

Exercise in Youth: Investing in a Healthier Future

Egbart Dekker
The Netherlands Heart Foundation
Den Haag, The Netherlands

It is my privilege to welcome you to the 11th Symposium on Pediatric Work Physiology. The title stresses the preoccupation not only with the health, but with the healing and perhaps the preventive aspects of physical exercise and sports. Sports and exercise can, of course, be viewed from a much broader aspect. Humans were made to move and to play. The passive enjoyment of the competitive play of others is also built into our genes. We have a record of its popularity from the dawn of Western history. The first records of the victors on the holy fields of Olympia marked the beginning of the Greek calendar. Furthermore, the Roman emperors knew that the stability of the state depended on the staging of spectacles of several forms of competition. We find examples like these in almost all primitive cultures, often having a profound religious meaning linked with the survival of the population. Sociologists have argued that this is intimately related to ritualizing our one most dangerous innate tendency: intraspecies aggression. Linked with those large scale tribal contests were mass festivites in which the victors were hailed, and food and drink and the use of psychoactive drugs—alcohol and tobacco, among others—played a conspicuous role.

The health aspects of sports in youth have dimensions far broader than those of its physiological consequences per se. They are imbedded in a culture—they are part of a subculture that has consequences for the health and life styles of the coming generations. The sports environment, aglow with its mythical young heroes, is an anvil on which many of the tastes, values, and habits of future generations are forged. But who directs the hammer? If industry did not try to grasp it, it would not know its business. I don't blame it. But who else?

The medical community and sports physiologists as are gathered here today perhaps might be the persons to formulate explicit statements concerning the goals to which the community should strive in sports. Are the simple fun of it and its other psychological values sufficient justification for the expenditures, or is there indeed a more narrowly defined health implication?

It is almost axiomatic that sports are good for you. I happen to share that view. However, this firm conviction may have impeded well controlled experimental research that in other fields have been found a prerequisite for well-founded judgments. Instead, to a great extent we have relied on nonexperimental observations. With comparative ease these bring to light some negative aspects such as the 23% cumulative incidence of sports injuries per year in active sports participants, totaling 500,000 cases per year and contributing about 10 million days of sick leave in a population of 14 million in the Netherlands. The palpable mortal danger of some sports like motor racing or mountain climbing is part of the challenge, and the victory over death is part of the triumph. These risks are consciously accepted and are part of the attraction to both performers and the public alike and are, therefore, perhaps well worth taking.

But certainly those who engage in jogging and similar forms of strenuous exercise are not lured into these activities by the thrill of the danger of sudden death. Yet in some categories of age and exertion, the relative risk of sudden death during exercise may run up to 60 times that during everyday activities, as Vuori has calculated. It would be comforting if we had definite assurance that the risk is balanced by a preventive effect. Because the appreciation for the bliss of physical fitness is by no means universal among humans, progress in this field has been so slow that high drop-out rates have interfered with experimental intervention studies. Those who opt to discontinue physical exercise, therefore, are incomparable to those who participate. Inference about causality from such nonexperimental work is hazardous. We do not yet know for certain whether exercise prolongs life or whether those people fit for longevity exercise more.

Perhaps Miettinen's suggestion may help. If it were possible to set up a registry of people who have to quit sports because of a sports injury, and if they could be followed up for the occurrences of myocardial infarction resulting in sudden death, then using their more fortunate colleagues as a control, we might gain some insight.

Trusting that sports may be preventive, I have three other wishes to direct to the scientific community and perhaps to this audience: First, scientists must agree on some international standard to measure fitness at different ages in different countries and in different centuries so that we may validly compare and know what is happening here and abroad both now and in the future.

Second, physical education must be given in order to build regular exercise into the lifestyle of our youngsters instead of creating too much fascination with the spectator sports from which people withdraw at an early age. There is no virtue in the prevention of myocardial infarctions in children. Those occur at a later age.

Finally, sports medicine, as a supporter of health, must give proper attention to the importance of the other risk factors related to the lifestyles of those who are engaged in sports and of the huge crowds who watch them. Only if the overall lifestyles in sports are sound will the subculture contribute to the health of the nation. Physical exercise alone will not do the trick. Teaching children the skills of spectator sports will not notably increase lifespan.

These are the reflections I would like to leave with you at the beginning of this symposium.

Risk Indicators for Cardiovascular Disease in Relation to Physical Activity in Youth

Henry J. Montoye
University of Wisconsin, Madison, U.S.A.
Madison, Wisconsin USA

Coronary heart disease (CHD) and the underlying pathology, atherosclerosis, is now recognized as a pediatric problem. Many years ago, fatty streaks in the aortas of children were reported (Albert, 1939; Klotz & Manning, 1911; Zeek, 1930; Zinserling, 1925), but these observations went mostly unnoticed. Recent interest has confirmed and extended these observations (Strong & McGill, 1969). Probably the most comprehensive data were those collected under the International Atherosclerosis Project in which 23,000 sets of coronary arteries and aortas of subjects from 14 countries were analyzed (McGill, 1968). From these data it appears that fatty streaks are present by age 3 in the aortas of almost all children, regardless of geographical area. In the coronary arteries, fatty streaks are rare before age 10 but are frequent thereafter. There is a question whether the fatty streaks in the aortas of infants are of importance, but the presence of fatty streaks in the coronary arteries in children is correlated with the incidence of the raised lesions in middle age (McGill, 1969). The interest in childhood development of atherosclerosis was probably stimulated by the high percentage of advanced atherosclerosis in young men in the United States (Enos, Beyer, & Holmes, 1953; Glantz & Stembridge, 1959; McNamara, Molot, Stremple, & Cutting, 1971; Rigal, Lovell, & Townsend, 1960).

When it became apparent that it might be helpful to study children in order to reduce heart disease in adults, descriptive studies of risk factors in children appeared. Space does not permit a review of these studies, but there have been many. For example, Berenson (1980, p. 14) summarizes 15 studies of serum cholesterol in pediatric populations in nine countries in the world. It is interesting to note that the lowest concentration of cholesterol in the blood was that of the Tarahumara, a tribe of Indians who are known for their physical activity and leanness. Similarly, Knuiman and Hautvast (1980) of the Netherlands reported the results of measuring serum total and HDL-cholesterol in 7- and 8-year-olds from 16 countries, and Saris (1982) compared data on Dutch children with those of other children. Probably the largest of such studies of children in the United States are those in Bogalusa, Louisiana, (Frerichs, Srinivasan, Webber, & Berenson, 1976) and in Muscatine, Iowa, (Lauer, Connor, Leaverton, Reiter, & Clarke, 1975). In addition to blood lipids, most of these investigations of children also included blood pressure and body fatness. However, in other studies, serum uric acid and blood glucose have been reported (Balram & Fodor, 1983), as well as smoking habits (Durant, Linder, Harkness, & Gray, 1983; Feinlieb, Kannel, Garrison, McNamara, & Castelli, 1976; Green, 1980; Hurd, Johnson, Pechacek, Bast, Jacobs, & Luepker, 1980; Ibsen, Lous, & Andersen, 1982; Laakso, Rimpela, & Telama, 1979; Tell & Vellar, 1983; Tibblin, 1980; Williams, Carter, Arnold, & Wynder, 1979). Attempts have even been made to study type A behavior in children (Gerace, Smith, Christakis, Kafatos, Trakas, & Stangos, 1983; Hunter, Parker, Williamson, Weber, & Berenson, 1983; Nora, 1980). Studies have also begun on habitual physical activity in children (Durnin, 1971; Gilliam, Freedson, Greenan, & Shahraray, 1981; Laakso & Telama, 1981; LaPort et al., 1982; Rutenfranz, Berndt, & Knauth, 1974; Saris, 1982; Seliger, Trefny, Bartunkova, & Pauer, 1974), but methods still have much to be desired.

In recent years, "tracking" of the most common CHD risk factors has been reported (Berenson, 1980, pp. 394-395; Berenson, Srinivasan, & Webber, 1980; Cresanata, Webber, Srinivasan, & Berenson, 1983; Costello, Disney, Dodson, & Bush, 1983; Feinlieb, Garrison, & Havlik, 1980; Lauer & Clarke, 1980; Linder & DuRant, 1982). Tracking refers to the consistency of the risk factor over time. In general, children who are at the high end of the distribution continue to retain their relative position as they grow older. To my knowledge, this has not been studied as far as physical activity is concerned.

Risk factors in children are more prevalent in countries where the incidence of coronary heart disease in adults is high (Connor, 1981; Kannel, 1976). Even in the same country, the presence of risk factors was correlated with CHD mortality of different regions (Balram & Fodor, 1983). In general, risk factors in children are higher if their parents' risks are also greater or if a parent died from CHD at a young age (Feinlieb, 1976; Glueck, Fallat, Tsang, & Buncher, 1974; Ibsen, Lous, & Andersen, 1982; Linder, & DuRant, 1982). I'm aware of only one study in which physical activity of children of fathers who died at a young age from CHD was compared with the activity of other children. In this case, the activity of both groups of children was not significantly different (Ibsen et al., 1982).

In general, CHD risk factors are only moderately correlated in families (Berenson, 1980; Cresanta, Baugh, Voors, Webber, & Berenson, 1983; Deutscher, Epstein, & Kjelsberg, 1966; Feinlieb, 1980; French, Dodge, & Kjelsberg, 1967; Higgins, Kjelsberg, & Metzner, 1967; Johnson, Epstein, & Kjelsberg, 1965; Montoye, Metzner, & Keller, 1975; Namboodiri et al., 1983). This list of references is not exhaustive, but it illustrates the point.

Risk Factors and Habitual Physical Activity

There have been many studies in which risk factors for coronary heart disease have been compared in groups of *adults* who vary in their habitual physical activity. With the exception of one risk factor, body fatness, the investigations of this kind in *children* are rare. With regard to obesity or body fatness, generally it has been demonstrated that fat children are less active than lean children. A few examples of such studies are Ishiko, Ikeda, and Enomoto (1968); Johnson, Burke, and Mayer (1956); Parizkova (1974); Saris, Binkhorst, Cramwinckel, Van Der Veen-Hezemans, and Van Waesbergae

(1979); and Stefanki, Heald, and Mayer (1956). However, there have been a few reports in which leaner children were not more active, as pointed out in the review by Thompson, Jarvie, Lahey, and Cureton, (1982).

Only a few investigations of the relationship of blood pressure to habitual physical activity in children have been reported. Fixler (1978) found no significant relationship of blood pressure to habitual physical activity in 8th-grade children (about 13 years of age). Similarly, Kemper (1980) reported that the blood pressure of active 13-to-14-year-old boys was not significantly different from that of less active boys of the same age. He used a questionnaire and pedometers to measure physical activity. Aerobic power was significantly higher in the active boys.

Smoking in children as related to habitual physical activity has also received only limited attention. In a survey of 2,831 Finnish children, Laakso, Rimpela, and Telama (1979) found that a significantly higher percentage of inactive boys and girls smoked daily than did the more active children. The data were collected by questionnaire. One must wonder if all the children who smoke admit this fact; perhaps smoking practices in children should be assessed by biochemical methods.

Blood lipids in children have been studied a little more extensively, but the numbers of subjects were still small. Table 1 contains a summary of investigations comparing active and inactive children. Differences in blood lipids are not impressive, although there is a tendency for active children to have higher HDL-cholesterol and ratio of HDL-C to total cholesterol. Unlike some studies in adults, the influence of body fatness in the activity-blood lipid relationships has not been removed. Methods of measuring physical activity in children leave something to be desired. It is possible that the differences in blood lipids between active and inactive children would be greater if the classification by activity were more accurate.

Risk Factors and Physical Fitness

Another approach is to assess the relationship of physical fitness to risk factors for CHD. However, a low score on a fitness test does not necessarily mean inactivity. If the studies by Klissouras (1971, 1972, 1973) and Klissouras, Pirnay, and Petit (1973) are to be accepted, physical fitness is mainly inherited. Nevertheless, one's fitness can be improved with an increase in exercise training, and children who are more active tend to be capable of a greater work capacity. Even though there are problems in measuring fitness in children, the difficulties are not as great as those encountered in trying to assess physical activity. Most investigators would expect risk factors to be more closely related to an estimate of the circulatory-respiratory capacity, namely $\dot{V}O_2$ max, than to other aspects of fitness, for example, strength and balance. However, in some instances, it is not possible to measure $\dot{V}O_2$ max, and another measurement is used, for example, work capacity, heart rate response to a standard exercise, and PWC_{170}.

Body fatness has long been known to be inversely related to $\dot{V}O_2$ max or working capacity in children. A few typical investigations are Fraser, Phillips, and Harris (1983); Gilliam, Katch, Thorland, and Weltman (1977); Mocellin and Rutenfranz (1971); Montoye (1975, p. 98); Parizkova, Vaneckova, Sprynardva, and Vamberova (1971); Saris (1982); Williams, Carter, Arnold, and Wynder (1979); and Wilmore and McNamara (1979).

Table 2 contains a summary of studies of the relationship of resting blood pressure

Table 1
Habitual Physical Activity and Blood Lipids in Children Literature Review

Subjects and Age (yrs)	Serum Total Cholesterol mmol/l	HDL Cholesterol mmol/l	HDL-C/Total C	Serum Total Triglycerides mmol/l	Reference
Adolescents, 13-14	Act. vs Inact., NS				Kemper (1980)[a]
27 active boys, 8-11	3.73 NS	1.20 NS	0.33 *	0.65 *	Thorland & Gilliam (1981)[b]
28 inactive boys, 8-11	3.85	1.11	0.29	0.85	
197 children,					Viikari et al. (1981)
12 least active, 12	4.61 NS	1.35 NS	0.30 NS	0.79 NS	
14 most active, 12	5.12	1.53	0.30	0.94	
85 swimmers, 8-16		1.69 **			Birk et al. (1982)[c]
12 controls, 8-16		1.45			
9 trained boys, 11-13	4.8 NS	1.7 **	0.35 NS	0.73 NS	Välimäki et al. (1980)
11 untrained boys, 11-13	4.4	1.3	0.30	0.98	
7 trained girls, 11-13	4.5 NS	1.6 *	0.36 NS	0.68 **	
4 untrained girls, 11-13	4.2	1.3	0.31	1.11	
33 active children, 7-15			0.33 *		Durant et al. (1983)
66 inactive children, 7-15			0.31		

[a]Body fatness not significantly different; [b]Diets were similar: inactive were fatter; [c]Fatness and HDL-C inversely correlated; *$p<.05$; **$p<.01$.

Table 2

Physical Fitness vs. Blood Pressure in Children
Literature Review

Subjects and Age (yrs)	Physical Fitness Measure	Blood Pressure	Correlation Coefficient	Reference
95 boys, 8-12	$\dot{V}O_2$ max	Systolic	−.21*	Wilmore & McNamara (1974)
95 boys, 8-12	$\dot{V}O_2$ max	Diastolic	−.16	
755 boys, 9-18	Speed in 600 yard run	Systolic	−.35 to +.37[bc]	Montoye, p. 107 (1975)
749 boys, 9-18		Diastolic	−.20 to +.10[b]	
629 girls, 9-18		Systolic	−.16 to +.20[b]	
626 girls, 9-18		Diastolic	−.24 to +.27[bc]	
101 boys, 8-18	PWC_{150}	Systolic	.13[a]	Boulton (1981)
96 girls, 8-18	PWC_{150}	Systolic	−.15[a]	

[a]Partial r, effect of height, weight, fatness and pubertal stage removed.
[b]Ten age specific partial r's, effect of weight and height removed.
[c]One partial r of ten statistically significant $p<.05$.
*$p<.05$.

and physical fitness measurements. If the effects of body fatness are removed in some way, there appears to be little or no relationship between physical fitness and blood pressure. Of course, it is possible that one's physical fitness as a child could be related to one's blood pressure later in life, but apparently, this has not been studied. In Tecumseh High School in Michigan children were allowed to select physical education, band, art, or music as one of their courses. The more physically fit selected physical education, but the systolic and diastolic blood pressures of this group were not statistically different from those who elected one of the other courses (Montoye, 1975, p. 108).

Tables 3a and 3b contain a summary of studies in which the physical fitness of children was compared with their serum total cholesterol. In the modified Harvard Step Test, a high score (i.e., heart rate) indicates poor fitness. Clearly, regardless of how the work or cardiovascular-respiratory capacity is estimated, it is not correlated with serum total cholesterol, particularly when the effect of body fatness is removed. As with blood pressure, children in Tecumseh High School who selected physical education did not have different concentrations of total cholesterol in their blood than those who elected another subject (Montoye, 1975, p. 163). Table 4 indicates there also is little or no relationship between physical fitness and serum triglycerides.

Whereas HDL-cholesterol has generally been reported to be higher in more fit adults (Howley, Gayle, Montoye, Painter, Fleshood, Endress & Sundahl, 1982), Tables 5a and 5b indicate no strong evidence that this holds true for children. That fitness and HDL-C is related is suggested, but the relationship is not impressive. When a ratio is formed by dividing the HDL-C by total cholesterol, a statistically significant relationship generally exists, the ratio being higher in more fit children (Table 6). Because of a tendency for LDL-C to be lower and for HDL-C to be higher in more fit children, the ratio HDL-C/TC differentiates better between fit and unfit children. However, fatness is known to be related to total cholesterol and LDL-C, and the effects of fatness were not removed in the data in Table 6. Whether or not this would affect the relationship is not known. In one sense, it is academic; if exercise reduces body fatness which in turn reduces total cholesterol or LDL-C, exercise may indeed be the important variable.

Glucose tolerance and serum uric acid are sometimes also considered risk factors for CHD. The relationship of these variables to physical fitness is shown in Tables 7 and 8. A high score for glucose tolerance (i.e., a high concentration of glucose 1 hour after a glucose challenge) is an indication of poor tolerance. Serum uric acid concentration does not appear to be related to physical fitness, but there is a suggestion that poor fitness and poor glucose tolerance are related, albeit weakly. As with several other risk factors, glucose tolerance and serum uric acid were no different in children who elected physical education in high school from those who elected other courses (Montoye, 1975, page 146 & 167).

Effects of Exercise Training on Risk Factors

Another approach in studying the relationship of coronary risk factors is an experimental one; namely, increasing the amount of exercise in children and measuring change, if any, in risk factors. That an increase in physical activity, particularly in obese children, can cause a reduction in fatness is well known (Brownell & Kaye, 1982; Fisher & Brown, 1982; Parizkova, 1963, 1982; Parizkova, Vaneckova, Sprynarova, &

Table 3a

Physical Fitness vs. Serum Total Cholesterol in Children
Literature Review

Subject and Age (yrs)	Physical Fitness Measure	Correlation Coefficient	Reference
95 boys, 8-12	$\dot{V}O_2$ max	−.18	Wilmore & McNamara (1974)
699 boys, 9-18	Speed in	−.36 to +.25[a,b]	Montoye, p. 165 (1975)
564 girls, 9-18	600 yd run	−.37 to +.14[a]	
869 boys, 10-19	Modified Harvard	−.08 to +.18[c]	Montoye et al. (1976)
791 girls, 10-19	Step Test	−.02 to +.11	
47 children 7-12	$\dot{V}O_2$ max	−.04	Gilliam et al. (1977)
285 boys, 10-19	$\dot{V}O_2$ max	.08[d]	Montoye, Block & Gayle (1978)
44 girls, 10-19	$\dot{V}O_2$ max	−.06[d]	
20 boys, 11-13	Bicycle Erg. Perf.	.35	Välimäki et al. (1980)
11 girls, 11-13	work/body wt.	.19	

[a] Age-specific partial r's, effect of weight and height remove.
[b] Two partial r's of ten were statistically significant, $p<.05$.
[c] Partial r's in 2 year-age groups, effect of skinfolds removed.
[d] Partial r, effect of age, weight, and skinfolds removed.

Table 3b
Physical Fitness vs. Serum Total Cholesterol in Children Literature Review

Subjects and Age (yrs)	Physical Fitness Measure	Mean Cholesterol mmol/l Fit >75 Percentile	Mean Cholesterol mmol/l Unfit <25 Percentile	Significance of Difference	Reference
171 children, 4-6	PWC$_{170}$	4.72	4.82	NS	Saris et al. (1979)
54 children, 8-12					
2658 children, 10-15	Modified Harvard Step Test	4.01	4.16[a]	$p<.05$	Williams et al. (1979)
372 boys, 6	$\dot{V}O_2$ max	4.0	4.3	$p<.01$	Saris (1982)
339 girls, 6		4.4	4.1	$p<.05$	
427 boys, 8		4.3	4.3	NS	
447 girls, 8		4.3	4.6	$p<.05$	
368 boys, 10		4.4	4.5	NS	
426 girls, 10		4.7	4.7	NS	

[a]Below 17 percentile rather than below 25 percentile.

Table 4

Physical Fitness vs. Serum Triglycerides in Children
Literature Review

Subjects and Age (yrs)	Physical Fitness Measures	Correlation Coefficient	Reference
95 boys, 8-12	$\dot{V}O_2$ max	−.23*	Wilmore & McNamara (1974)
47 children, 7-12	$\dot{V}O_2$ max	−.30	Gilliam et al. (1977)
285 boys, 10-19	$\dot{V}O_2$ max	.05[a]	Montoye, Block, & Gayle (1978)
44 girls, 10-19	$\dot{V}O_2$ max	−.05[a]	
20 boys, 11-13	Bicycle Erg. Perf. work/body wt.	−.13	Välimäki et al. (1980)
11 girls, 11-13		−.83**	

	Mean Triglycerides mmol/l		
	Fit >75 Percentile	Unfit <25 Percentile	Significance of Difference
171 children, 4-6	PWC_{170} 0.86	0.82	NS
54 children, 8-12	PWC_{170} 1.07	0.84	NS

Saris et al. (1979)

[a]Partial r, effect of age, weight, and skinfolds removed.
*$p<.05$.
**$p<.01$.

Table 5

Physical Fitness vs. HDL-Cholesterol in Children
Literature Review

Subjects and Age (yrs)	Physical Fitness Measures	Correlation Coefficient	Reference
20 boys, 11-13	Bicycle Erg. Perf. work/body wt.	.53*	Välimäki et al. (1980)
11 girls, 11-13	Bicycle Erg. Perf. work/body wt.	.51	
53 obese children, 7-14	Bicycle Erg. Perf.	Boys, .20 Girls, .48*	Ylitalo (1981)
51 children, 6-12	$\dot{V}O_2$ max	Not related[a]	Sady et al. (1981)

Subjects and Age (yrs)	Physical Fitness Measures	Mean HDL-C mmol/l		Significance of Difference	Reference
		Fit >75 Percentile	Unfit <25 Percentile		
171 children, 4-6	PWC_{170}	1.35	1.32	NS	Saris et al. (1979)
54 children, 8-12		1.37	1.35	NS	
372 boys, 6	$\dot{V}O_2$ max	1.4	1.4	NS	Saris (1982)
339 girls, 6		1.5	1.3	$p<.01$	
427 boys, 8		1.4	1.4	NS	
447 girls, 8		1.4	1.4	NS	
368 boys, 10		1.5	1.4	NS	
426 girls, 10		1.5	1.3	$p<.01$	

[a]Partial r, effect of fatness removed, not satistically significant.
*$p<.05$.

Table 6

Physical Fitness vs. HDL-Cholesterol/Total Cholesterol Ratio in Children
Literature Review

Subjects and Age (yrs)	Physical Fitness Measures	Correlation Coefficient		Reference
20 boys, 11-13	Bicycle Erg. Perf. work/body wt.	.20		Välimäki et al. (1980)
11 girls, 11-13	Bicycle Erg. Perf. work/body wt.	.37		
53 obese children, 7-14	Bicycle Erg. Perf.	Boys, .47* Girls, .24		Ylitalo (1981)

		Mean HDL-C/TC			
		Fit <75 Percentile	Unfit <25 Percentile	Significance of Difference	
342 boys, 6	$\dot{V}O_2$ max	0.36	0.35	$p<.05$	Saris (1982)
339 girls, 8		0.34	0.32	$p<.01$	
427 boys, 8		0.34	0.32	$p<.05$	
447 girls, 8		0.33	0.30	$p<.01$	
368 boys, 10		0.34	0.31	$p<.01$	
426 girls, 10		0.32	0.28	$p<.001$	

*$p<.05$.

Table 7
Physical Fitness vs. Glucose Tolerances in Children Literature Review

Subjects and Age (yrs)	Physical Fitness Measures	Correlation Coefficient	Reference
725 boys, 9-18 583 girls, 9-18	Speed in 600 yd run	−.20 to +.18[a] −.39 to +.12[a,b]	Montoye, p. 166 (1975)
848 boys, 10-19 759 girls, 10-19	Modified Harvard Step Test	+.06 to +.15[b,c] +.08 to +.23[c,d]	Montoye, Block, Keller, & Willis (1977)
274 boys, 10-19 41 girls, 10-19	$\dot{V}O_2$ max $\dot{V}O_2$ max	−.02[e] −.35[e]	Montoye, Mikkelsen, Block, & Gayle (1978)

[a]Age specific partial r's, effect of weight and height removed.
[b]One partial r of ten statistically significant, $p<.05$.
[c]Partial r's in 2 year-age groups, effect of skinfolds removed.
[d]Two partial r's of ten statistically significant $p<.05$.
[e]Partial r, effect of age, weight, and skinfolds removed.

Table 8

Physical Fitness vs. Serum Uric Acid in Children
Literature Review

Subjects and Age (yrs)	Physical Fitness Measures	Correlation Coefficient	Reference
536 boys, 9-18 454 girls, 9-18	Speed in 600 yd run	−.26 to +.21[a] −.38 to +.15[a]	Montoye, p. 147 (1975)
789 boys, 10-19 710 girls, 10-19	Modified Harvard Step Test	.01 to .17[bc] .00 to .11[b]	Montoye et al. (1975)
274 boys, 10-19 41 girls, 10-19	$\dot{V}O_2$ max $\dot{V}O_2$ max	.02[d] .40[d]**	Montoye, Mikkelsen, Block, & Gayle (1978)

[a] Age specific partial r's, effects of weight and height removed, one statistically signigicant, $p<.05$.
[b] Partial r's in 2-year age groups, effect of skinfolds removed.
[c] Two partial r's of five, statistically significant $p<.05$.
[d] Partial r, effects of age, weight, and skinfolds removed.
**$p<.01$.

Vamberova, 1971; Thompson, Jarvie, Lahey, & Cureton, 1982; Vlasek, Hart, & Seitz, 1983).

In their review, Pate and Blair (1978) concluded that significant changes in blood pressure following an exercise program have not been demonstrated in children. Linder, DuRant, & Mahoney (1983) exercised 25 white males, age 11-to-17, 30 min/day, 4 days/week for 8 weeks. Although their physical working capacity increased, their blood pressure did not change significantly when compared to 25 control subjects. However, Fisher and Brown (1982) reported a significant decrease in diastolic blood pressure in 9 or 10 seventh-graders (about age 12-13) who exercised 30 min/day, 5 days/week for 12 weeks. These subjects also increased their endurance on a treadmill test. The control group did not change in either blood pressure or work capacity.

Tables 9 and 10 contain the results of studies of changes in blood lipids when children undertook an exercise program. The experiment by Widhalm, Maxa, and Zyman (1978) involved 7 boys and 7 girls age 11-to-13 who were obese, averaging 28% overweight. Several characteristics of the study make the results difficult to interpret. In the first place, there was no control group. Second, in addition to increasing their exercise, the children were placed on a diet of 1,000 kcal/day. Finally, this regimen was followed for only 3 weeks, rather a short time for an exercise-training experiment. Both total cholesterol and the low-density lipoprotein fraction decreased. However, the children lost on the average 4.7 kg of body weight. Under these conditions it is difficult to determine if exercise training is responsible for the change. Details of the exercise program were not given and it is not known if there was an increase in work capacity of the children.

The training program in the study by Gilliam and Burke (1978) lasted twice as long (6 weeks). The subjects were 14 girls, age 8-to-10, and they exercised for 40 min/day, 6 days/week. There was no change after 6 weeks in total cholesterol but HDL-C and the ratio of HDL-C to total cholesterol increased significantly, which is a frequent finding in studies of adults. Unfortunately, a control group was not studied simultaneously, and it was not reported whether or not there was a significant change in body fatness or work capacity.

In the study by Linder, DuRant, Grey, and Harkess (1979) 103 black children, age 7-to-15 years, were assigned at random to either an exercise or control group. The exercise program lasted 4 weeks, but no other details were given. No significant changes in any blood lipids were observed. In a later study. Linder, DuRant, and Mahoney (1983) compared 25 boys, age 11-to-17 years, who exercised aerobically 4 days/week, for 8 weeks with a control group of 25 boys of the same age. The exercise group improved in work capacity, whereas the control group did not. There was no evidence that body fatness changed in either group, nor was there a significant change in any of the blood lipids (Tables 9 & 10). In the study by Fisher and Brown (1980), 38 seventh graders (age 12-to-13) were randomly assigned to an exercise, exercise and diet, diet only, or a control group. The first two groups participated in 30 min/day, 5 days/week of "vigorous" physical activity. After 12 weeks total cholesterol and body fatness decreased and work capacity increased in the first two groups. The "exercise only" group also increased in HDL-C and HDL-C/total cholesterol ratio. The only change in the diet group was a significant decrease in total cholesterol. The control group did not change in any of the measurements.

The effects of exercise training on blood glucose and glucose tolerance in normal adults have been studied a number of times with inconclusive results. These investiga-

Table 9

The Effect of Exercise Training on Serum Total and HDL-Cholesterol in Children Literature Review[a]

Total Cholesterol mmol/l		HDL-Cholesterol mmol/l		HDL-C/TC		Reference
Before	After	Before	After	Before	After	
5.63	4.33**	1.79	1.59	—	—	Wildhalm et al. (1978)
3.59	3.38	0.78	0.94*	0.22	0.29*	Gilliam & Burke (1978)
No sig. change		No sig. change		No sig. change[b]		Linder et al. (1979)
Decrease of 0.74*		Increase of 0.31*		Increase of 0.70*		Fisher & Brown (1980)
3.84	3.81	1.07	0.97	0.42	0.37	Linder et al. (1983)

[a] See text for details of studies.
[b] This ratio was LDL-C/HDL-C.
*$p < .05$ for change, before vs. after.
**$p < .01$ for change, before vs. after.

Table 10
The Effect of Exercise Training on Serum Triglycerides and LDL-C and VLDL-C in Children Literature Review[a]

Total Triglycerides mmol/l		LDL-C mmol/l		VLDL-C mmol/l		Reference
Before	After	Before	After	Before	After	
1.10	1.22	3.46	1.96**	0.12	0.30*	Widhalm et al. (1978)
No sig. change		No sig. change		No sig. change		Linder et al. (1979)
1.05	1.05	2.43	2.52	0.40	0.37	Linder et al. (1983)

[a] See text for details of studies.
*$p<.05$ for change, before vs. after.
**$p<.01$ for change, before vs. after.

tions have been reviewed elsewhere (Montoye, Block, Metzner & Keller, 1977). To my knowledge, similar studies have not been done in normal children. For many years, exercise has been one of the treatment modalities in diabetes (Montoye et al., 1977), and it is known that the insulin requirment is reduced if a program of regular exercise is followed. Diabetic control appears to improve with exercise (Ludvigsson, 1980). However, there is little data in the literature on the long range effects of training with adequate controls, even among diabetic children (Koivisto & Groop, 1982).

Conclusions

The results presented in this review are disappointing. However, one should keep in mind that in adults, also, the results of research-relating habitual physical activity or physical fitness to most CHD risk factors is equivocal. It is true, of course, that active adults are generally leaner, and that increasing one's exercise usually results in some loss in body fat. On the other hand, differences between active and inactive people are not so apparent with regard to other risk factors such as blood pressure, serum total cholesterol or triglycerides, glucose tolerance, serum uric acid, or blood clotting or lysis time. The one exception appears to be serum HDL-cholesterol and its percentage of total cholesterol, both of which seem to be higher in active adults. Physical fitness for muscular work in adults has not been shown to be an important correlate of CHD risk factors; again with the exceptions of body fatness and possibly HDL-C and HDL-C/TC. It should not be surprising, therefore, that the relationship of physical activity or physical fitness to CHD risk factors in children appears to be unimpressive.

It might be that CHD risk factors simply are not closely related to exercise habits or work capacity. It is possible, for example, that in human beings, exercise does not have a profound effect on the development of atherosclerosis, but that a program of vigorous activity may permit some people to live longer with atherosclerosis.

But before we settle on this conclusion, we should more closely examine the "state of the art" in research with children. There are many difficulties in the assessment of habitual physical activity in adults, but these difficulties are even greater with children. Among adults, one's occupation frequently accounts for much of the variation in habitual physical activity among men and women. However, in children, it is the use of their leisure time which determines how active they are, and this activity is more difficult to assess than occupational activity. Also, during much of the year when a child's life is more regimented in school, there may be less opportunity for variation in physical activity. In addition, as we grow older, the environment has more time to exert its influence on the CHD risk factors, resulting in a greater variance in these measures among adults. Thus, the smaller variance in physical activity and risk factors in children make it more difficult to show a correlation between the two.

Exercise may require a long period of time to produce an effect on risk factors. A 10- or 12-year-old boy or girl has not lived long enough to have exercised regularly and strenuously for very long. Some adults, on the other hand, have exercised for many years; for example, the tennis players we studied (Howley et al., 1982) had been playing regularly for 40 years and had significantly higher HDL-cholesterol than age-matched controls.

Time works in another way. Perhaps risk factors and physical fitness in children are determined primarily by inheritance and family environment. As children grow older and leave home, the new environment outside the home is able to exert greater influence. This is related to the smaller variance in children discussed above. The result is greater difficulty in demonstrating an effect of exercise in children.

What can be suggested for future research? Certainly we should continue to study the effects of exercise on risk factors in children for several reasons. In the first place, with regard to some risk factors, there is a paucity of data on children in the literature. Second, the numbers are still small in some analyses. Third, the statistical analyses in many instances are not as complete in children: for example, removing the influence of body fatness or other confounding variables. Fourth, our methods of measuring habitual physical activity and physical fitness in children must be improved.

Perhaps we should not expect much effect of physical activity if the risk factor (blood pressure, cholesterol, etc.) is normal. It might be better to single out those children with high values and study the effects of exercise on this population.

Finally, I would like to suggest what is, in my opinion, a more fundamental question than any of the others; namely, can physical educators influence children to remain active in later life, and if so, how? As far as I know, this question has not been studied with an appropriate research design.

References

ALBERT, Z., (1939). Die Veranderungen der Aorta bei Kindern und ihr Verhaltnis zur Atherosklerose. *Virchow's Archiv fur Pathologische Anatomie und Physiologie*, **303**, 265-279.

BALRAM, B.C., & Fodor, J.G. (1983). Coronary heart disease risk factors in Newfoundland children. *CVD Epidemiology Newsletter*, No. 33, p. 53.

BERENSON, G.S. (1980). *Cardiovascular risk factors in children*. Oxford: Oxford University Press.

BERENSON, G.S., Srinivasan, S.R., & Webber, L.S. (1980). Prognostic significance of lipid profiles in children. In R.M. Lauer, & R.B. Shekelle (Eds.), *Childhood prevention of Atherosclerosis and hypertension*, pp. 75-86. New York: Raven Press.

BIRK, T., Quan, A., Dillingham, C., Schroeder, R., & Fahey, T. (1981). *Plamsa HDL-cholesterol and body composition of swimmers aged 8-16 years*. Presented at annual meeting, American Alliance for Health, Physical Education, Recreation and Dance, Boston, MA.

BOULTON, J. (1981). Nutrition in childhood and its relationships to early somatic growth, body fat, blood pressure, and physical fitness. *Acta Paediatrica Scandinavica*, Suppl. 284, 1-85.

BROWNELL, K.D., & Kaye, F.S. (1982). A school-based behavior modification, nutrition education, and physical activity program for obese children. *American Journal of Clinical Nutrition*, **35**, 277-283.

CONNOR, W.E. (1980). Cross-cultural studies of diet and plasma lipid and lipoproteins. In R.M. Lauer & R.B. Shekelle (Eds.), *Childhood prevention of atherosclerosis and hypertension*, pp. 99-111. New York: Raven Press.

COSTELLO, C., Disney, G., Dodson, W., & Bush, M. (1983). Longitudinal study of the incidence and persistence of obesity in girls from ages 9-to-16 years. *Federation Proceedings*, **42**, 535. (Abstract)

CRESANTA, J.L., Baugh, J.G., Voors, A.W., Webber, L.S., & Berenson, G.S. (1983). Parent-child interactions of cardiovascular disease risk factors in a biracial community—the Bogalusa heart study. *CVD Epidemiology Newsletter*, No. 33, p. 41.

CRESANTA, J.L., Webber, L.S., Srinivasan, S.R., & Berenson, G.S. (1983). Tracking of lipoprotein cholesterol in children over a six year period. *CVD Epidemiology Newsletter*, No. 33, p. 41.

DEUTSCHER, S., Epstein, F.H., & Kjelsberg, M.O. (1966). Familial aggregation of factors associated with coronary heart disease. *Circulation*, 33, 911-924.

DURANT, R.H., Linder, C.W., Harkess, J.W., & Gray, R.G. (1983). The relationship between physical activity and serum lipids and lipoproteins in black children and adolescents. *Journal of Adolescent Health Care*, 4, 55-60.

DURNIN, J.V.G.A. (1971). Physical activity of adolescents. *Acta Paediatrica Scandinavica*, Suppl. 217, 133-135.

ENOS, W.F., Jr., Beyer, J.C., & Holmes, R.H. (1953). Pathogenesis of coronary disease in American soldiers killed in Korea. *Journal of the American Medical Association*, 152, 1090-1093.

FEINLEIB, M., Garrison, R.J., & Havlik, R.J. (1980). Environmental and genetic factors affecting the distribution of blood pressure in children. In R.M. Lauer & R.B. Shekelle (Eds.), *Childhood prevention of atherosclerosis and hypertension*, pp. 271-279. New York: Raven Press.

FEINLEIB, M., Kannel, W.B., Garrison, R.J., McNamara, P., & Castelli, W.P. (1976). Relation of parental history of coronary heart disease to risk factors in young adults. *Circulation*, 54(2), 52. (Abstract).

FISHER, H.G., & Brown, M. (1982). The effects of diet and exercise on selected coronary risk factors in children. *Medicine and Science in Sports and Exercise*, 14, 171. (Abstract)

FIXLER, D.E. (1978). Epidemiology of childhood hypertension. In W.B. Strong (Ed.), *Atherosclerosis: Its pediatric aspects*, Chapter 9. New York: Grune and Stratton.

FRASER, G.E., Phillips, R.L., & Harris, R. (1983). Physical fitness and blood pressure in school children. *Circulation*, 67, 405-412.

FRENCH, J.G., Dodge, H.J., & Kjelsberg, M.O. (1967). A study of familial aggregation of serum uric acid levels in the population of Tecumseh, Michigan, 1959-60. *American Journal of Epidemiology*, 86, 214-224.

FRERICHS, R.R., Srinivasan, S.R., Webber, L.S., & Berenson, G.S. (1976). Serum cholesterol and triglyceride levels in 3,446 children from a biracial community: The Bogalusa heart study. *Circulation*, 54, 302-309.

GARN, S.M., Bailey, S.M., & Higgins, I.T.T. (1980). Effects of socioeconomic status, family line, and living together on fatness and obesity. In R.M. Lauer & R.B. Shekelle (Eds.), *Childhood prevention and atherosclerosis and hypertension*, pp. 187-204. New York: Raven Press.

GERACE, T., Smith, J.C., Christakis, G., Kafatos, A., Trakas, D., & Stangos, L. (1983). Prevalence of type A in young males in rural and urban mainland Greece and Crete. *CVD Epidemiology Newsletter*, No. 33, p. 16.

GILLIAM, T.B., & Burke, M.B. (1978). Effects of exercise on serum lipids and lipoproteins in girls, ages 8-to-10 years. *Artery*, 4, 203-213.

GILLIAM, T.B., Freedson, P.S., Geenan, D.L., & Shahraray, B. (1981). Physical activity patterns determined by heart rate monitoring in 6-to-7 year-old children. *Medicine and Science in Sports and Exercise*, 13, 65-67.

GILLIAM, T.B., Katch, V.L., Thorland, W., & Weltman, A. (1977). Prevalence of coronary heart disease risk factors in active children, 7-to-12 years of age. *Medicine and Science in Sports*, **9**, 21-25.

GLANTZ, W.M., & Stembridge, V.A. (1959). Coronary artery atherosclerosis as a factor in aircraft accident fatalities. *Journal of Aviation Medicine*, **30**, 75-89.

GLUECK, C.J., Fallat, R.W. Tsang, R., & Buncher, C.R. (1974). Hyperlipemia in progeny of parents with myocardial infarction before age 50. *American Journal of Diseases of Children*, **127**, 70-75.

GREEN, D.E. (1980). Beliefs of teenagers about smoking and health. In R.M. Lauer & R.B. Shekelle (Eds.), *Childhood prevention of atherosclerosis and hypertension*, pp. 223-228. New York: Raven Press.

HIGGINS, M.W., Kjelsberg, M., & Metzner, H. (1967). Characteristics of smokers and nonsmokers in Tecumseh, Michigan, I. The distribution of smoking habits in persons and families and their relationship to social characteristics. *American Journal of Epidemiology*, **86**, 45-59.

HOWLEY, E.T., Gayle, R.C., Montoye, H.J., Painter, P., Fleshhood, L., Endres, J., & Sundahl, L. (1982). HDL-Cholesterol in senior tennis players. *Scandinavian Journal of Sports Science*, **4**, 44-48.

HUNTER, S.M., Parker, F., Williamson, D., Webber, L.S., & Berenson, G.S. (1983). Type A behavior pattern and observed hyperactivity in children—Bogalusa heart study. *CVD Epidemiology Newsletter*, No. 33, p. 42.

HURD, P.D., Johnson, C.A., Pechacek, T., Bast, L.P., Jacobs, D.R., & Luepker, R. (1980). Prevention of cigarette smoking in seventh grade students. *Journal of Behavioral Medicine*, **3**, 15-28.

IBSEN, K.K., Lous, P., & Andersen, G.E. (1982). Coronary heart risk factors in 177 children and young adults whose fathers died from ischemic heart disease before age 45. *Acta Paediatrica Scandinavica*, **71**, 609-613.

ISHIKO, T., Ikeda, N., & Enomoto, Y. (1968). Obese children in Japan. *Research Journal of Physical Education*, **12**, 168-174.

JOHNSON, B.C., Epstein, F.H., & Kjelsberg, M.O. (1965). Distributions and family studies of blood pressure and serum cholesterol levels in a total community—Tecumseh, Michigan. *Journal of Chronic Diseases*, **18**, 147-160.

JOHNSON, M.L., Burke, B.S., & Mayer, J. (1956). Relative importance of inactivity and overeating in the energy balance of obese high school girls. *American Journal of Clinical Nutrition*, **4**, 37-44.

KANNEL, W.B. (1976). Prospects for prevention of atherosclerosis in the young. *Australian and New Zealand Journal of Medicine*, **6**, 410-419.

KEMPER, H.C.G. (1982). Growth and health of adolescents. *Geneeskunde en Sport*, **13**, 18. Quoted by Saris, W.H.M. *Aerobic power and daily physical activity in children*, p. 10. Nijmegen, The Netherlands: Krips.

KLISSOURAS, V. (1973). Prediction of potential performance with reference to heredity. *Journal of Sports Medicine and Physical Fitness*, **13**, 100-107.

KLISSOURAS, V. (1972). Genetic limit of functional adaptability. *International Zeitschrift für Angewante Physiologie*, **30**, 85-94.

KLISSOURAS, V. (1971). Heritability of adaptive variation. *Journal of Applied Physiology*, **31**, 338-344.

KLISSOURAS, V., Pirnay, F., & Petit, M. (1973). Adaptations to maximal effort: Genetics and age. *Journal of Applied Physiology*, **35**, 228-293.

KLOTZ, O., & Manning, M.F. (1911). Fatty streaks in the intima of arteries. *Journal of Pathology and Bacteriology*, **16**, 211-220.

KNUIMAN, J.T., & Hautvast, J.G.A.J. (1980). Serum total and HDL cholesterol in schoolboys from 16 countries. *CVD Epidemiology Newsletter*, No. 29, 86.

KOIVISTO, V.A., & Groop, L. (1982). Physical training in juvenile diabetes. *Annals of Clinical Research*, Suppl. 34, **14**, 74-79.

LAAKSO, L., Rimpela, M., Telama, R. (1979). Relationship between physical activity and some health habits among Finnish youth. *Schriftenreihe des Bundesintituts für Sportwissenschaft*, **36**, 76-81.

LAPORTE, R.E., Cauley, J.A. Kinsey, C.M., Corbett, W., Robertson, R., Black-Sandler, R., Kuller, L.H., & Falkel, J. (1982). The epidemiology of physical activity in children, college students, middle-aged men, menopausal females, annd monkeys. *Journal of Chronic Diseases*, **35**, 787-795.

LAUER, R.M., & Clarke, W.R. (1980). Immediate and long-term prognostic significance of childhood blood pressure levels. In R.M. Lauer & R.B. Shekelle (Eds.), *Childhood prevention of atherosclerosis and hypertension*, pp. 281-290. New York: Raven Press.

LAUER, R.M., Connor, W.E., Leaverton, P.E., Reiter, M.A., & Clarke, W.R. (1975). Coronary heart disease risk factors in school children: The Muscatine study. *Journal of Pediatrics*, **86**, 697-700.

LINDER, C.W., & DuRant, R.H. (1982). Exercise, serum lipids, and cardiovascular disease-risk factors in children. *Pediatric Clinics of North America*, **29**, 1341-1354.

LINDER, C.W., DuRant, R.H., Gray, R.G., & Harkess, J.W. (1979). The effect of exercise in serum lipid levels in children. *Clinical Research*, **27**, 797. (Abstract)

LINDER, C.W., DuRant, R.H., & Mahoney, O.M. (1983). The effect of physical conditioning on serum lipids and lipoproteins in white male adolescents. *Medicine and Science in Sports and Exercise*, **15**, 232-236.

LUDVIGSSON, J. (Ed.) (1980). Physical exercise in the treatment of juvenile diabetes mellitus, *Acta Paediatrica Scandinavica*, Suppl. No. 283, 1-122.

MCGILL, H.C., Jr. (1968). The geographic pathology of atherosclerosis. *Laboratory Investigation*, **18**, 463-502.

MCNAMARA, J.J., Molot, M.A., Stremple, J.F., & Cutting, R.T. (1971). Coronary artery disease in combat casualties in Vietnam. *Journal of the American Medical Association*, **216**, 1185-1187.

MOCELLIN, R., & Rutenfranz, J. (1971). Investigations of the physical working capacity of obese children. *Acta Paediatrica Scandinavica*, Suppl. 217, 77-79.

MONTOYE, H.J. (1975). *Physical activity and health: An epidemiologic study of an entire community*. Englewood Cliffs, NJ: Prentice-Hall, Inc.

MONTOYE, H.J., Block, W., & Gayle, R. (1978). Maximal oxygen uptake and blood lipids. *Journal of Chronic Diseases*, **31**, 111-118.

MONTOYE, H.J., Block, W., Keller, J.B., & Willis, P.W., III. (1977). Glucose tolerance and physical fitness: An epidemiologic study in an entire community. *European Journal of Applied Physiology*, **37**, 237-242.

MONTOYE, H.J., Block, W., Keller, J.B., & Willis, P.W., III. (1976). Fitness, fatness, and serum cholesterol: An epidemiologic study in an entire community. *Research Quarterly, 47,* 400-408.

MONTOYE, H.J., Block, W.D., Metzner, H., & Keller, J.B. (1977). Habitual physical activity and glucose tolerance: Males age 16-to-64 in a total community. *Diabetes,* **26,** 172-176.

MONTOYE, H.J., Frantz, M.E., Kozar, A.J., & Johnson, B.C. (1974). Relation of certain measurements to physical fitness and participation in physical education. *Physical Educator,* **31,** 3-7.

MONTOYE, H.J., Metzner, H.L., & Keller, M.O. (1975). Familial aggregation of strength and heart rate response to exercise. *Human Biology,* **47,** 17-36.

NAMBOODIRI, K., Morrison, J., Green, P., Kaplan, E., Glueck, C.J., & Rifkind, B. (1983). *CVD Epidemiology Newsletter,* No. 33, p. 29.

NORA, J.J. (1980). Identifying the child at risk for coronary heart disease as an adult: A strategy for prevention. *Journal of Pediatrics,* **97,** 706-714.

PARIZKOVA, J. (1982). Physical training in weight reduction of obese adolescents. *Annals of Clinical Research,* **34,** 63-68.

PARIZKOVA, J. (1974). Particularities of lean body mass and fat development in growing boys as related to their motor activity. *Acta Paediatric Belgica,* Suppl. 28, 233-243.

PARIZKOVA, J. (1963). Impact of age, diet, and exercise on man's body composition. *Annals New York Academy of Science,* **110,** 661-674.

PARIZKOVA J., Vanneckova, M., Sprynarova, S., & Vamberova, M. (1971). Body composition and fitness in obese children before and after special treatment. *Acta Paediatrica Scandinavica,* Suppl. 217, 80-85.

PATE, R.R., & Blair, S.N. (1978). Exercise and the prevention of atherosclerosis: Pediatric implications. In W.B. Strong (Ed.), *Atherosclerosis: Its pediatric aspects,* pp. 251-286. New York: Grune & Stratton.

RIGAL, R.D., Lovell, F.W., & Townsend, F.M. (1960). Pathologic findings in the cardiovascular systems of military flying personnel. *American Journal of Cardiology,* **6,** 19-25.

RUTENFRANZ, J., Berndt, I., & Knauth, P. (1974). Daily physical activity investigated by time budget studies and physical performance capacity of schoolboys. *Acta Paediatrica Belgica,* Suppl. 28, 79-86.

SADY, S.P., Berg, K., Beal, D., & Smith, J.L. (1981). Relation between high density lipoprotein cholesterol and body fatness or aerobic power in 6-to-12 year old boys and girls. *Medicine and Science in Sports and Exercise,* **13,** 106. (Abstract)

SARIS, W.H.M. (1982). *Aerobic power and daily physical activity in children.* Nijmegen, The Netherlands: Krips.

SARIS, W.H.M., Binkhorst, R.A., Cramwinckel, A.B., Van Der Veen-Hezemans, A.M., & Van Waesberghe, F. (1979). Evauluation of somatic effects of health education program for schoolchildren. *Bibliotheca Nutrito et Dieta (Basel),* **27,** 77-84.

SELIGER, V., Trefny, Z., Bartunkova, S., & Pauer, M. (1974). The habitual activity and physical fitness of 12-year-old boys. *Acta Paediatrica Belgica,* **25,** Suppl. 54-59.

SING, C.F., Orr, J.D., & Moll, P.P. (1980). Review of factors that predict serum cholesterol in the general population. In R.M. Lauer & R.B. Shekelle (Eds.), *Childhood prevention of atherosclerosis and hypertension,* pp. 87-97. New York: Raven Press.

STEFANKI, P.A., Heald, F.P., & Mayer, J. (1959). Caloric intake in relation to energy output in obese and non-obese adolescent boys. *American Journal of Clinical Nutrition*, **7**, 55-62.

STRONG, P., & McGill, H.C., Jr. (1969). The pediatric aspects of atherosclerosis. *Journal of Atherosclerosis Research*, **9**, 251-265.

TELL, G.S., & Vellar, O.D. (1983). CVD risk factors related to pubertal development: The Oslo youth study. *CVD Epidemiology Newsletter*, No. 33, p. 21.

TIBBLIN, G. (1980). Raising a smoke-free generation in Sweden. In R.M. Lauer & R.B. Shekelle (Eds.), *Childhood prevention of atherosclerosis and hypertension*l, pp. 453-458. New York: Raven Press.

THOMPSON, J.K., Jarvie, G.J., Lahey, B.B., & Cureton, K.J. (1982). Exercise and obesity: Etiology, physiology, and intervention. *Psychological Bulletin*, **91**, 55-79.

THORLAND, W.G., & Gilliam, T.B. (1981). Comparison of serum lipids between habitually high and low active pre-adolescent males. *Medicine and Science in Sports and Exercise*, **13**, 316-321.

VÄLIMÄKI, I., Hursti, M.L., Pihlaskoski, L., & Viikari, J. (1980). Exercise performance and serum lipids in relation to physical activity in schoolchildren. *International Journal of Sports Medicine*, **1**, 132-136.

VIIKARI, J., Välimäki, I., Telama, R., & Siren-Tiusanen, H. (1981). Atherosclerosis precursors in Finnish children: Physical activity and plasma lipids in 3-year-old and 12-year-old children. Presented at Pediatric Work Physiology Congress X, Joutsa, Finland.

VLASEK, I.W., Hart, S.S., & Seitz, G. (1983). Fatness changes in adolescent summer campers. *Medicine and Science in Sports and Exercise*, **15**, 180. (Abstract)

WIDHALM, K., Maxa, E., & Zyman, H. (1978). Effect of diet and exercise upon cholesterol and triglyceride content of plasma lipoproteins in overweight children. *European Journal of Pediatrics*, **127**, 121-126.

WILLIAMS, C.L., Carter, B.J., Arnold, C.B., & Wynder, E.L. (1979). Chronic disease risk factors among children. The "know your body" study. *Journal of Chronic Diseases*, **32**, 505-513.

WILMORE, J.H., & McNamara, J.J. (1974). Prevalence of coronary heart disease risk factors in boys, 8-to-12 years of age. *Journal of Pediatrics*, **84**, 527-533.

YLITALO, V. (1981). Treatment of obese schoolchildren. *Acta Paediatrica Scandinavica*, Suppl. 290, 1-108.

ZEEK, P. (1930). Juvenile arteriosclerosis. *Archives of Pathology*, **10**, 417-446.

ZINSERLING, W.D. (1925). Untersuchungen über Atherosklerose. 2. Über die Aortaverfettung bei Kindern. *Vierchow's Archiv für Pathologische Anatomie und Physiologie*, **255**, 677-705.

Children With Cardiac Disease and Exercise

Rolf Mocellin
Abteilung Kinderkardiologie der Universitäts-Kinderklinik
Freiburg, Federal Republic of Germany

Since Adams and Duffie (1961) published their data related to physical working capacity of children with heart disease, many authors have tried to quantify the functional ability of children with different cardiac malformations. The results were by no means consistent, and it is rather difficult to obtain an adequate idea of the cardiovascular performance capacity of children with cardiac disease by studying the literature.

There is, however, agreement in that exercise ability is always diminished in the presence of a right-to-left shunt, even if merely apparent with exercise and not at rest. In contrast, children with a left-to-right shunt at the ventricular or atrial levels or with stenotic malformations of the right or left ventricular outflow tract were also found to have normal test results (Kramer & Lurie, 1964), but were generally disabled (Goldberg, Weiss, & Adams, 1966). A more detailed analysis of some hemodynamic aspects seemed to reveal that elevation of pulmonary pressure in children with ventricular septal defects was regularly combined with a decrease in cardiovascular ability, and that the extent of disability in patients with right or left ventricular outflow tract obstruction depended on the pressure gradient measured at rest (Adams & Duffie, 1961; Duffie & Adams, 1963; Kjelsberg, 1959). These findings however, though highly suggestive, could not be confirmed by others (Mocellin, Rutenfranz, & Bühlmeyer, 1982; Thorén, 1967).

The reasons for the striking differences resulting from different investigations are manifold: In view of the great variability of aerobic capacity in a normal population, ranging from 30 to 60 ml/min kg $\dot{V}O_2$, it is not at all surprising that discrimination between children with and without cardiac malformations is rather difficult, at least in the individual. Also when dealing with a group of children suffering from the same cardiac malformation, discrimination from normal individuals is difficult because there is a strong tendency of the heart muscle to compensate for the specific defect as far as possible. As the heart muscle is healthy in children, unlike the situation encountered in adults with coronary heart disease, it may overcome a mild to moderate pulmonary stenosis or an atrial septal defect by right ventricular hypertrophy or dilatation, reestablishing a rather normal functional ability.

Additional difficulties in differentiation of what is normal or pathological originate from methodological errors. Adams, Linde, and Miyake (1961) propagated a geometric digressive relationship between body surface area and W_{170} as being valid for normal children and suggested its suitability for comparison of children with cardiac defects. From a theoretical point of view, however, a geometrical progressive relationship between body surface area and W_{170} is to be expected, and this has been verified by other investigators (Rutenfranz & Mocellin, 1968). It is easy to appreciate that comparisons are not possible if the reference standard is invalid.

Another principle to be taken into consideration when comparisons are made between standardized values and values of children with cardiac malformations is that body height and body weight parallel each other only to a certain degree. The consequence is that relationships between weight and cardiovascular performance capacity, when established in consecutive age groups, show a tendency to overlap (see Figure 1). For example, in the group of 12- to 15-year-old children, the upper part of the relation between weight and W_{170} is made up of children whose height has not kept up with their weight, whereas the lower part of the regression in this age group and in the others is represented by children whose height retardation is less pronounced than is their weight retardation. The reason for this is that weight and height are not only interdependent to a certain degree, but also age-dependent. That means that older children are more fit than younger children of the same weight or of the same height, as can be likewise seen in Figure 1. This also means that standardization of normal values in relation to parameters of body development is only meaningful if age is taken into consideration; that is, standardization must be performed separately for each age group and, naturally, separately for boys and girls (see Table 1), as already proposed by Åstrand (1952), but not always observed by his successors.

Another problem, which was extensively discussed during the first International Symposium on Paediatric Work Physiology at Dortmund is the validity of indirect methods,

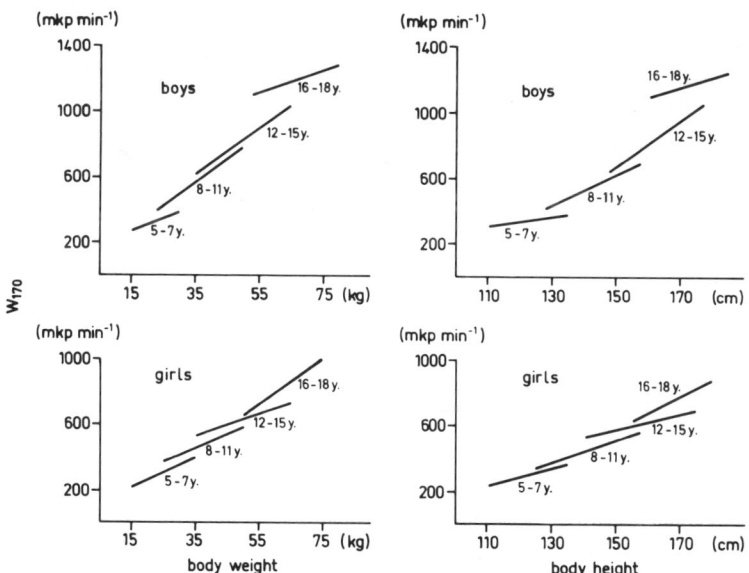

Figure 1—Relationships between body weight or body height, respectively, and W_{170} in boys and girls of different age groups.

Table 1

Absolute and Relative Standard Values of the W_{170} Evaluated at a Stepwise Increasing Load in Boys and Girls

Age (yrs)	Boys W_{170}[a] (Watt)	W_{170}/BH[b] (Watt/cm)	Girls W_{170} (Watt)	W_{170}/BH (Watt/cm)
5.5	35	0.30	28	0.25
6.5	42	0.35	33	0.28
7.5	50	0.39	39	0.31
8.5	58	0.44	45	0.35
9.5	67	0.48	52	0.38
10.5	75	0.53	59	0.42
11.5	84	0.57	67	0.46
12.5	96	0.63	77	0.50
13.5	112	0.71	85	0.53
14.5	131	0.79	89	0.56
15.5	145	0.85	92	0.57
16.5	155	0.90	94	0.58
17.5	161	0.92	95	0.58
18.5	162	0.93	95	0.58

[a]W_{170} = the work rate at a heart rate of 70 bmp.
[b]BH = body height.

as for example W_{170}, in the assessment of cardiovascular performance capacity. Criticism against the applicability of indirect methods was based upon three main arguments: (a) Comparisons of measurements performed using different types of ergometers are impossible because of the different calibrations; (b) Measurement of the physical load is not a sufficient basis for the estimation of oxygen uptake in view of the interindividual differences in mechanical efficiency; (c) Indirect methods start from the principle of a constant maximal heart rate, whereas in children and adolescents maximal heart rate may differ from about 180 to about 210 beats/min. The W_{170} is the indirect method most widely used. It has been compared with the maximal oxygen uptake in children with cardiac diseases on the assumption that maximal oxygen uptake represents a direct measurement of cardiovascular performance capacity. This seemed to be justified when bearing in mind that cardiovascular performance capacity is directly related to the capacity of the organism to transport oxygen. The W_{170}-values as well as the maximal $\dot{V}O_2$--values were related to standard values for the different age groups of boys and girls.

As to the W_{170} standard values referred, they were determined by Mocellin, Rutenfranz, and Singer (1971) and Mocellin, Sebening, and Bühlmeyer (1972). The reference values of $\dot{V}O_2$ max were based on a mean value of 45 ml/min•kg body weight which appears to be valid for boys of all age groups according to a review of literature by Eriksson (1972). Taking into account normal values of weight and height for the different age groups, it is possible to calculate the absolute and relative (body height squared) (Van Dubeln & Eriksson, 1972) standard values of $\dot{V}O_2$ max for boys of different age groups (see Table 2). In order to obtain standard values of $\dot{V}O_2$ max for girls, investigations were reviewed in which authors had compared the $\dot{V}O_2$ max for boys and girls

Table 2

Absolute and Relative Standard Values of Aerobic Capacity in Relation to Sex and Age

Age (yrs)	Boys		Girls	
	$\dot{V}O_2$ max[a] (l/min)	$\dot{V}O_2$ max/BH²[b] (l/min/m²)	$\dot{V}O_2$ max (l/min)	$\dot{V}O_2$ max/BH² (l/min/m²)
6.5	1.04	0.71	0.93	0.66
7.5	1.17	0.72	1.03	0.66
8.5	1.29	0.74	1.14	0.67
9.5	1.41	0.75	1.24	0.67
10.5	1.53	0.76	1.35	0.67
11.5	1.65	0.77	1.47	0.67
12.5	1.81	0.79	1.62	0.68
13.5	2.05	0.81	1.73	0.69
14.5	2.32	0.84	1.80	0.70
15.5	2.55	0.88	1.86	0.71
16.5	2.71	0.91	1.87	0.71
17.5	2.81	0.93	1.87	0.71

[a] $\dot{V}O_2$ max = aerobic capacity.
[b] $\dot{V}O_2$ max/BH² = aerobic capacity/per square of body height.

in different age groups. Figure 2 represents the height-related $\dot{V}O_2$ max values of girls of different age groups as a percentage of the corresponding values of boys as reported by Åstrand (1952), Bar-Or et al. (1971), Knuttgen (1967), Lange-Andersen and Ghesquierre (1973), Lange-Andersen, Seliger, Rutenfranz, and Mocellin (1974), Mácek et al. (1973), Mocellin and Wasmund (1973), Seliger et al. (1971) and Skinner et al. (1971). The values of height-related $\dot{V}O_2$ max of the girls were calculated from the corresponding values for boys given in Table 2, and the corresponding absolute and weight-related $\dot{V}O_2$ max-values for the different age groups of girls were derived, taking into account normal values of height and weight. The values of $\dot{V}O_2$ max for girls thus obtained are likewise represented in Table 2.

It may appear complicated to compare W_{170} and $\dot{V}O_2$ max on the basis of individual values related to standard values instead of merely starting from the individual values without taking into account their relation to the corresponding standard values. But the advantage of the former method is to eliminate the tendency to create correlations as a result of combining data from children of different ages and different somatic development.

Table 3 shows the results of a comparison of 20 boys and 23 girls with pre- and postoperative heart malformations, aged 6-to-16 years. Considering exclusively the relative values, only 18 to 37% of the variance of the $\dot{V}O_2$ max is accounted for by the W_{170}. This means that an estimation of the cardiovascular performance capacity in the individual is not sufficient by measuring only W_{170}.

The question emerging from this result was: To what extent is the indirect measurement of cardiovascular performance capacity impeded by differences in the individual

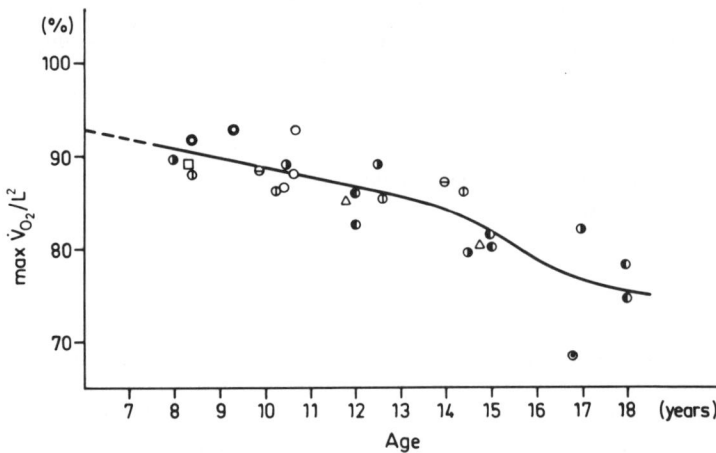

Figure 2—Maximal oxygen uptake related to square of body height ($\dot{V}O_2$ max/H^2) of girls as percentage of boys of equal age according to different authors (O Åstrand [1952]; □ Bar-Or et al. [1971]; ⊙ Knuttgen [1967]; ⊖ Lange-Andersen & Ghesquierre [1973]; OLange-Andersen, Seliger, Rutenfranz, & Mocellin [1974]; OMácek et al. [1973]; O Rutenfranz & Mocellin [1968]; △ Seliger et al. [1971]; O Skinner et al. [1971].

Table 3

Relationship Between W_{170} and $\dot{V}O_2$ max in Boys and Girls With Different Pre- and Postoperative Cardiac Malformations

	Boys $n=20$ 6-16 years		Girls $n=23$ 6-16 years	
	r	r^2	r	r^2
W_{170} (Watt): $\dot{V}O_2$ max (l/min)	0.67	0.45	0.74	0.55
W_{170}^a (% AS): $\dot{V}O_2$ max (% AS)	0.61	0.37	0.44	0.19
W_{170}^b (% HS): $\dot{V}O_2$ max (% HS)	0.59	0.35	0.42	0.18

[a]% AS = percent of age standard.
[b]% HS = percent of height standard.

maximal heart rate? To answer this, the differences of $\dot{V}O_2$ max and W_{170}, both in percent of the expected values according to height, were if related to the corresponding values of maximal heart rate, as demonstrated in Figure 3 (Mocellin & Bastanier, 1976). The correlation coefficient of 0.47 was significantly different from zero. Therefore, at least a certain part of the differences between indirectly and directly measured physical performance capacity could be attributed to differences in individual maximal heart rate. As seen in Figure 3, the difference of the relative values of $\dot{V}O_2$ max and W_{170} assumes a negative value at lower maximal heart rates and a positive

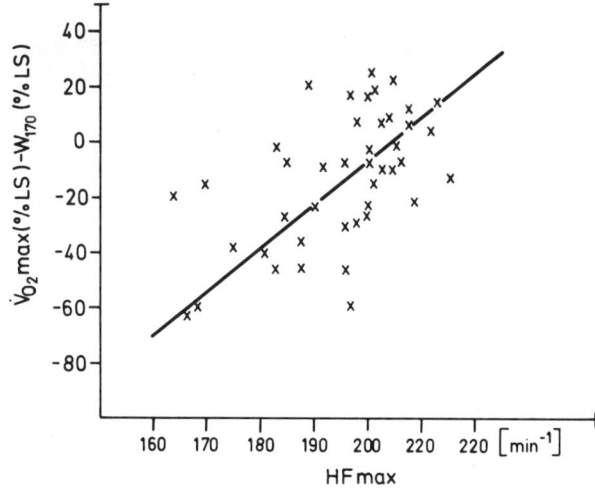

Figure 3—Difference of maximal oxygen uptake ($\dot{V}O_2$ max) and W_{170}, both in percent of expected values according to body height (% LS), in relation to maximal heart rate in 43 children with different pre- and postoperative cardiac malformations.

value at higher maximal heart rates. This implies that by using W_{170}, the cardiovascular performance capacity is overestimated at lower heart rates, whereas it is underestimated at higher maximal heart rates.

Another problem emerging from this investigation was to explain the differences between the simple mean values of W_{170} and $\dot{V}O_2$ max when related to the expected values (see Table 4). For instance, $\dot{V}O_2$ max of boys, when related to the expected values according to height, was 85%, whereas the corresponding value of W_{170} was 100%. This led us to the question of the validity of standard values. When these standard values of W_{170} were elaborated (Mocellin, Rutenfranz, & Singer, 1971) a special type of ergometer was employed with a relatively low gyrating mass. The ergometer used when performing these investigations (Mocellin & Bastanier, 1976) was calibrated with the same machine used for the calibration of the other ergometer, but had a higher gyrating mass. Perhaps the higher mechanical efficiency brought about by the greater gyrating mass was the reason for the inconsistencies mentioned. The present view is that it is not advisable to use one type of ergometer for measuing W_{170} and rely on standard values elaborated with another type of ergometer. Since indirect methods have been shown to be invalid, at least for children with cardiac diseases, direct measurement of $\dot{V}O_2$ max in these children seems to be necessary in order to provide relevant information concerning functional ability of the cardiovascular system.

Concerning the solution of methodological problems, cardiac surgery has advanced substantially, and most of the children with more severe types of cardiac malformations have been operated upon. The method was established, but there were only a few subjects available. Actually, cardiac surgery of most of the hemodynamically relevant heart malformations is at present performed in infancy or at least before school age, that is, at an age when determination of functional ability by means of ergometry is not yet possible, and when participation in sport events has not yet begun. For ex-

Table 4

Mean Values and Standard Deviations of $\dot{V}O_2$ max and W_{170}
in Boys and Girls With Different Cardiac Malformations

	Boys $n=20$ 6-16 years		Girls $n=23$ 6-16 years	
	M	S	M	S
$\dot{V}O_2$ max[a] (% AS)	81	19	89	13
$\dot{V}O_2$ max[b] (% HS)	85	16	90	13
W_{170} (% AS)	97	31	104	27
W_{170} (% HS)	100	32	100	28

[a]% AS = percent of age standard.
[b]% HS = percent of height standard.

ample, this is valid for the large ventricular septal defect, Fallot's tetralogy; transposition of the great arteries, including those cases with additional ventricular septal defect or left ventricular outflow tract obstruction; coarctation of the aorta; large persistent ductus arteriosus Botalli; severe pulmonary stenosis with intact ventricular septum; and complete atrioventricular defect. The question arising in these patients, therefore, is merely whether normal or approximately normal functional capacity has been achieved by the operation, and what kind of residual malformation may perhaps be responsible for limitations of the functional capacity after the operation. Cardiac malformations sometimes not yet operated on at school age comprise hemodynamically less severe malformations as, for instance, the small or medium-sized ventricular septal defect, the mild or moderate pulmonary stenosis, the atrial septal defect, the partial anomalous pulmonary venous connection, the coarctation with good collaterals, and the small persistent ductus arteriosus Botalli. Many of these children need no operation at all, and their functional ability does not differ from those of healthy children. Thus, there are no objections to their participations in sporting events. In other children of these groups of cardiac malformations, cardiac surgery is needed. The decision to perform surgery in these cases in which there are no complaints or symptoms is based on our knowledge of the natural history of the disease derived from earlier observations, when cardiac surgery was not yet available. Functional ability in these children generally turns out to be in the normal range so that there is no reason for limiting their participation in school sports either.

Patients with aortic stenosis cannot be allowed to participate in sporting events because of the risk of sudden death. This danger increases with the degree of the stenosis and is imminent, especially in cases showing a strain pattern in the ECG. Patients with a gradient of more than 50 mmHg will be operated on, and their physical activity should be restricted before operation. Children with a gradient of less than 50 mmHg need no operation. In spite of their relatively low risk for sudden death, strenuous activities should not be encouraged, but school sports may perhaps be permitted.

The number of patients with cyanotic heart disease not yet operated on at school age is relatively small and comprises complex malformations with cyanosis, where either additional pulmonary stenosis is present or palliative banding of the pulmonary artery has been performed during infancy. Venous admixture to the arterial blood increases with exercise, resulting in a further decrease of arterial oxygen content. Maximal oxygen uptake is in the range of about 30 to 50% of normals (Cumming, 1980; de Knecht & Binkhorst, 1980). Training is not possible except for the motor performance capacity. Thus, mechanical efficiency can be improved, resulting in an elevated load for the same oxygen uptake in certain types of physical activity.

As cardiac performance capacity is not substantially impeded in many patients with congenital heart disease undergoing cardiac surgery, an operation will not always bring about a direct increase in functional ability of the cardiovascular system. However, prognosis concerning physical working capacity will be better the more complete the correction of a malformation of the heart or of the vessels. A complete correction is possible, for example, in patients with patent ductus arteriosus, with coarctation of the aorta, and with atrial and ventricular septal defects.

For patients with valvular disease, the prospects after operation are less satisfactory. After valvotomy of a pulmonary stenosis there may be some degree of pulmonary incompetence; however, this usually does not have a significant influence on the child's working capacity. Yet a residual gradient, when combined with inadequate compliance of the right ventricle, may lead to a decrease in stroke volume during work. This happened in 3 out of 20 investigated children with this malformation after surgery (Bastanier, Kaltwasser, & Mocellin, 1977). When cardiovascular performance capacity in these children is significantly reduced, reoperation must be considered.

After valvotomy of an aortic stenosis, especially when performed in a considerably malformed valve, aortic insufficiency is generally present. It may even happen that functional disability is more pronounced after operation than it had been before. In these cases, valve replacement must be considered.

When dealing with the assessment of cardiovascular performance capacity in operated children, more detailed information concerning cardiac output, stroke volume, and pressure gradients may be needed. These are generally only obtained by means of a central venous catheter and arterial cannulation during exercise. It must be carefully considered whether the information to be obtained justifies the application invasive methods. On the other hand, comparability should be provided concerning cardiac output or stroke volume in different age groups of boys and girls if a meaningful interpretation of the values is to be realized. Otherwise, findings such as low cardiac output in relation to measured $\dot{V}O_2$ max (James, 1983) may turn out to be misinterpretations based on incorrect assumptions concerning the normal relationships of $\dot{V}O_2$ and cardiac output in children of different ages and sex.

The maximal values of cardiac output for boys and girls of any age can be calculated from the corresponding values of $\dot{V}O_2$ max if the maximal arteriovenous oxygen difference $AVDO_2$ max is known. For children of more than 10 years of age $AVDO_2$ max can be assumed to be about 13.5 ml/100 ml (Ekblom et al., 1968; Eriksson, Grimby, & Saltin, 1971; Eriksson & Koch, 1973; Saltin et al., 1968). In younger children, $AVDO_2$ max must be assumed to be somewhat lower because of the lower hemoglobin. However, for calculation of maximal cardiac output, this small discrepancy was ignored, and we started from a constant $AVDO_2$ max of 13.5 ml/100 ml for all age groups. The resulting values are presented in Table 5, together with the corresponding values of stroke volume, calculated by assuming that a mean maximal heart rate of 200 beats/min is valid for all age groups. The relative values given in Table 5 were evaluated

Table 5
Absolute and Relative Standard Values of Maximal Cardiac Output and Stroke Volume During Exercise in Relation to Sex and Age

Age (yrs)	Boys				Girls			
	$^a\dot{Q}$ max (l/min)	$^b\dot{Q}$ max/BH^2 (l/min/m²)	^{c}SV (ml)	^{d}SV/BH^3 (ml/m³)	$\dot{Q}$ max (l/min)	$\dot{Q}$ max/BH^2 (l/min/m²)	SV (ml)	SV/BH^3 (ml/m³)
6.5	7.7	5.3	39	21.9	6.9	4.9	35	20.4
7.5	8.7	5.4	43	21.1	7.6	4.9	38	19.5
8.5	9.6	5.4	48	20.4	8.4	5.0	42	19.0
9.5	10.4	5.5	52	19.9	9.2	5.0	46	18.4
10.5	11.3	5.6	57	19.7	10.0	5.0	50	17.6
11.5	12.2	5.7	61	19.3	10.9	5.0	55	16.8
12.5	13.4	5.8	67	19.0	12.0	5.0	60	16.3
13.5	15.2	6.0	76	18.9	12.8	5.1	64	16.1
14.5	17.2	6.3	86	19.0	13.3	5.2	67	16.2
15.5	18.9	6.6	94	19.3	13.8	5.3	69	16.3
16.5	20.1	6.7	100	19.5	13.9	5.3	69	16.2
17.5	20.8	6.9	104	19.7	13.9	5.2	69	16.2

$^a\dot{Q}$ max = maximal cardiac output.
$^b\dot{Q}$ max/BH^2 = maximal cardiac output/squared body height.
^{c}SV = stroke volume.
^{d}SV/BH^3 = stroke volume/cubic body height.

with regard to body height square ($\dot{Q}max/BH^2$) and body height cubed (SV/BH^3) following a suggestion of Eriksson (1972).

Before giving an example of how these values can be applied for evaluating the cardiovascular performance capacity of children with heart disease, brief mention will be made of submaximal cardiac output. At equal relative loads—for instance, at equal percentages of $\dot{V}O_2$ max—arteriovenous oxygen difference displays similar values in children of different age groups. Hence, it follows that the $\dot{V}O_2$ max and cardiac output from children of different ages parallel each other, which has also been established empirically by different authors (Bar-Or, Shephard, & Allen, 1971; Eriksson, Grimby, & Saltin, 1971; Eriksson & Koch, 1973; Godfrey, Davies, Wozniak, & Barnes, 1971; Mocellin, Sebening, & Bühlmeyer, 1973).

In Figure 4 (Mocellin, 1982) the maximal mean values of $\dot{V}O_2$ max (see Table 2) and cardiac output (see Table 5) are located along a line connecting all values with an arteriovenous oxygen difference of 13.5 ml/100 ml, the value which had been used as stated previously, for calculation of the mean maximal cardiac output values form mean $\dot{V}O_2$ max values. The figure contains also the regression between $\dot{V}O_2$ and cardiac output derived from values of Ekblom, Åstrand, Saltin, Stenberg, & Wallström (1968) and valid for male adults, calculated using the equation.

$$\dot{Q} \text{ (l/min)} = 5.1 + 5.8\ \dot{V}O_2 \text{ (l/min)}.$$

Parallel to this regression and starting from the respective mean maximal values, the regressions of five groups of boys have been drawn according to the considerations

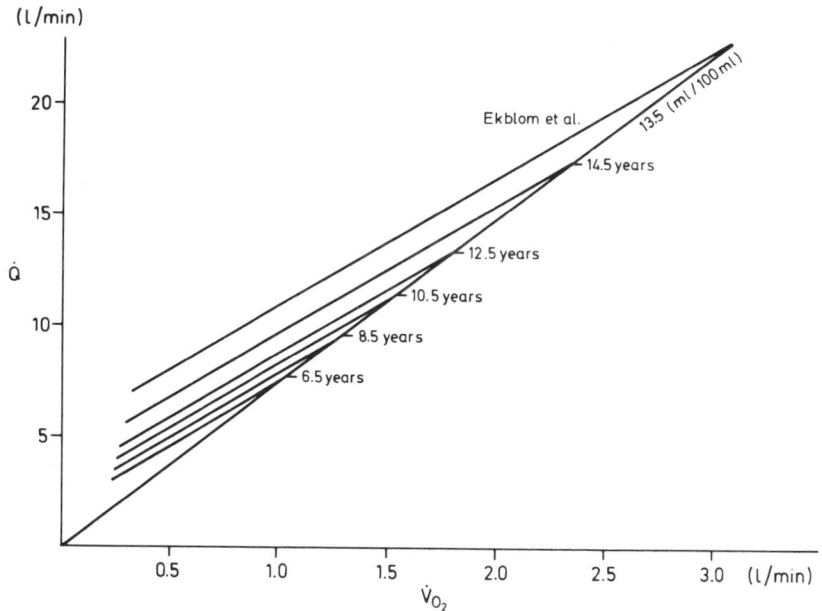

Figure 4—Regression lines between oxygen uptake ($\dot{V}O_2$) and cardiac output ($\dot{Q}$) in boys of different age groups (for details see text).

pointed out. The intercept of each regression can be easily calculated (Mocellin, 1982). The different intercepts of the corresponding regressions for boys and girls of all age groups are represented in Table 6. By subtracting the respective intercept from a measured value of cardiac output at rest and during exercise the influence of age and sex on the measured values can be eliminated; thus, this makes it possible to compare individuals of different ages and sex. The corresponding standard regression valid for all age groups of boys and girls then is

$$\dot{Q}_{corr} \text{ (l/min)} = 5.8 \ \dot{V}O_2 \text{ (l/min)}.$$

A typical example for the application of this kind of relation is given in Figure 5. The values of cardiac output measured at rest and during submaximal and maximal exercise in 21 boys and girls from 7.9 to 17.3 years of age with Falot's tetralogy who had undergone surgical repair were corrected for the age-depending intercepts (see Table 6) and related to the corresponding oxygen uptake (Mocellin, Bastanier, Hofacker, & Bühlmeyer, 1976).

The regression line represents, rather than the result of plotting the single values as might be supposed, the standard regression already mentioned. The distribution of the corrected values around the standard regression appears completely normal, indicating normal cardiac output in relation to measured $\dot{V}O_2$ max in these children. Aerobic capacity and maximal cardiac output were, however, not normal in these children as might be supposed from Figure 5. In Figure 6, the individual values for maximal oxygen uptake, expressed in percentage of expected values for children of the same height, are related to the age of the patients at the time of operation. An above average cardiovascular performance capacity was found only in three of the children. Mean aerobic capacity of all children was 85% of normal values according to height standards.

Table 6

Intercepts of the Regression Lines Between Oxygen Uptake and Cardiac Output in Boys and Girls

Age (yrs)	Boys a (l/min)	Girls a (l/min)
6.5	1.7	1.5
7.5	1.9	1.7
8.5	2.1	1.8
9.5	2.3	2.0
10.5	2.5	2.2
11.5	2.7	2.4
12.5	2.9	2.6
13.5	3.3	2.8
14.5	3.7	2.9
15.5	4.1	3.0
16.5	4.4	3.0
17.5	4.6	3.0

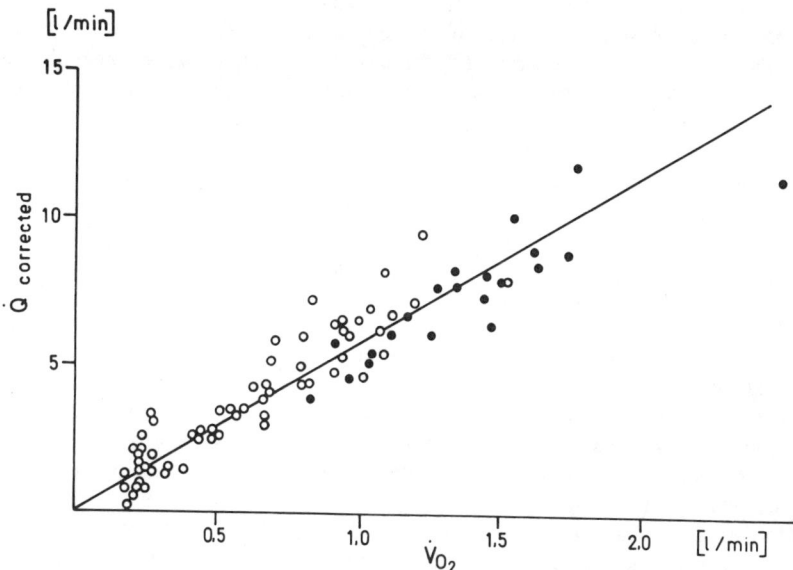

Figure 5—Cardiac output ($\dot{Q}_{corr}$) in relation to oxygen uptake ($\dot{V}O_2$) at rest (O) and during submaximal (O and maximal (●) work load in 21 children and adolescents with tetralogy of Fallot after surgical repair (for details see text).

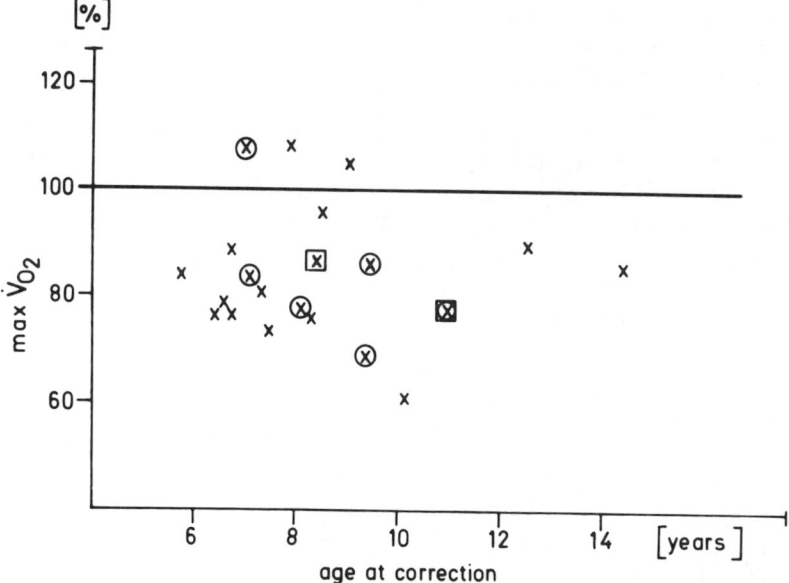

Figure 6—Maximal oxygen uptake (% of height standard) related to the age at correction in 21 children and adolescents with tetralogy of Fallot afte surgical repair (O children with former Blalock-Taussig-anastomosis; □ children with outflow patch).

Table 7 shows that the reduction of aerobic capacity was related to a similar reduction of maximal cardiac output and of stroke volume. The normal submaximal output could be explained by the fact that the reduced stroke volume was compensated for by a relatively high heart rate at submaximal levels resulting in a normal cardiac output at submaximal work (see Figure 5). During maximal exercise, however, the heart rate did not exceed that of healthy children and the reduced stroke volume resulted in a diminished maximal cardiac output and, consequently, in a reduction of maximal oxygen uptake. Further investigations showed that the reduction of stroke volume was mostly combined with an elevated end diastolic pressure in the right ventricle so that impaired filling of the right ventricle, rather than a residual gradient, seemed to be the reason for the reduced stroke volume.

Contrary to children with tetralogy of Fallot, who have been extensively investigated after corrective surgery, there is relatively little information on the functional capacity of children after the Senning- or Mustard-procedure in transposition of the great arteries, after the Fontan-procedure in tricuspid atresia or single ventricle, after surgical correction of a complete AV-defect in infancy as done nowadays. This is partly due to the fact that in most centers where functional studies could be performed, the patients are not yet at the age where precise testing is possible. There is, however, even a lack of information concerning the functional results of valvotomies performed in children with aortic stenosis, sometimes complicated by aortic incompetence postoperatively.

In view of the residual functional and anatomical disorders of the heart present in many children, after surgery, especially in tetrology of Fallot, but also after Senning- (Mocellini et al., 1982) and Mustard-procedures (Jarmaki & Conent, 1974) in children with transposition of the great arteries; or after Fontan-procedures in childen with tricuspid atresia (Mocellin, Henglein, & Bühlmeyer, 1981) it seems rather difficult to advise a child how to behave with regard to physical activity. However, some investigations have been performed (Goldberg et al., 1981; Ruttenberg, Adams, Orsmond, Couke, & Fisher, 1983) demonstrating significant improvement in maximum work capacity after 6- to 9-weeks of training in children following repair of tetralogy of Fallot, ventricular septal defect, aortic stenosis, and transposition of the great arteries. Interestingly, no significant difference was noted in maximum oxygen uptake before and after training, and the higher work load performed had to be attributed to a significant improvement in the efficiency of performance. Thus, no training effect on the car-

Table 7

Maximal Oxygen Uptake, Stroke Volume During Exercise, and Maximal Cardiac Output Values of 21 Children and Adolescents With Tetralogy of Fallot After Surgical Repair

	M	S
$\dot{V}O_2$ max[a] (% HS)	84.6	12.4
SV max (% HS)	88.5	16.3
$\dot{Q}$ max (% HS)	83.4	13.3

% HS = percent of height standard.

diovascular system itself could be observed, and the higher mechanical efficiency noted after training may be regarded as the effect of improved coordination of movements, that is, better motor performance capacity. Similar results have also been described in healthy children following a submaximal training program (Bar-Or & Zwiren, 1973; Mocellin & Wasmund, 1973). In conclusion, submaximal training in children after repair of cardiac defects has a positive influence on their capacity to perform work, despite the lack of increase of aerobic capacity.

References

ADAMS, F.H., & Duffie, E.R. (1961). Physical working capacity of children with heart disease. *J. Lancet,* **81,** 493.

ADAMS, F.H., Linde, L.M., & Miyake, H. (1961). The physical working capacity of normal school children. I. California. *Pediatrics,* **28,** 55.

ÅSTRAND, P.-O. (1952). Experimental studies of physical working capacity in relation to sex and age. Copenhagen: Munksgaard.

BAR-OR, O., Shephard, R., & Allen, C. (1971). Cardiac output of 10- to 13-year-old boys and girls during submaximal exercise. *Journal of Applied Physiology,* **30,** 219.

BAR-OR, O., Skinner, J.S., Bergsteinova, V., Shearburn, C., Royer, D., Bell, W., Haas, J., & Buskirk, E.R. (1971). Maximal aerobic capacity of 6- to 15-year-old girls and boys with subnormal intelligence quotients. *Acta Paediatrica Scandinavia,* (Suppl. 217), 108.

BAR-OR, O., & Zwiren, L.D. (1973). Physiological effects of frequency and content variation of physical education classes and of endurance conditioning on 9- to 10-year-old females and males. In *Pediatric Work Physiology: Proceedings of the 4th International Symposium,* p. 199. Tel Aviv, Israel: Wingate Institute.

BASTANIER, C., Kaltwasser, B., & Mocellin, R. (1977). Postoperative Belastungsuntersuchungen bei Kindern und Jugendlichen mit valvulärer Pulmonalstenose. [Postoperative investigations of exercise in children and adolescents with pulmonary stenosis]. *Z. Kardiol,* **66,** 587.

CUMMING, G.R. (1980). Maximal treadmill endurance times of children with heart defects compared to those of normal children. In K. Berg & B.O. Eriksson (Eds.), *Children and exercise IX ,* (pp. 354). Baltimore: University Park Press.

DE KNECHT, S., & Binkhorst, R.A. (1980). Physical characteristics of children wtih congenital heart diesease: Body characteristics and physical working capacity. In K. Berg, & B.O. Eriksson (Eds.), *Children and exercise IX,* (pp. 333-346). Baltimore: University Park Press.

DUFFIE, E.R., & Adams, F.H. (1963). The use of the working capacity test in the evaluation of children with congenital heart disease. *Pediatrics,* **32,** 757.

EKBLOM, B., Åstrand, P.-O., Saltin, B., Stenberg, J., & Wallström, B. (1968). Effect of training on circulatory response to exercise. *Journal of Applied Physiology,* **24,** 518.

ERIKSSON, B.O. (1972). Physical training, oxygen supply and muscle metabolism in 11-to-13 year old boys. *Acta Physiologica Scandinavia,* (Suppl. 384).

ERIKSSON, B.O., Grimby, G., & Saltin, B. (1971). Cardiac output and arterial blood gases during exercise in pubertal boys. *Journal of Applied Physiology,* **31,** 348.

ERIKSSON, B.O., & Koch. G. (1973). Effect of physical training on haemodynamic response during submaximal and maximal exercise in 11- to 13-year old boys. *Acta Physiologica Scandinavia*, **87**, 27.

GODFREY, S., Davies, C.T.M., Wozniak, E., & Barnes, C.A. (1971). Cardio-respiratory response to exercise in normal children. *Clinical Science*, **40**, 419.

GOLDBERG, B., Fripp, R.R., Lister, G., Loke, J., Nicholas, J.A., & Talner, N.S. (1981). Effect of physical training on exercise performance of children following surgical repair of congenital heart disease. *Pediatrics*, **68**, 691.

GOLDBERG, S.J., Weiss, R., & Adams, F.H. (1966). Comparison of the maximal endurance of normal children and patients with congenital cardiac disease. *Journal of Pediatrics*, **69**, 46.

JAMES, F.W. (1983). Exercise testing: In F.H. Adams, & G.C. Emmanouilides (Eds.), *Heart Disease in Infants, Children, and Adolescents*, (p. 107). Baltimore: Williams and Wilkins.

JARMAKANI, J., & Canent, R.V. (1974). Pre- and postoperative right ventricular function in children with transposition of the heart vessels. *Circulation*, **50** (Suppl. 11), 39.

KJELLBERG, S.R., Mannheimer, E., Rudhe, U., & Jonsson, B. (1959). Diagnosis of congenital heart disease. Chicago: Yearbook Publishers.

KNUTTGEN, H.G. (1967). Aerobic capacity of adolescents. *Journal of Applied Physiology*, **22**, 655.

KRAMER, J.D., & Lurie, P.R. (1964). The maximal exercise in children. *American Journal Dis. Child.*, **108**, 283.

LANGE-ANDERSEN, K., & Ghesquierre, J. (1973). Sex differences in the development of physical performance capacity during the puberty growth spurt period in a population unit at the west coast of Norway. In V. Seliger (Ed.), *Physical Fitness*, p. 55. Praha: Universita of Karlova.

LANGE-ANDERSEN, K., Seliger, V., Rutenfranz, J., & Mocellin, R. (1974). Physical performance capacity of children in Norway. Part I. Population parameters in a rural inland community with regard to maximal aerobic power. *European Journal of Applied Physiology*, **33**, 177.

MÁCEK, M., Cermák, V., Handzo, P., Horák, J., Jirka, Z., Rous, J., Seliger, V., & Ulbrich, J. (1973). Comparison between 12- 15- and 18-year-old groups of country and urban boys and girls. In V. Seliger (Ed.), *Physical fitness*. Praha: Universita Karlova.

MOCELLIN, R. (1982). Ergometrie im Kindesalter. [Ergometry in childhood]. *Herz* **7**, 42.

MOCELLIN, R., & Bastanier, C. (1976). Zur Frage der Zuverlässigkeit der W_{170} als Maß der körperlichen Leistungsfähigkeit bei der Beurteilung von Kindern mit Herzkrankheiten. [On the validity of W_{170} for estimation of physical working capacity in children with cardiac diseases]. *European Journal of Pediatrics*, **122**, 233.

MOCELLIN, R., Bastanier, C., Hofacker, W., & Bühlmeyer, K. (1976). Exercise performance in children and adolescents after surgical repair of tetralogy of Fallot. *European Journal of Cardiology*, **4**, 367.

MOCELLIN, R., Henglein, D., & Bühlmeyer, K. (1982). Ventrikelfunktion vor und nach Senning-Operation bei Patienten mit Transposition der großen Arterien. [Ventricular function before and after Senning-operation in patients with transposition of the great arteries]. *Herz*, **7**, 267.

MOCELLIN, R., Rutenfranz, J., & Bühlmeyer, K. (1970). Untersuchungen über die körperliche Leistungsfähigkeit Heransachsender. IV. Die Leistungsfähigkeit von Kindern und Jugendlichen mit angeborenen und erworbenen Herzfehlern. [Investigations on the physical working capacity of adolescents. IV. The performance capacity of adolescents with heart defects]. Z. Kinderheilk, **108**, 265.

MOCELLIN, R., Rutenfranz, J., & Singer, R. (1971). Zur Frage von Normwerten der körperlichen Leistungsfähigkeit (W_{170}) im Kindes- und Jugendalter. [On normal values of physical working capacity (W_{170}) in children and adolescents]. Z. Kinderheilk, **110**, 140.

MOCELLIN, R., Sebening, W., & Bühlmeyer, K. (1972). Zur Beurteilung der körperlichen Leistungsfähigkeit bei Kindern und Jugendlichen mit operierten Herzfehlern. [On the estimation of physical working capacity in children and adolescents with operated cardiac defects]. Z. Kinderheilk, **112**, 281.

MOCELLIN, R., Sebening, W., & Bühlmeyer, K. (1973). Herzminutenvolumen und Sauerstoffaufnahme in Ruhe und während submaximaler Belastungen bei 8 - 14jährigen Kindern. [Cardiac output and oxygen uptake at rest and during submaximal load in 8- to 14-year-old children]. Z. Kinderheilk, **114**, 323.

MOCELLIN, R., Silber, S., Sauer, U., & Bühlmeyer, K. (1981). Comparison of radionuclide and angiographic ventriculography in children with tricuspid atresia and in children with anomalous origin of the left coronary artery from the pulmonary artery. (Abstract). *First International Symposium on Nuclear Cardiology* (Abstracts). Tel Aviv, Israel.

MOCELLIN, R., & Wasmund, U. (1973). Investigations of the influence of a running training programme on the cardiovascular and motor performance capacity in 53 males and females of a second and third grade primary school class. In *Pediatric work physiology: Proceedings of the 4th International Symposium*, p. 279. Tel Aviv, Israel: Wingate Institute.

RUTENFRANZ, J., & Mocellin, R. (1968). Untersuchungen über die körperliche Leistungsfähigkeit Heranwachsender. I. Bezugsgrößen und Normwerte. [Investigations on the physical working capacity of adolescents. I. Normal values]. Z. Kinderheilk, **103**, 109.

RUTTENBERG, H.O., Adams, T.D., Orsmond, G.B., Couke, R.K., & Fisher, A.G. (1983). Effects of exercise training on aerobic fitness in children after open heart surgery. *Pediatric Cardiology*, **4**, 19.

SALTIN, B., Blomquist, G., Mitchel, J.H., Johnson, R.L., Wildenthal, K., Chapman, C. (1968). Response to exercise after bedrest and training. *Circulation*, **38**, (Suppl. 7).

SELIGER, V., Cermák, V., Handzo, S., Horák, J., Jirka, Z., Mácek, M., Pribil, M., Rous, J., Skranz, O., Ulbricht, J., & Urbanek, J. (1971). Physical fitness of the Czechoslovak 12- to 15-year-old population. *Acta Paediatrica Scandinavica*, (Suppl. 217), 37.

SKINNER, J.S., Bar-Or, O., Bergsteinova, V., Bell, C.W., Royer, D., Buskirk, E.R. (1971). Comparison of continuous and intermittent tests for determining maximal oxygen intake in children. *Acta Paediatrica Scandinavica*, (Suppl. 217), 24.

THORÉN, C. (1967). Die körperliche Leistungsfähigkeit bei verschiedenen angeborenen Herzfehlern. [The physical working capacity in different congenital heart malformations]. *Ärztl. Jugendk.*, **58**, 397.

VAN DÖBELN, W., & Eriksson, B. (1972). Physical training, maximal oxygen uptake and dimensions of the oxygen transporting and metabolizing organs in boys 11-to-13 years of age. *Acta Paediatrica Scandinavia*, **61**, 653.

Ventilatory Anaerobic Threshold in Children With Atrial or Ventricular Septal Defects

Tony Reybrouck, Maria Weymans,
Hugo Stijns, and Luc Van der Hauwaert
University of Leuven
Leuven, Belgium

Patients with atrial septal defects (ASD) or ventricular septal defects (VSD) have been shown to have a reduced exercise performance capacity (Cumming, 1978; Frick & Punsar, 1967; Goldberg, Weiss, & Adams, 1966) both before and after surgical correction (Cumming, 1978; Petersson, 1967).

Recently the exercise intensity at which the pulmonary ventilation ($\dot{V}_E$) ceases to increase in a linear fashion in relation to oxygen uptake ($\dot{V}O_2$) has been considered to be a sensitive criterion of submaximal exercise performance capacity in healthy adults (Wasserman, 1982), in healthy children (Reybrouck, Weymans, Ghesquiere, Van Gerven, & Stijns, 1982), and in children with congenital heart disease (Reybrouck et al., in press). Because of the reported coincidence of the nonlinear increase in $\dot{V}_E$ and lactate with increasing $\dot{V}O_2$ (Wasserman, Whipp, Koyal, & Beaver, 1973), this threshold has been identified as the "ventilatory anaerobic threshold." It has been shown to be a sensitive criterion of exercise performance (Reybrouck et al., 1984).

The aim of the present study was to investigate the exercise performance in children with ASD or VSD as compared to normal children with emphasis on the onset of anaerobic metabolism during graded exercise.

Methods

Children ($N=62$) with congenital heart disease (CHD) varying in age from 5 to 15.3 years (median age, 10.1 years) were studied. Five patients had ASD, 30 had VSD. Nine were examined on the average 2 years and 8 months after closure of an ASD; and 18 subjects were examined on the average 3 years and 6 months after closure of a VSD. In 19 of the 35 children who were not operated on, cardiac catheterization was performed previously. For the children with ASD, the pulmonary-to-systemic flow ratio at cardiac catheterization varied from 1.1 to 2.0 (mean = 1.4) and for VSD 1.1 to 3.0 (mean = 1.4). For comparison, 97 healthy age-matched children (49 boys and

48 girls) were also studied. They were grouped according to age: 6 to 7 years ($n=29$), 11 to 12 ($n=29$) and 14 to 15 ($n=39$). The healthy children were randomly selected at the School of Public Health (Leuven) at the occasion of a routine medical school examination. A written informed consent was obtained from the parents of the children.

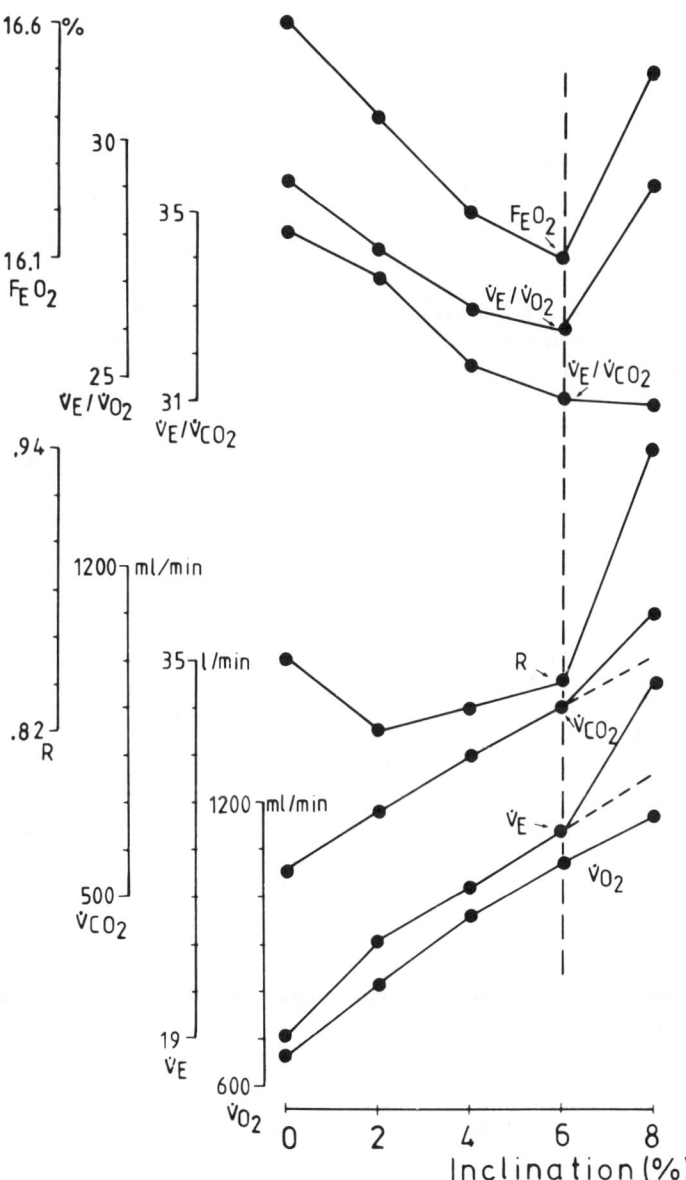

Figure 1—Changes in respiratory variables below and above the ventilatory anaerobic threshold during graded exercise in one representative child.

Exercise tests were performed on a treadmill. The speed was set at 4.8 km/hr for children younger than 6 years of age and at 5.6 km/hr for children aged 6 years and more. The inclination of the belt was increased stepwise by 2% every minute (Chandramouli, Ehmke, & Lauer, 1973) until a heart rate of 170 beats per min was reached. Heart rate was measured from the ECG. Oxygen uptake ($\dot{V}O_2$) and carbon dioxide output ($\dot{V}CO_2$) were measured by the open circuit method from the volume of expired air ($\dot{V}_E$), which was collected every minute in Douglas bags. The O_2 concentration was analyzed by a paramagnetic O_2 analyzer and the CO_2 concentration by an infrared CO_2 analyzer. The $\dot{V}_E$ was determined by a dry gas meter. The exercise capacity of the patients was estimated by the ventilatory anaerobic threshold (VAT) during graded exercise. The VAT was determined graphically as the highest exercise intensity at which the $\dot{V}_E$ failed to increase linearly with increasing $\dot{V}O_2$. Above this threshold, an exponential increase is observed for the $\dot{V}_E$. This onset of hyperventilation was futher checked by: (a) a systematic increase in the $\dot{V}_E/\dot{V}O_2$ without an increase in the $\dot{V}_E/\dot{V}CO_2$ (Caiozzo, et al., 1982), (b) a nonlinear increase in $\dot{V}CO_2$, and (c) an excessive rise of the respiratory gas exchange ratio (R) (Reybrouck, Weymans, Ghesquiere, Van Gerven & Stijns, 1982; Wasserman, Whipp, Koyal, & Beaver, 1973). A typical example is shown in Figure 1. The VAT was expressed as ml $O_2 \cdot min^{-1} \cdot kg^{-1}$. To assess the habitual level of physical activity of the healthy children and the patients, a standardized questionnaire was used. The questionnaire was very reproducible (r = .99). In this way, information was obtained on the number of hours of sports participation at school and during leisure time, recreational exercises, leisure time activities, and how the patients moved to and from school to home. The number of hours of physical activity were cumulated as a score.

The data were reported as the mean and the standard error of the mean. For the normal values, the 95% confidence limits were also reported. For comparison of the number of subnormal values in different subgroups a chi-square test was applied and an analysis of variance (ANOVA) was performed where appropriate.

Results

In the healthy children, aged 6 to 7, 11 to 12 and 14 to 15 years, the VAT was reached by the boys at 33.5 ± 0.97 ml $O_2 \cdot min^{-1} \cdot kg^{-1}$, 35.1 ± 1.47, and 29.5 ± 1.06 and by the girls at 29.3 ± 0.77, 29.7 ± 1.20, and 24.1 ± 0.69, respectively. A significantly ($p < .05$) lower VAT was found for the girls compared to the boys at every age.

When compared with age- and sex-matched normal children, subnormal values (below the 95% confidence limits) were found for the VAT in 4 of 5 (80%) of the children with ASD and in 24 of 30 (80%) of the children with VSD (see Figures 2A & B). In the group of patients who were examined after surgical correction 6 of 9 (67%) for ASD and 14 of 18 (78%) for VSD were below this normal limit (see Figures 2A & B). No significant differences existed between patients with ASD and VSD nor between the operated or nonoperated patients. When expressed as a percentage of the normal value found in age- and sex-matched children, the VAT in children with unoperated ASD and VSD was reached at 88.5 ± 5.5%, and 81.5 ± 4.0%, respectively. In operated children, the VAT was reached at 86 ± 3.2% for those with ASD, and 88.2 ± 3.7% for those with VSD. No significant difference was found between these groups. However, when compared with normal values, the VAT was significantly lower than the value found in age- and sex-matched normal children. This was also found in patients who were operated on as well as those who were not.

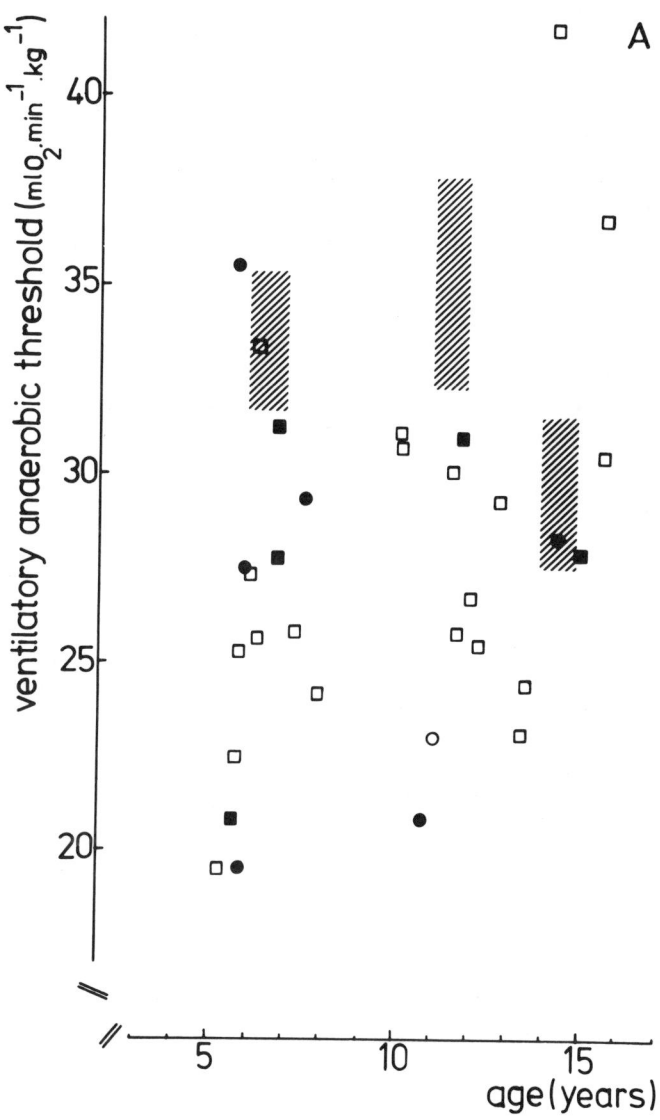

Figure 2A: Boys—The ventilatory anaerobic threshold in children with ASD or VSD, or in postoperative ASD and VSD patients. The shaded area represents the 95% confidence limits for healthy children. The O represents patients with ASD and □ VSD. Closed symbols refer to patients who underwent operations.

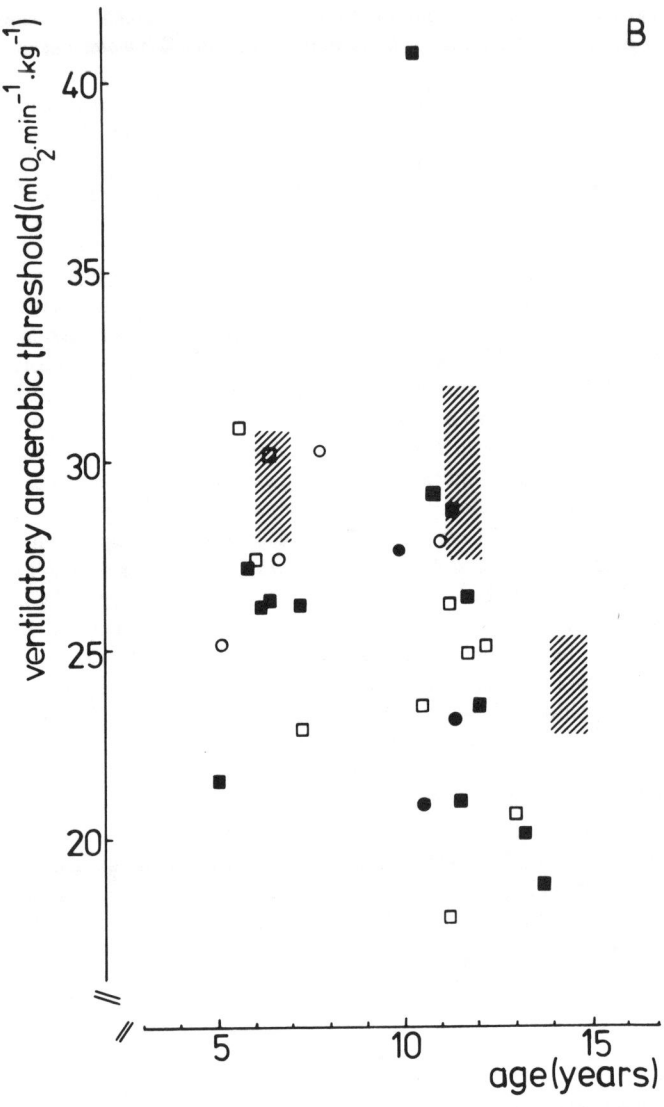

Figure 2B: Girls.

In children with right ventricular systolic pressure (RVSP) in excess of 30 mm HG at the time of cardiac catheterization, the VAT tended to be lower (84.7 ± 4.6% of the normal values) when compared to the VAT of those with RVSP below 30 mm Hg (99.5 ± 9.67% of the normal values) (.05<p< .10) (see Table 1).

In the children with ASD or VSD whether operated on or not, their habitual level of physical activity was significantly (p< .05) lower than the value in age and sex matched normal children (see Table 2).

Table 1

Ventilatory Anaerobic Threshold (% of normal values)

<30 mm Hg RVSP[a]		>30 mm Hg RVSP
N = 6		12
M = 23.8		36.8
S = 99.5 ± 9.7	.05<P< .10	84.7 ± 4.6

[a]RVSP = Right ventricular systolic pressure.
S = Percentage of normal values.

Table 2

The Habitual Level of Physical Activity in Children With Congenital Heart Diseases Compared to Normal Children

Sex	Habitual Level of Physical Activity		F
	Normals	Patients	
Boys	5.0 ± 0.35	2.8 ± 0.29	16.56 ($p< .005$)
Girls	4.0 ± 0.28	2.8 ± 0.23	9.14 ($p< .005$)

Discussion

In the pediatric age group, maximal exercise tests to evaluate the cardiorespiratory performance capacity are largely dependent on the motivation of the child, which is a highly variable factor. Therefore, submaximal exercise tests are advantageous for clinical exercise testing in children with CHD. One exercise procedure which has been used frequently is the exercise capacity or PWC_{170} (Duffie & Adams, 1963; Mocellin & Bastanier, 1976). Recently, however, the "ventilatory anaerobic threshold" has been shown to be a more sensitive criterion for studying endurance capacity in adults (Weltman, Katch, Sady, & Freedson, 1978) and in children with congenital heart disease (Reybrouck et al., 1984).

The finding of a subnormal exercise performance capacity in children with ASD or VSD is in agreement with previous reports (Cumming, 1974, 1980; Petersson, 1967), although a larger portion of subnormal values was observed in the present study than in the series by Cumming (1974, 1980). Cumming (1980) reported a maximal endurance time during graded treadmill exercise below the 10th percentile of the normal values in 22% of his patients with moderate VSD and in 27% of his patients with moderate ASD. In postoperative patients, these values were 32% for VSD and 44% for ASD. In the present study, a considerably larger portion of patients had subnormal values (below the 95% confidence limits for normal children): 67% for ASD and 80% for VSD; and 67% and 78% for ASD or VSD, postoperatively. As the VAT has been shown to be a more sensitive measure of exercise performance capacity in children with CHD compared to the PWC_{170} (Reybrouck et al., 1984), it is likely that the VAT is also a more sensitive measure than the maximal endurance time during a graded treadmill run.

The early onset of hyperventilation during graded exercise in children with ASD or VSD suggests an early accumulation of lactate during graded exercise. In ASD, this low anaerobic threshold may result from a hypokinetic circulation during exercise due to a diminished left ventricular stroke volume (Epstein et al., 1973; Jonsson, 1973; Petersson, 1967). Similarly, in children with VSD, a decreased left ventricular function can be expected to contribute to subnormal exercise performance as has been reported in adults with VSD (Jablonsky et al., 1983). The lower VAT in children with the higher RVSP confirms observations of Frick and Punsar (1967) for the PWC_{150} in adult patients with left-to-right shunts. They reported normal values for the PWC_{150} in patients with RVSP below 50 mm Hg, but subnormal values in those whose RVSP exceeded 50 mm Hg. The latter group also had an increased pulmonary vascular resistance.

After corrective surgery, the VAT in the patients in this study was also subnormal and did not show any significant difference from children who were not operated on. In a postoperative hemodynamic study, 6 to 16 years after surgery in children who were operated on for VSD between the ages of 5 and 13 years, left ventricular response to exercise was still abnormal, and a low maximum work load for the group as a whole has been reported (Hallidie-Smith, Wilson, Hart, & Zeidifard, 1977).

A decreased cardiorespiratory endurance capacity in children with left-to-right shunts may also result to some extent from a lack of physical activity, as children with CHD are often overprotected for physical activity (Strong & Alpert, 1982). If hypoactivity is a major factor leading to submaximal performance capacity, physical activity must be strongly encouraged, unless specifically contraindicated, which is very exceptional in the pediatric age group (Bar-Or, 1982).

References

BAR-OR, O. (1982). Clinical implications of pediatric exercise physiology. *Annals of Clinical Research*, **14**, (Suppl. 34), 97-106.

CAIOZZO, V.J., Davis, J., Ellis, J.F., Azus, J.L., Vandagriff, R., Prietto, C.A., & McMaster, W.A. (1982). Comparison of gas exchange indices used to detect the anaerobic threshold. *Journal of Applied Physiology*, **53**, 1184-1189.

CHANDRAMOULI, B., Ehmke, D.A., & Lauer, L.M. (1973). Exercise-induced electrocardiographic changes in children with congenital aortic stenosis. *Journal of Pediatrics*, **87**, 725-730.

CUMMING, G.R. (1978). Maximal exercise capacity of children with heart defects. *American Journal of Cardiology*, **42**, 613-619.

CUMMING, G.R. (1980). Maximal treadmill endurance times of children with heart defects compared to those of normal children. In K. Berg & B.O. Eriksson (Eds.), *Children and exercise IX*, (pp. 354-368). Baltimore: University Park Press.

DUFFIE, E.R., & Adams, F.H. (1963). The use of working capacity tests in the evaluation of children with congenital heart disease. *Pediatrics*, **32**, 757-768.

EPSTEIN, S.E., Beiser, G.D., Goldstein, R.E., Rosing, D.R., Redwood, D.R., & Morrow, A.G. (1973). Hemodynamic abnormalities in response to mild and intense upright exercise following operative correction of an atrial septal defect or Tetralogy of Fallot. *Circulation*, **47**, 1065-1075.

FRICK, N.H., & Punsar, S. (1967). Physical fitness of patients with left-to-right shunts. In M.J. Karvonen & H.J. Barry (Eds.), *Physical activity and the heart*, (pp. 42-50). Springfield, IL: Charles C. Thomas Publishers.

GOLDBERG, S.J., Weiss, R., & Adams, F.H. (1966). A comparison of the maximal endurance of normal children and patients with congenital heart disease. *The Journal of Pediatrics*, **69**, 46-55.

HALLIDIE-SMITH, K.A., Wilson, R.S.E., Hart, A., & Zeidifard, E. (1977). Functional status of patients with large ventricular septal defect and pulmonary vascular disease 6 to 16 years after surgical closure of their defect in childhood. *British Heart Journal*, **39**, 1093-1101.

JABLONSKY, G., Hilton, J.D., Liu, P.P., Morch, J.E., Druck, M.N., Bar-Shlomo, B.Z., & McLaughlin, P.R. (1983). Rest and exercise ventricular function in adults with congenital ventricular septal defects. *American Journal of Cardiology*, **51**, 293-298.

JONSSON, B. (1973). Circulatory adaptation to exercise in congenital heart disease. *Proceedings of the Association of European Paediatric Cardiologists*, **9**, 2-8.

MOCELLIN, R., & Bastanier, C. (1976). Zur Frage der Zuverlässigkeit des W_{170} als Mass der Körperlichen Leistungsfähigkeit bei der Beurteilung von Kindern mit Herzkrankheiten (On the validity of W_{170} as a measure of physical performance capacity in the assessment of children with heart disease). *European Journal of Pediatrics*, **122**, 223-239.

PETERSSON, P.O. (1967). Atrial septal defect of secundum type. *Acta Paediatrica Scandinavica*, (Suppl. 174).

REYBROUCK, T., Weymans, M., Ghesquiere, J., Van Gerven, D., & Stijns, H. (1982). Ventilatory threshold in kindergarten children during treadmill exercise. *European Journal of Applied Physiology*, **50**, 79-86.

REYBROUCK, T., Weymans, M., Stijns, H., De Belva, A., Allegaert, M., & Van der Hauwaert, L. (1984). Ventilatory thresholds as an estimate of cardiorespiratory performance capacity in children with congenital heart disease. In *Proceedings of the III International Congress of Auxology*. New York & London: Plenum Press.

STRONG, W.B., & Alpert, B.S. (1982). The child with heart disease: Play, recreation, and sports. *Current problems in pediatrics*. Chicago, IL: Year Book Medical Publishers.

WASSERMAN, K. (1982) Physiology of gas exchange and exertional dyspnea. *Clinical Science*, **61**, 7-13.

WASSERMAN, K., Whipp, B.J., Koyal, S.N., & Beaver, W.L. (1973). Anaerobic threshold and respiratory gas exchange during exercise. *Journal of Applied Physiology*, **35**, 236-243.

WELTMAN, A., Katch, V., Sady, S., & Freedson, P. (1978). Onset of metabolic acidosis (anaerobic threshold) as a criterion measure of submaximal fitness. *Research Quarterly*, **49**, 218-227.

Dynamic Exercise in Children With Sickle Cell Anemia and Sickle Cell Trait

Ian C. Balfour, William B. Strong, Wesley Covitz, and Bruce S. Alpert
Medical College of Georgia, Augusta, Georgia, U.S.A.

Physical activity and exercise are important for the normal growth and development of children. Children with sickle cell anemia have significant impairment of their exercise tolerance, caused in part by their anemia and the cardiac dysfunction associated with this disease. The purpose of this article is to describe the response to exercise of children with hemoglobins SS and AS and also to describe left ventricular function in individuals with SS hemoglobin.

Methods

Exercise stress tests were performed on 47 children (28 male and 19 female) aged 5 to 18 years (mean = 10.3 years) who had sickle cell anemia (SS), and 48 children (25 male and 23 female) aged 4 to 21 years (mean = 11.6 years) with sickle cell trait (AS) (see Table 1). The SS patients and AS subjects had their hematologic studies (hemoglobin, hematocrit, hemoglobin electrophoresis) performed by the Comprehensive Sickle Cell Center of the Medical College of Georgia. The exercise data of the SS and AS subjects were compared to that of 170 healthy black volunteers (HB) (Strong, Spencer, Miller, & Salebhai, 1978) 74 males and 96 females, aged 7 to 14 years (mean = 10 years).

The exercise tests were performed with the subjects seated upright on a mechanically braked cycle ergometer (Monark). "Resting heart rate" was obtained with the individual sitting on the cycle ergometer prior to testing. It might better be called the preexercise heart rate rather than implying a basal state. The subjects' EKGs (leads X, Y, and Z) were monitored continuously, with blood pressure and heart rate measurements and EKG tracings ($\dot{V}_5$) being recorded at 3-min intervals. All subjects were exercised to exhaustion, that is, maximum voluntary effort (MVE). The exercise protocol for the SS and AS group has been published previously. (Alpert et al., 1981; Alpert, et al., 1982).

Table 1

Means (± Standard Deviations) of Ages and Hematology of Groups of Subjects

	Normals	AS[a]	SS[b]		
			N	B	I
Number	170	48	24	16	7
Age (years)	10.1 ± 2.1	11.6	10.5 ± 2.8	9.2 ± 2.5	12.0 ± 2.6
Hematocrit or Hemoglobin (g/dl)	36.4 ± 2%	[c]	8.1 ± 1.0	8.2 ± 1.1	7.2 ± 0.4

[a]AS—Sickle trait subjects.
[b]N, B, I—Sickle cell subjects grouped by EKG: N = non-ischemic; B = Borderline equivocal for ischemia; I = ischemic.
[c]The Human Assurance Committee of the Medical College of Georgia did not approve hemoglobin measurements in AS patients, as their hemoglobins are generally accepted as being the same as those of normal black children with hemoglobin AA.

Radionuclide stress tests (Covitz et al., 1983) were performed on 22 patients (11 male and 11 female) aged 10 to 22 years (mean = 15.3 years). Twelve subjects served as the control group. The controls were evaluated because of chest pain of unknown etiology, or as part of a postoperative evaluation. They all had normal exercise tests and cardiac catherization data. The nuclear stress tests were performed with the patients seated upright on a mechanically-braked cycle ergometer (Monark). The workloads used were derived in a similar manner as in the non-nuclear tests (Alpert et al., 1981; Strong et al., 1978).

The radionuclide data were collected with a portable gamma camera (Technicare Sigma 420) interfaced with a portable computer (Medical Data Systems). A Brattle physiologic gate was used to trigger the system. Gated equilibrium studies (MUGA) were performed at rest and during the last 2 min of each 3-min exercise state. Technetium-99m albumin (0.3 m Ci/kg) was administered just before positioning the patient on the bicycle. A high sensitivity parallel hole collimator was placed within 2 cm of the chest. The patients were maintained in the proper left anterior obliquity (by using an adjustable wedge mold and harness) so that the collimator was perpendicular to the interventricular septum (see Figure 1). Ejection fraction and end-diastolic counts were determined at rest and during each exercise stage. Changes in end-diastolic counts from rest were assumed to reflect changes in ventricular volume, and changes in counts ejected/minute to reflect changes in cardiac output. Wall motion abnormalities were detected by viewing the cineangiographic format of the equilibrium studies, and by overlaying edge images from end-systole and end-diastole.

All subjects were evaluated for the presence of ischemia by EKG during the tests. The P-R isoelectric line was used, as it has been found that this decreases the number of false positives (see Figure 2). All protocols were approved by the Human Assurance Committee of the Medical College of Georgia.

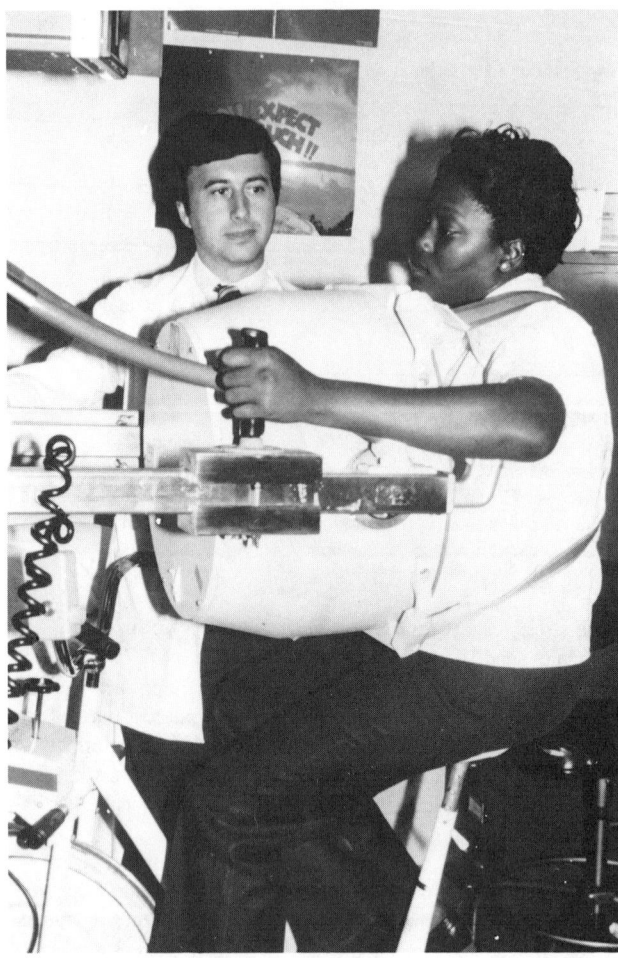

Figure 1—Procedure for the radionuclide test.

Results

For the purpose of analyzing the data, the SS subjects were assigned to subgroups according to their exercise EKG into those with a normal EKG (*N*) and those with borderline evidence of ischemia (*B*) and those with definite ischemia (*I*). The P-R isoelectric line was used to determine the J point and ST depression as work of Thapar, Strong, Miller, Leatherbury, and Salebhai (1978) on healthy black children has shown that those patients exhibiting J point displacement with a downsloping ST segment, or J point displacement with a flat ST segment, or a normal J point with a downsloping ST segment were regarded as exhibiting definite ischemia. A normal J point with a flat ST segment, or a displaced J point with a upsloping ST segment was regarded as being borderline or equivocal for ischemia (see Figure 3). Using these criteria, 15% of the SS patients had definite ischemia (*I*), 34% had borderline ischemia (*B*), and 51% had

Method of Measuring the "J" Point

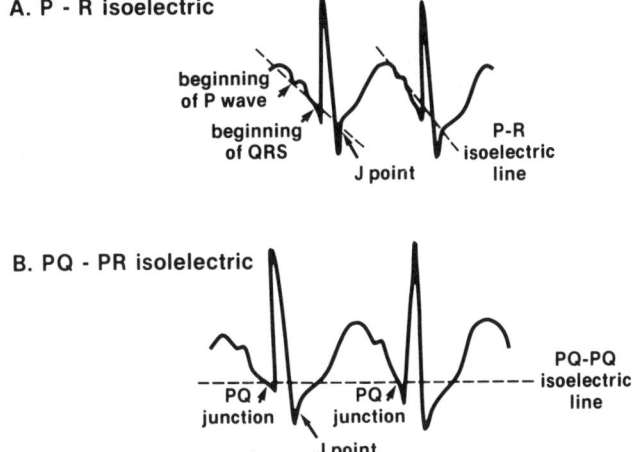

Figure 2—The PR isoelectric vs. the P-P isoelectric for determination of the isoelectric line. Because of baseline variation and the T_a, PR isoelectric is considered to be preferable in children, especially as they approach maximum effort and begin to "strain" during the last stage of exercise.

Pediatric Electrocardiographic Response to Exercise

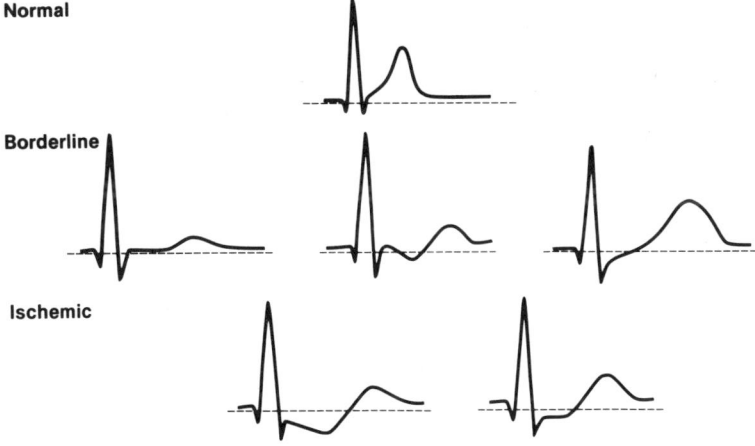

Figure 3—Examples of the interpretation of an ischemic response—definite, probable or borderline, and possible. The normal response would have no J point depression and the ST segment slope would be positive as in Figure 2 (P-R isoelectric).

a normal EKG (*N*) during their stress tests. In the HB group, none had definite ischemia and 2.6% had borderline ischemia.

Heart Rate

Preexercise heart rate (see Table 2) was not different between the healthy controls and the subjects with sickle trait (87 ± 13 vs. 87 ± 16 beats/min). There was a significant difference between the HB subjects and the children with sickle cell anemia (93 ± 12 beats/min p_3 .01). At maximum voluntary effort, the respective heart rate values for the HB, AS and SS groups were 191 ± 10, 181 ± 14, and 180 ± 10 beats/min. The latter mean values being significantly different from that of the control group (p_3 .0001).

Blood Pressure

Resting (i.e., preexercise, seated on the cycle ergometer) systolic blood pressure (SBP) was comparable in the 3 groups being 103 ± 13 for the HB, 115 ± 16 for the AS and 99 ± 17 mm Hg for the SS children (see Table 2). The healthy black children had the greatest rise of SBP, 51 ± 16.5 mm Hg. The maximum SBP developed by this group was 158 ± 20 mm Hg. The mean for the subjects with AS increased almost a much, 48 mm Hg, to a peak SBP of 163 ± 26 mm Hg, which was not statistically different than the HB group. One AS subject had a peak SBP of 252/95 mm Hg. The

Table 2

Comparisons of Exercise Variable Among Groups
(Means ± Standard Deviations)

Variable	Control Group HB	AS[a]	SS[b]	P*
N	170	48	47	
H R Resting (beats/min)	87 ± 13	87 ± 16	93 ± 12	
HR Maximum (beats/min)	191 ± 10	181 ± 14	181 ± 10	< .001
S B P Resting (mm Hg)	103 ± 13	115 ± 16	99 ± 12	NS
S B P Max (mm Hg)	158 ± 20	163 ± 26	122 ± 40	< 0.0001
PWCI (kg m/min/kg)	15.6 ± 3.5	12 ± 2.3	N^b 11.8 ± 2.4 B^b 11.1 ± 3.3 I^b 9.5 ± 2.6	< 0.01

[a] AS—Sickle trait subjects.
[b] N, B, I—Sickle cell subjects grouped by EKG: N = non-ischemic; B = borderline for ischemia; I = ischemic.

patients with SS had the lowest SBP change of only 23 mm Hg, peaking at 122 ± 40 mm Hg. The patients with the ischemic ECG changes rose 28 mm Hg, while those with borderline or nonischemic ECG responses rose 34 mm Hg and 31 mm Hg respectively. The differences were significant between the major groups and also between one of the SS subgroups (N and B vs. D p_s .01).

Physical Working Capacity Index (PWCI)

As might be expected, the children with less hemoglobin were able to perform less work (see Table 2). The mean PWCI of the HB was 15.6 ± 3.5 kgm/min/kg. The AS subjects performed intermediate levels of work, that is, 12 ± 2.3 kgm/min/kg, and the patients with SS performed the least work. The difference between the HB and AS was significant at the $p< .0005$ level. Based upon their ECG response, the SS patients performed work as follows: $N = 11.8 ± 2.4$, $B = 11.1 ± 3.5$, and $D = 9.5 ± 2.6$ kgm/min/kg. The differences of the PWCI between subgroups was significantly different $p< .01$. Ear oximetry performed during the exercise tests of the AS patients did not detect any evidence of oxygen desaturation.

Radionuclide Data

End Diastolic Volume. Four of the 22 patients exhibited EKG evidence of ischemia during their nuclear stress tests. These 4 patients also exhibited wall motion abnormalities. In the SS group, left ventricular end-diastolic volume at maximum exercise was found to be less when compared to the resting value (controls = 1.00 ± 0.10, $N = 0.94 ± 0.03$, $I = 0.85 ± 0.09$; $p< 0.06$) (see Table 3). Left ventricular end-diastolic volume is here expressed as a fraction of the same measurement at rest. There was a statistically significant difference between control and SS subjects.

Table 3

Means (± Standard Deviations) for Radionuclide Data

Variable	Controls	P^b	N^a	I^a	$P*^c$
Left ventricular diastolic volume at maximal exercise[d]	1.00 ± 0.10	< 0.10	0.94 ± 0.03	0.85 ± 0.09	NS
Maximal ejection fraction	0.81 ± 0.07	< 0.001	0.73 ± 0.08	0.62 ± 0.06	< 0.05
Maximal cardiac output	2.80 ± 0.26	< 0.00001	2.30 ± 0.30	1.60 ± 0.40	< 0.005

[a]N, I—Sickle cell subjects grouped by EKG: N = non-ischemic; I = definitely ischemic.
[b]P—Significant differences between control group and sickle patients.
[c]$P*$—Significant differences between N and I.
[d]±—Expressed as a multiple or fraction of the same measurement at rest.

Ejection Fraction. The HB sickle cell patients demonstrated a rise in the ejection fraction with progression of the exercise test. In contrast, ejection fraction was found to decline at maximal exercise in those SS patients with evidence of ischemia when their exercise values were compared to their resting values (HB = 0.81 ± 0.07, $N = 0.73 \pm 0.08$, $I = 0.62 \pm 0.06$, $p < .001$ and $< .02$ for significant differences between SS and HB, and between N and I, respectively. These data are presented in Table 3.

Cardiac Output (Counts Per Minute). The HB had the greatest increase in cardiac output (counts ejected per minute) during exercise when compared to the number of counts ejected per minute at rest (HB = 2.80 ± 0.26, SS (N) = $2.30 \pm .30$, and SS (I) = 1.60 ± 0.40. These values were significant at the p_3 .0005 level (see Table 3).

Discussion

Sickle cell patients were found to have significant impairment of their exercise tolerance in this investigation. Cardiac and noncardiac factors (e.g., anemia and poor growth and development) contribute to this exercise intolerance. The cardiac causes of the poor exercise capability include the volume overload from the anemia, as determined echocardiographically and by radionuclide imaging, (Varat, Adolph, & Fowler, 1972) and the cardiac dysfunction (Balfour et al., in press; Rees et al., 1978) associated with the disease. Those sickle cell patients with the lowest hemoglobins developed ischemia during exercise, and performed the poorest during exercise. The cardiac performance in these patients may be related to the imbalance of the myocardial oxygen supply and the demand that exists in these patients, with the ischemic patients being the most affected. Oxygen carrying capacity is reduced in sickle cell patients because of the anemia present. With exercise and an increase in myocardial oxygen demand, the demand may exceed the supply.

The SS patients also demonstrated impaired cardiac function: (a) low maximum workload, (b) impaired blood pressure, and (c) poor heart rate response. In the radionuclide studies, left ventricular end-diastolic volume decreased with progression of the exercise test. Normally, left ventricular volume increases with increasing severity of exercise, as venous return increases (Bar-Shlomo et al., 1982). A decrease in ventricular volume suggests that the left ventricles of these subjects become less compliant and more difficult to fill when increasing demands are placed on the myocardium. The ischemic patients were more severely affected, as they demonstrated a fall in ejection fraction, suggesting that compliance was even more reduced in the ischemic group. The reduced filling in these subjects is even more significant in view of the increased preload in anemic subjects (Varat, Adolph, & Fowler, 1972) which would tend to result in increased ventricular filling pressures and cause increased ventricular filling.

Subjects with sickle trait also demonstrated impaired performance on exercise. The cause of this is not known at this time. Sickling of red cells does not occur in individuals with sickle trait under normal barametric conditions; this probably does not explain the abnormal exercise performance in these subjects.

Of paramount importance is the fact that no child with sickle cell anemia developed a crisis secondary to maximum voluntary effort. It is believed, therefore, that there is no support for placing arbitrary activity restrictions on children with sickle cell anemia. It reinforces the principle of allowing them to do what they are comfortable doing.

References

ALPERT, B., Flood, N., Strong, W., Blair, J., Walpert, J., Levy, A. (1982). Responses to exercise in children with sickle cell trait. *American Journal of Diseases of Children*, **136**, 1002-1004.

ALPERT, B., Gillman, P., Strong, W., Ellison, M., Miller M., McFarlane, J., & Hayashidera, T. (1981). Hemodynamic and ECG responses to exercise in children with sickle cell anemia. *American Journal of Diseases of Children*, **135**, 362-366.

BALFOUR, I., Covitz, W., Davis, H., Rao, P., Strong, W., Alpert, B. (1984). Cardiac size and function in children with sickle cell anemia. *American Heart Journal*, **108**, 345-350.

BAR-SHLOMO, B., Druck, M., March, J., Jablonsky, G., Hilton, D., Feiglin, D., & McLaughlin, P. (1982). Left ventricular function in trained and untrained healthy subjects. *Circulation*, **65**, 484-488.

COVITZ, W., Eubig, C., Balfour, I., Jerath, R., Alpert, B., Strong, W., & DuRant, R. (1983). Exercise-induced cardiac dysfunction in sickle cell anemia—a radionuclide study. *The American Journal of Cardiology*, **51**, 570-575.

REES, A., Stefadouros, M., Strong, W., Miller, M., Gilman, P., Rigby, J., & McFarlané, J. (1978). Left ventricular performance in children with homozygous sickle cell anemia. *British Heart Journal*, **40**, 690-696.

STRONG, W., Spencer, D., Miller, M., & Salehbhai, M. (1978). The physical working capacity of healthy black children. *The American Journal of Diseases of Children*, **132**, 244-248.

THAPAR, M., Strong, W., Miller, M., Leatherbury, L., & Salebhai, M. (1978). Exercise electrocardiography of healthy black children. *American Journal of Diseases of Children*, **132**, 592-595.

VARAT, M., Adolph, R., & Fowler N. (1972). Cardiovascular effects of anemia. *American Heart Journal*, **83**, 415-426.

Comparison of Nine Exercise Tests Used in Pediatric Cardiology

Gordon R. Cumming and Steve Langford
University of Manitoba
Winnipeg, Manitoba, Canada

Pediatric exercise laboratories still have not adopted a standard test protocol, and, consequently, heart rate and exercise capacity data from various centers are difficult to compare. Nine tests that have been used for the exercise testing of children with heart disease were carried out in random order by 13 girls and 10 boys, and comparative information is presented on maximal oxygen uptake, work time, and rate of increase of $\dot{V}O_2$ and maximal heart rate.

Subjects

Six girls and 6 boys, aged 9 to 10 years, were recruited from a nearby elementary school (Grade 4), and 7 boys and 8 girls, aged 12 to 13 years, were recruited from a nearby junior high school (Grade 7). The subjects were paid a stipend as an incentive and 23 subjects completed all nine tests. Four subjects were drop outs early in the study and their results have not been included. The subjects were volunteers selected from a class list prepared by their teachers; they lived near the hospital, and the testing was performed out of school hours in a hospital laboratory. There was no history of significant illness or injury in any of the children. Their heart sounds, blood pressures, and electrocardiograms were normal; further medical examination was not carried out. The subjects' anthropometric data are listed in Table 1. Informed school board, school, subject, and parental consents were obtained. The subjects were not engaged in organized sports activities other than their regular twice weekly, 45-min physical education classes.

Methods

The nine tests were performed according to a random numbers table. The children first visited the laboratory and were familiarized with each test modality and with the oxygen uptake apparatus. All exercise tests were carried out in an air conditioned

Table 1

Anthropometric Data

	Group I 9-10 yrs		Group II 12-13 yrs	
	Females	Males	Females	Males
N	5	5	8	5
Age (yrs)	9.6 ± 0.5	9.8 ± 0.5	12.8 ± 0.5	12.6 ± 0.5
Height (cm)	136 ± 10	139 ± 7	151 ± 8	152 ± 5
Weight (kg)	35 ± 10	34 ± 10	47 ± 6	45 ± 9
Skinfolds[a] (mm)	38 ± 14	28 ± 14	38 ± 12	30 ± 37
Fat[b] (%)	22 ± 5	11 ± 5	22 ± 2	13 ± 9
FEV_1 (l)	1.9 ± 0.4	2.1 ± 0.1	2.5 ± 0.3	2.5 ± 0.2
FVC (l)	2.6 ± 0.6	2.5 ± 0.1	2.9 ± 0.4	3.0 ± 0.3
PEFR (l•min^{-1})	114 ± 52	278 ± 34	294 ± 39	289 ± 26
BSA (m²)	1.2 ± 0.20	1.1 ± 0.13	1.4 ± 0.13	1.4 ± 0.14

[a]Sum of 4 skinfolds
[b]% of body weight
BSA = body surface area

FEV_1 = forced expiratory volume in 1.0 sec
FVC = forced vital capacity
PEFR = peak expiratory flow rate

laboratory at 19° C temperature and 40% relative humidity. The children fasted at least 2 hours before testing. Heart rate was monitored by ECG lead CM5. A continuous record of oxygen uptake was obtained using a flow through method and a face mask (Kappagoda & Linden, 1972). $\dot{V}O_2$ by this method agreed within 1.0 ml•kg^{-1} $\dot{V}O_2$ determined by one-way expiratory valve air collection in 16 subjects tested in the same laboratory.

All tests were carried out by the same experienced exercise technician (S.L.). The children were encouraged to exercise until they could not do any more work because of severe fatigue. The subjective feeling of fatigue at the end point was quantified with the Borg system (Borg, 1970); the mean value was 18.6 with no difference between the various tests. Height without shoes, weight, and skinfold measurements (Durnin & Rahmon, 1967) were obtained at the initial visit to the laboratory. All tests were completed over a 4-week period.

Statistical analysis was carried out using a computer package allowing the results of the various tests to be compared by Dunhan, SNK, and Tukey scales.

Test Protocols (Summarized in Table 2)

The "W_{170} Protocol" (#1)

This consisted of 6 kpm/kg^{-1}•min^{-1} for 6 min, 13 kpm•kg^{-1}•min^{-1} for 6 min, then increments of 100 kpm•kg^{-1}•min^{-1} each minute until exhaustion. This protocol was designed to measure the work load that would produce a steady state heart rate of 170 beats•min^{-1} as used in Sweden (Adams, Bengtsson, Berven, & Wegelus, 1961;

Table 2
Test Results, Nine Different Exercise Tests

Parameter	Bicycle Ergometer Tests						Treadmill Tests		
	1	2	3	4	5	6	7	8	9
Protocols	W_{170}	Godfrey	James	Rapid Loading	By Wgt. Upright	By Wgt. Supine	Bruce	Short Bruce	Carolina Balke
Heart Rate beats/min^{-1}									
Rest	90±15	91±12	88±12	91±13	88±12	85±14	89±12	87± 7	88±17
2' Ex.	131±14	138±13	126±16	173±16	124±11	125±14	123±11	164±14	134±16
6' Ex.	135±14	176±14	159±14	—	157±17	148±17	144±13	—	160±16
Maximal	199± 5	195± 5	197± 7	192± 6	198± 5	182±11	204± 5	201± 6	198± 5
Recovery 2'	130±16	134±16	124±21	128±20	129±16	115±22	129±18	134±22	118±17
5'	113±12	113±12	114±11	113±11	113±12	109±17	114±11	117±11	111±12
Δ beats/min									
0-2 min	20	23.5	19.0	40.6	18.2	19.8	17.3	38.5	23.5
3-6 min	1.3	9.5	8.3	4.8	8.3	5.8	5.3	9.3	6.5
Oxygen Uptake ml·kg^{-1}·min^{-1}									
3' Ex.	21.1±2.0	22.0±4.3	19.5±4.4	35.7±7.2	18.5±3.1	17.6±3.1	18.4±2.2	30.3±2.7	20.3±1.7
6' Ex.	21.1±2.1	37.0±6.4	31.1±4.3	—	29.2±3.3	26.8±2.3	25.1±1.8	—	27.5±1.8
Maximal	47.4±8.2	47.9±8.3	48.5±7.2	48.2±8.3	47.4±7.0	40.4±7.4	54.0±7.6	52.9±7.7	48.2±6.6
Δ$\dot{V}O_2$ ml·kg^{-1}·min^{-1}									
3-6 min	0.2	5.0	3.7	4.0	3.3	3.0	2.3	7.7	2.7
Work time·min	14.9±1.5	8.5±1.5	10.2±1.4	5.1±0.6	11.3±1.5	10.1±1.5	12.8±1.5	7.0±1.5	12.8±1.9
Blood Pressure mm Hg									
Rest	109/59±12/13	108/58±17/12	106/59±13/11	105/60±13/11	104/58±13/13	111/63±16/14	110/59±15/13	106/59±11/ 9	107/56±11/13
Stage II Ex.	150/62±23/12	129/60±18/10	137/59±15/11	138/58±20/10	138/58±19/11	152/74±24/16	144/64±22/13	138/63±20/11	122/60±10/11
Postmaximal	144/53±18/ 9	143/55±28/12	144/54±19/12	144/56±20/11	140/54±22/12	163/63±19/11	158/63±18/14	156/62±20/10	149/64±16/ 9

Ex. = Exercise
± = Standard deviation

Bengtsson, 1956; Cumming, 1977a; Sjostrand, 1947; Wahlund, 1948). The 100 kpm•min⁻¹ incremental loading after the two steady stage loads was an expedient way of obtaining $\dot{V}O_2$ max and maximal work load (Cumming, 1977a), but this loading system did not take the subject's size into consideration.

Godfrey Progressive Protocol #2 (Godfrey, 1974)

Children under 125 cm tall started at 10 W (N 60 kpm•min⁻¹) and work was increased by 10 W every minute until fatigue. Children 125 to 150 cm tall started at 15 W (N 90 kpm•min⁻¹) and work rate was increased by 15 W every minute. This protocol is similar to that used by Wessell, Stent, Guerrero, and Paul (1976) who increased work load by 100 kpm•min⁻¹ every minute regardless of patient size. Children over 150 cm tall were given work increments of 20 W (N 125 kpm•min⁻¹). All work loads were only 1.0 min in duration so that there was insufficient time for any leveling off of the oxygen uptake or heart rate for any work load.

James Protocol #3 (James, 1978)

Children under 1.0 m² surface area worked at 200, 300, 500, 600, 700, 800, etc., kpm•min⁻¹, 3 min at each load, with continuous exercise. Children 1.0 to 1.19 m² worked at 200, 400, 600, 700, 800, 900, etc., kpm•min⁻¹, children over 1.19 m² worked at 200, 500, 800, 1000, 1200, 1400, 1600, etc., kpm•min⁻¹ also for 3 min at each work load. The children were urged to continue until exhausted.

Rapid Loading Protocol (#4)

Children under 1.0 m² cycled at work loads 100, 300, 500, 600, 700, 800, etc. kpm•min⁻¹ for 1 min for each load until voluntary fatigue. Children 1.0 to 1.2 m² worked at 100, 400, 600, 700, 800, 900, etc., kpm•min⁻¹ and children over 1.2 m² worked at 100, 500, 800, 1000, 1200, 1400, etc., kpm•min⁻¹. The work loads were the same as those advocated by Goldberg, Weiss and Adams (1966) but by mistake the loads were sustained for only 1 min each rather than for the 2 min used by Goldberg, Weiss, and Adams (1966).

Bicycle Ergometer Loading Based on Weight (#5)

A commonly used loading formula advocated by Macek and Vavra (1971) used work load increments based on weight. Instead of increments of 0.5 W•kg⁻¹ used by these workers, increments of 5 kpm•kg⁻¹ (0.82 W were used in this study. All work loads were of 3 min duration and exercise was continued until voluntary exhaustion.

Supine Ergometer Exercise (#6)

The same protocol as used for loading based on weight (#5) were performed supine.
All upright ergometer exercises were performed on the Elema ergometer (Holmgren & Mattson, 1954) calibrated at regular intervals (Cumming & Alexander, 1968). Cycling rate was maintained at 60 rev/min, saddle height was adjusted so that the legs were

almost fully extended. During the final exhausting work load, cycling rate was allowed to increase to 65 to 75 rev/min.

The Bruce Treadmill Protocol #7 (Bruce, Kusumi, & Hosmer, 1973)

This protocol was used starting at Stage I (1.7 miles/hr, 10% grade) and continuing until exhaustion with the 3 min loads and standard increments in grade and speed. Normal values for children were previously established (Cumming, Everatt, & Hastman, 1978) in this laboratory.

The Short Bruce Protocol (#8)

In this protocol exercise started at Stage III (3.4 miles/hr, 14% grade) and continued with the 3 min loads for Stages IV, V, and VI if the subject could manage. This was the same as protocol #7 (Bruce, Kusumi, & Hosmer, 1973) except that the first two stages were eliminated.

The Carolina Protocol #9 (Riopel, Taylor, & Hohn, 1979)

Treadmill speed was 3.5 miles/hr and grade increased by 2% each minute, following the protocol first used by Balke and Ware (1959). In the original description of this protocol for children some younger children were exercised at 2.5 or 3.0 miles/hr. All subjects in the present study walked at 3.5 miles/hr.

Results

The mean results for all subjects for all tests are shown in Table 2. Both mean maximal heart rates and mean $\dot{V}O_2$ max were significantly higher for the Bruce treadmill protocol (#7) than for the other tests. The shortened Bruce protocol (#8) was next with regard to both mean maximal heart rate and mean $\dot{V}O_2$ max, and differences with all the other tests were statistically significant ($p < .05$).

All of the upright bicycle tests were similar with regard to $\dot{V}O_2$ max and equal to the walking treadmill test (protocol #9). The mean maximal heart rates for the bicycle tests ranged from 192 to 198 beats•min^{-1}. The lowest rates were with the shortened Goldberg protocol (#4) followed by the Godfrey protocol (#2). The highest mean maximal heart rates were with the two bicycle protocols used by Cumming (1977) and Macek and Vavra (1971) #5.

Supine exercise gave considerably lower values for $\dot{V}O_2$ max and maximal heart rate compared to upright exercise in these children. Mean maximal heart rate was 10 beats•min^{-1} below that for the lowest of the upright ergometer protocols, and 22 beats•min^{-1} below that for the Bruce treadmill protocol. Mean $\dot{V}O_2$ max for supine work was 17% below the mean $\dot{V}O_2$ max for upright ergometer exercise, and mean $\dot{V}O_2$ max for the Bruce treadmill protocol was 35% greater than that recorded for supine ergometer exercise.

The mean maximal heart rate for the shortened Bruce protocol was 3 beats•min^{-1} lower than for the full Bruce protocol, and the mean $\dot{V}O_2$ max was 2% less. The subjects worked 0.2 min longer for the short protocol after adding the 6 min taken off the front end of the test. The rank order of endurance times for the short and regular Bruce protocols was a perfect fit.

The Rapid Loading and Godfrey ergometer protocols gave the shortest work times and the lowest mean maximal heart rates. The rate of rise of heart rate in the first 2 min of exercise was the highest for these 2 tests because of the higher rate of loading.

There were no significant differences in blood pressure responses among the nine tests, possibly because the ranges for pressure measurements were large. The highest mean exercise blood pressure occurred with supine exercise, followed by the Bruce test.

One encouraging finding about the study was the similarity in the rank orders for endurance times for the $\dot{V}O_2$ max for all of the tests. Table 3 shows the very high rank order correlations, all about 0.9, for $\dot{V}O_2$ max/per kg body weight and a lesser but highly significant rank order correlation of 0.63 for the endurance times. The older subjects tended to show higher correlation coefficients compared to the younger subjects for the rank orders for $\dot{V}O_2$ max and endurance time.

Normal values have been published for protocols 1, 2, 3, 5, 7, and 9, allowing a comparison of the relative fitness of the populations used to establish these normal values. In Table 4, the results of subjects in the present study are given as a percentage of the test scores reported.

The mean results in this study were the same as the normals published for this laboratory for the Bruce test (Cumming, Everatt, & Hastman, 1978) and were 25 to 39% higher than those found by Riopel, Taylor, and Hohn (1979) for their walking treadmill test. Except for the 9 to 10-year-old girls, our subjects did considerably more work than did the British subjects reported by Godfrey using the Godfrey protocol (1974). Our subjects recorded mean values very similar to the mean values found by James (1978) for his ergometer test (except our 9 to 10-year-old girls did 21% more work, and our 12 to 13-year-old girls did 7% less). For tests #1 (Cumming, 1977a), our volunteers performed about the same on the ergometer as earlier normal patients had.

Table 3
Kendall's Coefficients of Concordance.
Ranking of Subjects for Oxygen Uptakes and Endurance Times

Age Groups	$\dot{V}O_2$ Max		Work Time	
	W	χ^2	W	χ^2
9-11	.8443	60.79	.4692	33.78
12-13	.8943	96.58	.7218	76.99
All 9-13	.8919	168.88	.6306	119.0

W = Coefficient of Concordance
χ^2 = chi squared—all with $p < .01$

Table 4

Comparison to Normal Values Published for the Same Test[a]

Age	Sex	Cumming (8) Bicycle	Godfrey (9) Bicycle	James (11) Bicycle	Cumming (17) Bruce	Caolina (18) Balke
9-10	M	92	124	103	103	125
9-10	F	106	94	121	101	135
12-13	M	106	132	98	102	139
12-13	F	98	138	93	102	132

[a]Mean maximal work times or maximal work loads expressed as percent of published mean normal values.

Discussion

The results of this study help explain some of the differences in the results from the different laboratories that use different exercise tests.

For upright bicycle tests, work duration and maximal heart rate were directly related. Protocols that have shorter work times due to a more rapid increase in work load will show lower maximal heart rates. This may partially explain low maximal heart rates reported by some authors.

Maximal work time, maximal work load and $\dot{V}O_2$max were considerably lower for supine ergometer work compared to an identical protocol of upright ergometer work. The mean maximal heart rate for supine exercise in these children was similar to that previously reported for children with nearly normal hearts performing maximal supine exercise at the time of heart catheterization (Cumming, 1977b).

The Bruce treadmill protocols #7 and 8 had the children running at 7.0 and 8.2 k•h^{-1} and led to mean maximal heart rates 6 beats•min^{-1} more and $\dot{V}O_2$ max 11% more than the walking protocol (#9) at 5.8 k•h^{-1}. The low mean maximal heart rates found by Riopel, Taylor, and Hohn (1979) (as low as 180 beats•min^{-1} in some groups of children) must be attributed to an inability to obtain a near maximal effort from many of their subjects rather than entirely the use of a walking protocol. This would also account for our children doing up to 30% better than the children studied by Riopel, Taylor, and Hohn (1979) in terms of work time.

Despite test differences in rates of loading, the maximal heart rates, $\dot{V}O_2$ max, and the work times, the rank order of the test results for maximal work load or maximal oxygen uptake showed high correlations. This means that any of these tests applied consistently in any one laboratory may be used to measure comparative fitness for that test and comparative fitness for various groups of children. While we did not obtain a comparison of these tests in cardiac patients, it is likely that this maintenance of rank order should pertain to various patient groups the same as for normals. It must be appreciated that the work time with an endurance test, and to a lesser degree $\dot{V}O_2$ max, is dependent not only on the exercise capacity of the subject, but also on the subject's willingness to work for the test supervisor on any particular occasion. It is suspected that considerable differences exist in the level of encouragement given to children to work close to the point of physical exhaustion in various laboratories.

The results of present subjects can be used as human calibrators for published normal values of the different tests. The end points reached by our subjects were approximately equal to those of James (1978), better than those of Godfrey (1974), much better than those of Riopel, Taylor, and Hohn (1979), and similar to the subjects previously used for establishing normal values in this laboratory for both bicycle and treadmill (Cumming, 1977a; Cumming, Everatt, & Hastman, 1978). The lower work level attained in some of these normal series could be due to either or both of two factors: an actual difference in fitness in the populations tested, or technical differences in carrying out the tests. In some studies of children, it would appear that the investigators have fallen short of obtaining maximal efforts.

These differences emphasize the difficulties in using the normal standards obtained from one laboratory in another laboratory. Each laboratory needs to establish its own normal values and to continuously update these norms. If some laboratories are unable or unwilling to obtain near maximal efforts from normal children, they are even less likely to obtain a near maximal effort from children with health problems.

These comparative values cannot be used to compare the fitness of the entire populations where the studies were carried out, as the subjects available for establishing norms were not necessarily representative of the population at large: A proper comparison would require that the tests be administered by the same investigators.

Despite the consistent ranking of the 23 subjects' fitness values for 9 different exercise protocols, there is still a need for standardization of exercise protocols. The results of this study support the contention that if the heart and oxygen delivery system are to be fully stressed, a treadmill test is superior to the bicycle, and that the treadmill protocol should make the child run and not just walk. Tests can be standardized to some biologic end point. One such end point is maximal heart rate which is highest for a treadmill running test. The coefficient of variation and range of normal and maximal heart rate was also slightly smaller for the treadmill running than for the other tests.

All five of the upright ergometer tests gave mean $\dot{V}O_2$ max values that were within $1.0 \text{ ml} \cdot \text{kg}^{-1}$ of each other despite variable rates of loading and variable test duration. Where possible, $\dot{V}O_2$ max should be directly measured by acceptable techniques.

Prior studies in this laboratory (Cumming & Friesen, 1967) showed that a plateau in $\dot{V}O_2$ is demonstrable in less than 50% of children tested on 5 to 20 occasions on a bicycle ergometer, Åstrand (1952) and Cunningham and co-workers (1977) found that with treadmill exercise, $\dot{V}O_2$ reached a plateau in less than 50% of children; and only 50% of the children showing a plateau in an initial test showed a plateau in a second test. While theoretically the plateauing of $\dot{V}O_2$ is an end point, it would not seem to be useful in the routine clinical testing of children. For a single laboratory visit, one is forced to use the highest $\dot{V}O_2$ reached, without necessarily demonstrating a plateau. As treadmill running gave a 10% higher peak oxygen uptake than work on the cycle ergometer or for treadmill walking, it appears that a treadmill running test allowed the children to reach this physiologic end point more closely than did the other tests.

Patterson and Cunningham (1978) compared the response of 10 to 12-year-old-boys to maximal treadmill walking (3.4 miles/hr) and concluded that the walking test was inappropriate because of an 8% lower $\dot{V}O_2$ max and poorer reliability. This confirmed earlier studies in adults showing the superiority of running tests for the attainment of the highest oxygen uptake (Froelicher et al., 1974; McArdle, Katch & Pechor, 1973; Stamford, 1975).

We remain enthusiastic about using the Bruce protocol for children. The results also suggest that for children with normal exercise capacities, the Bruce protocol can be shortened by eliminating or rapidly passing through Stages I and II without sacrificing any of the discriminating powers of the test; this would still allow the same high level of maximal oxygen uptakes and maximal heart rates achieved with the full version of the test.

A collaborative World Health Study recommended using the treadmill for assessing aerobic power of children under 10 to 12 years of age (Shephard et al., 1978). In this study the results suggested that children 9 to 10 years of age were no different from children 12 to 13-years-old and likely all children should be tested on the treadmill. Unfortunately, a recent report by the American Heart Association (1982) accomplished nothing toward standardization of work procedures for children.

Summary and Conclusions

The random performance of six different maximal ergometer and three different maximal treadmill tests by 9 to 13-year-olds showed that the rank order for $\dot{V}O_2$ max or endurance times were very similar, but a treadmill test requiring the subject to run gave significantly higher values for $\dot{V}O_2$ max and heart rate and is the preferred test method. Comparison of normal values published for the various tests with the results of the subjects in the present study provided a human calibration comparison that showed a low performance of the children in a few laboratories, making it mandatory for all laboratories to establish and continuously update their own normal data.

References

ADAMS, F.H., Bengtsson, E., Berven, H., & Wegelius, C. (1961). The physical working capacity of normal school children II. Swedish city and country. *Pediatrics*, **28**, 243-257.

AMERICAN Heart Association. (1982). A.H.A. special report—Standards for exercise testing in the pediatric age group. *Circulation*, **66**, 1377A-1397A.

ÅSTRAND, P.O. (1952). Experimental studies of physical working capacity in relation to sex and age. Copenhagen: Munksgaard.

BALKE, B., & Ware, R.W. (1959). An experimental study of "physical fitness" of Air Force personnel. *U.S. Armed Forces Medical Journal*, **10**, 675-688.

BENGTSSON, E. (1956). The working capacity in normal children: Evaluation of submaximal exercise on the bicycle ergometer and compared with adults. *Acta Medica Scandinavica*, **154**, 91.

BORG, G. (1970). Perceived exertion as an indicator of somatic stress. *Scandinavian Journal of Rehabilitation Medicine*, **2**, 92-98.

BRUCE, R.A., Kusumi, F., & Hosmer, D. (1973). Maximal oxygen intake and nomographic assessment of functional aerobic impairment in cardiovascular disease. *American Heart Journal*, **85**, 545-562.

CUMMING, G.R. (1977a). Exercise studies in clinical pediatric cardiology frontiers of activity and child health. In H. Lavallee & R. Shepherd (Eds.), *Proceedings of the VIIth International Symposium of Paediatric Work Physiology*, (pp. 17-45). Ottawa: Editions du Pelican.

CUMMING, G.R. (1977b). Hemodynamics of supine bicycle exercise in normal children. *American Heart Journal*, **93**, 617-622.

CUMMING, G.R., & Friesen, W. (1967). Bicycle ergometer measurement of maximal oxygen uptake in children. *Canadian Journal of Physiology and Pharmacology*, **45**, 937-946.

CUMMING, G.R., & Alexander, W.D. (1968). The calibration of bicycle ergometers. *Canadian Journal of Physiology and Pharmacology*, **46**, 917-919.

CUMMING, G.R., Everatt, D., & Hastman, L. (1978). Bruce treadmill test in children. Normal values in a clinic population. *American Journal of Cardiology*, **41**, 69-75.

CUNNINGHAM, D.A., Van Waterschoot, B.M., Patterson, D.H., et al. (1977). Reliability and reproducibility of maximal oxygen uptake in children. *Medicine and Science in Sports*, **9**, 104-108.

DURNIN, J.V.G.A., & Rahman, M.M. (1967). The assessment of the amount of fat in the human body from measurements of skinfold thicknesses. *British Journal of Nutrition*, **21**, 681-689.

FROELICHER, V.F., Jr., Brammell, H., Davis, G., Noquera, I., Stewart, A. & Lancaster, M.C. (1974). A comparison of three maximal treadmill exercise protocols. *Journal of Applied Physiology*, **36**, 720-725.

GODFREY, S. (1974). Exercise testing in children. Philadelphia: W.B. Saunders.

GOLDBERG, S.J., Weiss, R.W., & Adams, F.H. (1966). A comparison of the maximal endurance of normal children and patients with congenital cardiac disease. *Journal of Pediatrics*, **69**, 46-55.

HOLMGREN, A., & Mattson, K.H. (1954). A new ergometer with constant load at varying pedalling rate. *Scandinavian Journal of Clinical Laboratory Investigations*, **6**, 137-140.

JAMES, F.W. (1978). Exercise testing in children and young adults. An overview. *Cardiovascular Clinics*, **9**, 187-203.

KAPPAGODA, C.T., & Linden, R.J. (1972). A critical assessment of an open circuit technique for measuring oxygen consumption. *Cardiovascular Research*, **6**, 589-598.

MACEK, M., & Vavra, J. (1971). Cardiopulmonary and metabolic changes during exercise in children 6-14 years old. *Journal of Applied Physiology*, **30**, 202-204.

MCARDLE, W.D., Katch, F.I., & Pechar, G.S. (1973). Comparison of continuous and discontinuous treadmill and bicycle tests for $\dot{V}O_2$ max. *Medicine and Science in Sports*, **5**, 156-160.

PATTERSON, D.H., & Cunningham, D.A. (1978). Maximal oxygen uptake in children—comparison of treadmill protocols at varied speeds. *Canadian Journal of Applied Sciences*, **3**, 188.

RIOPEL, D.A., Taylor, A.B., & Hohn, A.R. (1979). Blood pressure, heart rate, pressure rate product, and electrocardiographic changes in healthy children during treadmill exercise. *American Journal of Cardiology*, **44**, 697-704.

SHEPHARD, R.J., Allen, C., Benade, A.J.S., Davies, C.T.M., DiPrampero, P.E., Hedman, R., Merriman, J.E., Myrha, K., & Simmons, R. (1968). The maximum oxygen intake. An international reference standard of cardiorespiratory fitness. *Bulletin of the World Health Organization*, **38**, 757-764.

SJOSTRAND, T. (1947). Changes in the respiratory organs of workmen at an ore smelting works. *Acta Medica Scandinavica*, (Suppl. 196), p. 687.

STAMFORD, B.A. (1975). Maximal oxygen uptake during treadmill walking and running at various speeds. *Journal of Applied Physiology*, **39**, 386-389.

WAHLUND, H. (1948). Determination of physical working capacity. *Acta Medica Scandinavica*, **132** (Suppl. 215), p. 1.

WESSELL, H.U., Stent, R.L., Guerrero, L., & Paul, M.H. (1976). Postoperative exercise studies in Tetralogy of Fallot. In B.S.L. Kidd & R.D. Rowe (Eds.), *The child with congenital heart disease after surgery*, (p. 72). New York: Futura.

The Effects of Sprint Running on Cardiac Function During Recovery in 6- to 11-Year-Old Boys and Girls

Katsumi Asano and Naka Nakamura
University of Tsukuba
Ibaraki, Japan

Numerous studies of cardiac stroke volume during exercise have been reported. However, only a few investigations are available to elucidate stroke volume during recovery from exercise. Reindell, Roskamm, and Gerschuler (1962) postulated that stroke volume was higher during the recovery phase of exercise than during the exercise itself. Cumming (1972) found by direct measurement of cardiac output using a dilution technique that the highest stroke volume occurred during the first 2 min of recovery from the supine bicycle exercise in patients aged 7 to 54 years. But there have been no studies on cardiac function during recovery from upright exercise in healthy children.

Therefore, the present study was planned to investigate (a) whether sprint running in children causes an increase in the stroke volume during recovery from exercise, (b) the pattern of increase in stroke volume during recovery according to age and sex, and (c) the difference, if any, in the pattern of increase of stroke volume during recovery in the supine and the sitting positions.

Subjects and Methods

Subjects in this study were 36 healthy boys and girls, aged 6 to 11 years. Physical characteristics and 50 m sprint running performance are presented in Table 1. The subjects were thoroughly examined before the experiment, including history, examination of the heart and lungs, and ECG at rest and during exercise. All results were normal, so all subjects were regarded as healthy. All subjects performed two 50 m maximal sprint runs on separate days. The subjects rested for 10 min either in the sitting or supine position before and after each running exercise (see Figure 1). Heart rate was continuously recorded for 10 min at rest and from 15 s immediately after the running for 10 min during the recovery period for each experiment. Stroke volume and systolic time intervals were measured after 10 min of rest and every 15 s they were recorded beginning 15 s immediately after the run till 3 min of recovery and thereafter at 4 min,

Table 1
Physical Characteristics and Running Performance of Subjects

Subject		n	Age years mean (S.D.)	Height cm mean (S.D.)	Weight kg mean (S.D.)	B.S.A. m² mean (S.D.)	50m - run (1) m/s mean (S.D.)	(2) m/s mean (S.D.)
I	M	6	6.51 (0.26)	117.6 (1.7)	21.1 (1.2)	0.79 (0.05)	4.41 (0.23)	4.38 (0.16)
	F	6	6.54 (0.22)	116.3 (4.3)	21.8 (2.6)	0.81 (0.06)	4.16 (0.32)	4.12 (0.16)
II	M	6	7.56 (0.31)	119.8 (3.6)	23.8 (3.1)	0.86 (0.06)	4.75 (0.20)*	4.79 (0.22)**
	F	6	7.42 (0.32)	121.4 (4.0)	25.6 (4.2)	0.90 (0.08)	4.55 (0.21)*	4.54 (0.30)*
III	M	6	8.71 (0.32)	129.2 (4.2)	29.8 (7.1)	1.00 (0.12)*	4.89 (0.39)	5.21 (0.20)*
	F	6	8.67 (0.36)	127.8 (2.8)	25.7 (2.4)	0.93 (0.05)	4.97 (0.29)*	4.90 (0.46)
IV	M	6	9.81 (0.26)	132.6 (4.0)	28.5 (5.0)	1.00 (0.09)	5.08 (0.38)	5.01 (0.33)
	F	6	9.60 (0.28)	132.4 (9.9)	30.3 (7.6)	1.02 (0.16)	5.15 (0.28)	4.91 (0.39)
V	M	6	10.58 (0.27)	139.6 (5.2)	32.4 (5.8)	1.09 (0.11)	5.29 (0.24)	5.52 (0.40)
	F	6	10.57 (0.31)	137.4 (6.1)	33.7 (5.3)	1.10 (0.10)	5.21 (0.34)	5.15 (0.31)
VI	M	6	11.61 (0.34)	146.1 (6.9)	37.8 (5.0)	1.21 (0.11)	5.74 (0.35)*	5.78 (0.45)
	F	6	11.60 (0.28)	149.0 (2.9)	37.7 (3.7)	1.22 (0.07)	5.78 (0.14)**	5.58 (0.26)*

M: male; F: female; difference from each previous age: $-p < .05$, $**p < .01$, $***p < .001$; B.S.A.: Body Surface Area.

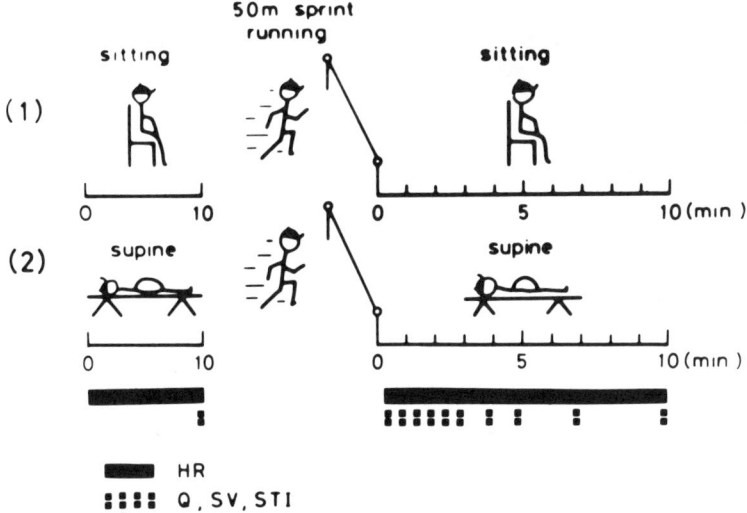

Figure 1—Experimental protocol (resting, running, and recovery at sitting and supine positions).

5 min, 7 min, and 10 min during recovery. Cardiac output was calculated by multiplying stroke volume by heart rate. For measurement of stroke volume and systolic time intervals, the derivative of thoracic impedance (dz/dt), electrocardiogram (ECG) and phonocardiogram (PCG) were recorded simultaneously in the supine and sitting positions during rest and recovery measurements with the subject in an end-expiratory apnea. Transthoracic electrical impedance was measured with a 4-electrode impedance cardiograph (IFM Minnesota Model 400, Instrumentation for Medicine Inc., Greenwich, CN). A constant sinusoidal alternating current of 4mA at a frequency of 100 KHZ was applied between the outer pair of four aluminum electrode tapes placed circumferentially around the subject's neck, thorax (just below the xiphosternal junction) and abdomen. The first derivative of the changes in impedance with respect to time which was picked up from the inner pair of electrodes, together with a ECG were recorded with high speed (100 mm/s) on a multichannel Rectigraph, Model 8K (SAN-EI Instrument Co., Japan). The thoracic impedance stroke volume was calculated from an average of six heart beats using the formula given by Kubicek, Karnegis, Patterson, Witsoe, and Mattson (1966):

$$\text{Stroke volume} = p\ (L/Z_0)\ T\ (dz/dt)\text{min},$$

where p indicates blood resistivity (taken as 135 ohm/cm), L is the shortest distance (cm) between the inner electrodes (mean of the front and back measurement), Z_0 is the basal thoracic impedance between the inner electrode (ohm), T is the ventricular ejection time (s), and (dz/dt)min is the value at the minimum peak value (ohm/s).

Even though impedance cardiography is an indirect method of assessing stroke volume, correlations of 0.90 and 0.89 have been found between stroke volume assessed by this method and dye cardiac output by others (Denniston et al., 1976) as well as by the present researchers (Asano & Hirakoba, 1984). The left ventricular ejection time (LVET) was determined as the time interval from the first crossing of the zero line by the dz/dt curve at the commencement of systole to either the second heart sound (S2) or the notch (X-point) which often occurs in the dz/dt tracing synchronous with the total electromechanical systole (QS2), which was measured from the onset of the QRS complex of ECG to the high frequency component of S2. The mean values obtained from at least six different heart cycles were used for the determination of QS2 and LVET.

Results

The heart rate, stroke volume, and cardiac output found in boys at rest and during the recovery phase in the sitting and supine position are presented in Figures 2 and 3. Subjects were divided to 3 groups so that each group consisted of 12 persons aged 6 to 7, 8 to 9, and 10 to 12 years of age. The sprint running exercise was a 50 m

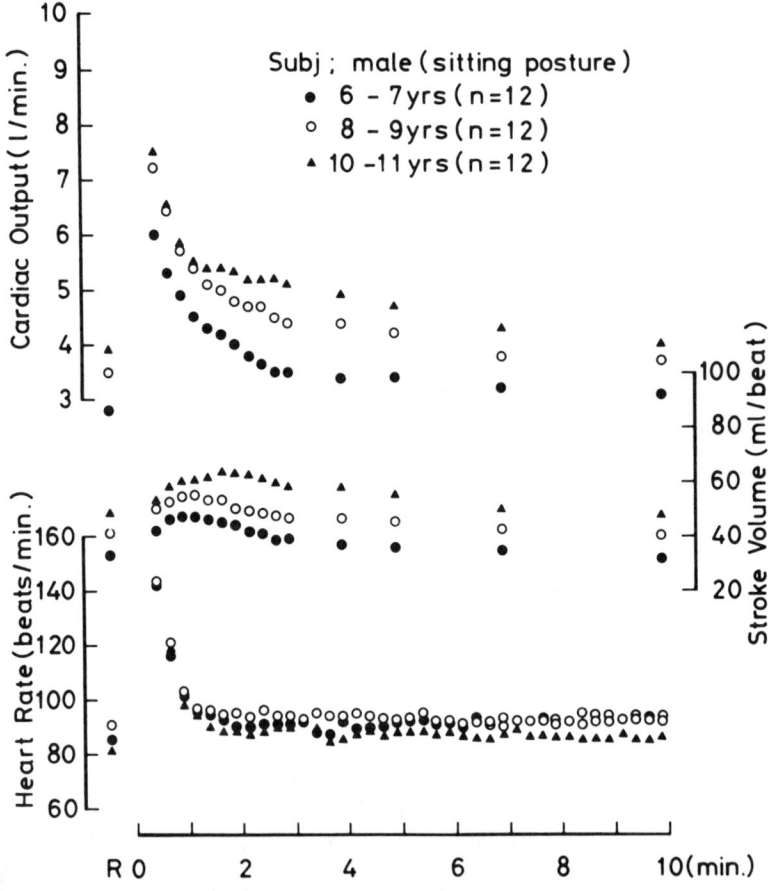

Figure 2—Changes in cardiac output, stroke volume, and heart rate at rest and recovery in sitting position of children aged 6-11 years (male).

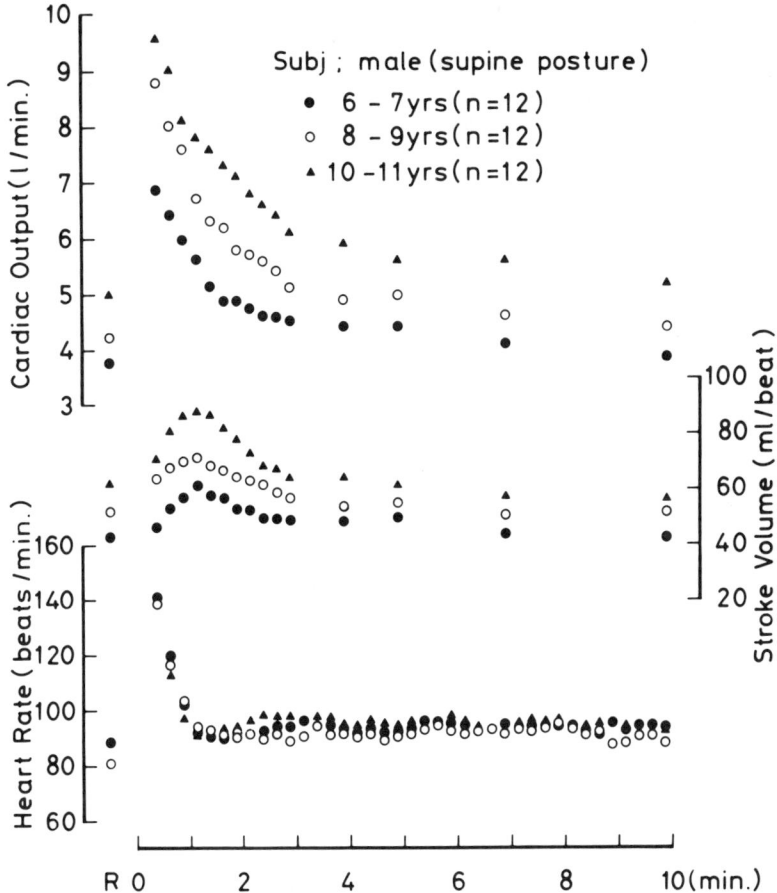

Figure 3—Changes in cardiac output, stroke volume, and heart rate at rest and recovery in supine position of children aged 6-11 years (male).

dash on the playground at school. Attempts were made to have the subjects run maximally. Running records ranged from 8.7 s (5.7 m/s) to 12.1 s (4.1 m/s) in all 3 age groups of both sexes. Maximal heart rate immediately after running at 15 s of recovery ranged from 141 to 151 beats/min in the sitting position and 135 to 141 beats/min in the supine position in all 3 age groups of both sexes. The mean recovery heart rate in all 3 age groups in the sitting and supine position decreased sharply during the first 60 s of recovery, almost reaching the resting values. However, of great interest is the observed significant transient increase in the mean stroke volume during the first approximately 1 min of recovery in all 3 age groups for subjects of both sexes in the sitting and supine positions. The increase began approximately 15 s after the exercise with peak values, shown at an average of 65 s, ranging from 45 to 90 s. After that, the stroke volume showed a gradual decrease and reached almost the resting values at 10 min of recovery. These tendencies were almost the same in all 3 age groups of both sexes. But the absolute values in the mean stroke volume showed higher values in the older age group than in the younger group of both sexes. It should be pointed out that the peak amplitude of absolute mean stroke volume during recovery showed higher values in the supine than in the sitting position in both sexes. There was an equal number of instances of peak stroke volume in heart rate ranges from 95 to 100 beats/min in all 3 age groups of both sexes. On the other hand, the mean recovery cardiac output exponentially decreased in all 3 age groups of both sexes, although the values tended to be higher in the older age groups than the younger groups. The absolute values in mean cardiac output showed higher values in the supine than in the sitting position in both sexes.

The percent change ($\Delta\%$) relative to the control resting values in heart rate, stroke volume, and cardiac output during recovery in the sitting and supine position in all 3 age groups of both sexes are presented in Figures 4 to 7. There were no sex and age group differences in the $\Delta\%$ of heart rate and cardiac output in the sitting and supine position. However, in the sitting position, the $\Delta\%$ of stroke volume in the 6- to 7-year-old group of both sexes was 45 to 48%, whereas the values in the 8- to 9- and 10-

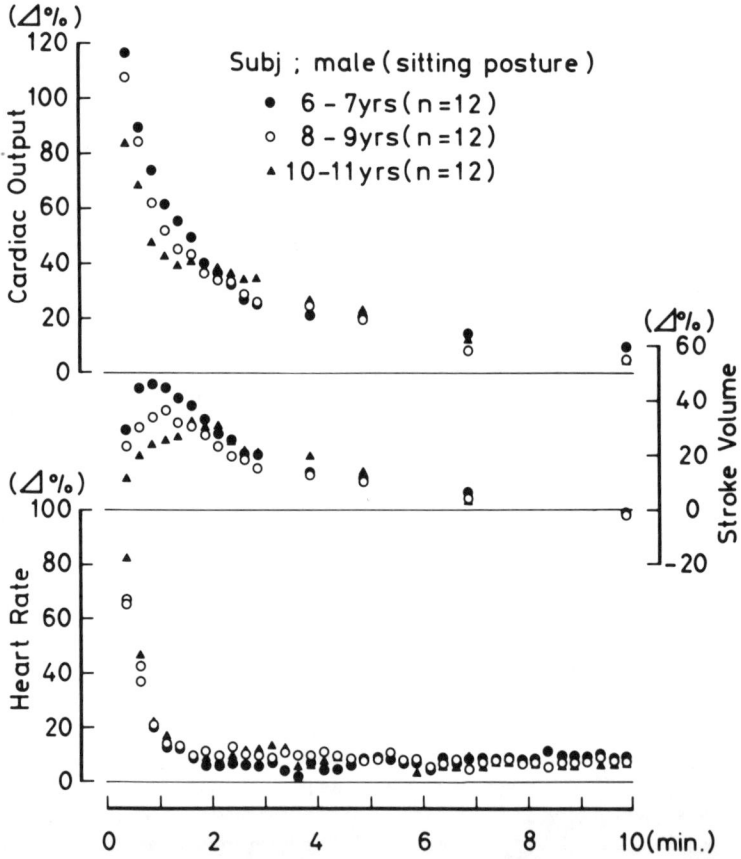

Figure 4—Percent changes in cardiac output, stroke volume, and heart rate during recovery compared to resting values in sitting position of children aged 6-11 years (male).

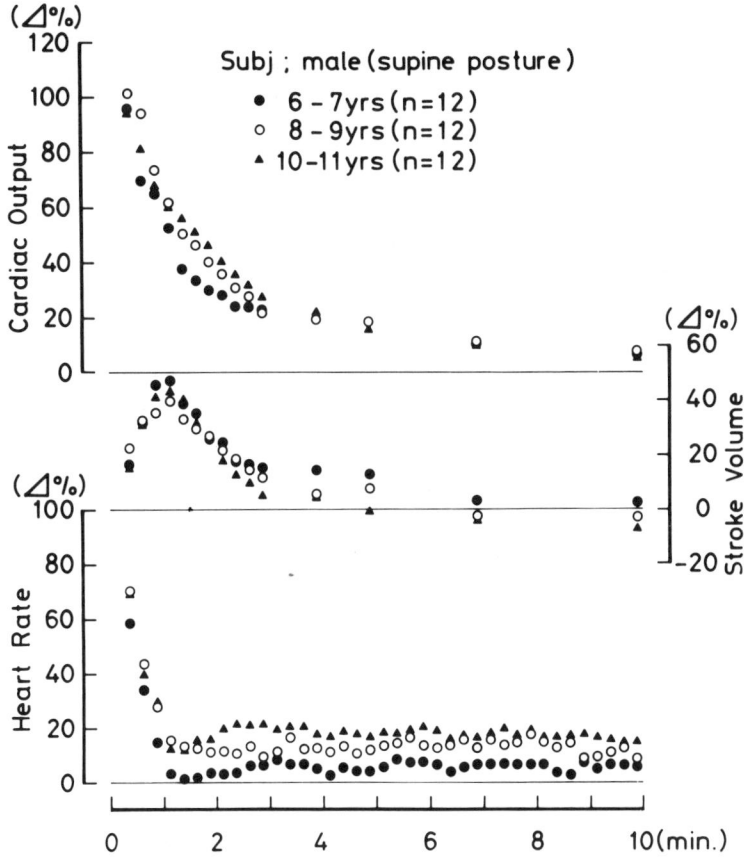

Figure 5—Percent changes in cardiac output, stroke volume, and heart rate during recovery compared to resting values in supine position of children aged 6-11 years (male).

to 11-year-old group showed 31 to 35% for both sexes. On the other hand, in the supine position, the Δ% of stroke volume in all 3 age groups showed almost the same mean values of 43% in boys and 39% in girls. Therefore, there were no siginificant differences in Δ% of stroke volume between each age group of both sexes, because increases of Δ% of stroke volume in the 8- to 9- and 10- to 11-year-old groups of both sexes occurred only in the supine position. The QS2, LVET, PEP, and PEP/LVET found in each age group of boys at rest and the recovery phase in the sitting and supine positions are presented in Figures 8 to 9.

The mean recovery QS2, LVET, and PEP in all 3 groups in the sitting and supine positions decreased sharply during approximately 30 s of recovery and showed a tendency of prolongation to 2 min recovery. The PEP/LVET ratio during recovery in boys of the 3 groups and girls of the 6- to 7- and 8- to 9-year-old age groups in the sitting position decreased during approximately 60 s of recovery and reached minimum values at the time when stroke volume during recovery showed a peak value. Thereafter, the values increased for 2 min of recovery. However, these tendencies were not evident

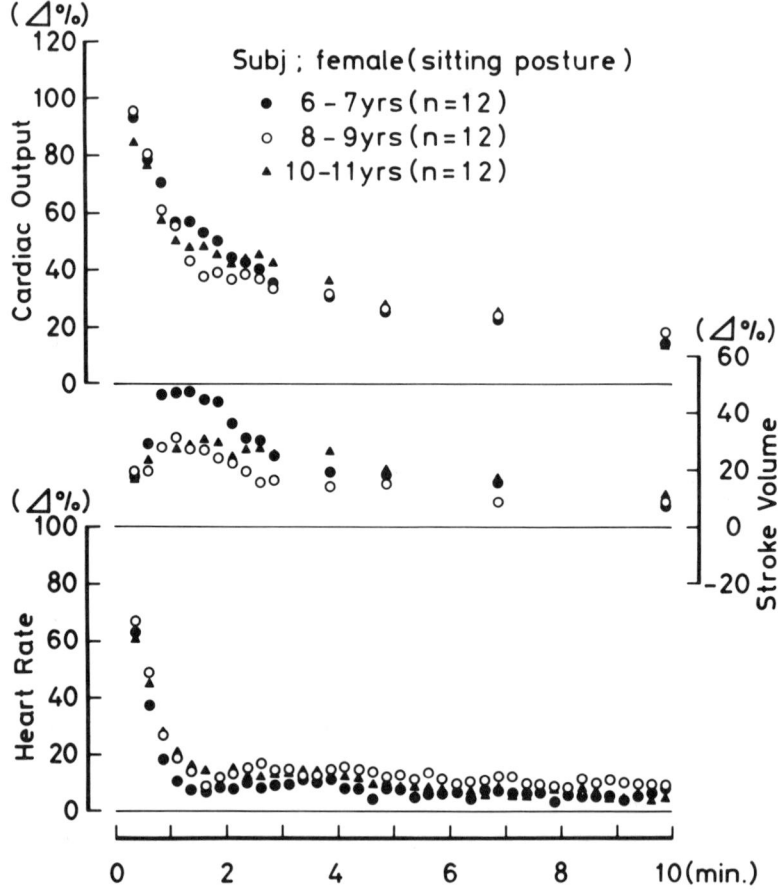

Figure 6—Percent changes in cardiac output, stroke volume, and heart rate during recovery comparing to resting values in sitting position of children aged 6-11 years (female).

in the supine position in all 3 age groups of both sexes. Marked differences in systolic time interval parameters during recovery between the sitting and supine position were found. The prolongation of LVET, the shortening of PEP, and the decrease of the PEP/LVET ratio were more characteristic in the supine than in the sitting position during recovery in all three age groups of both sexes.

Therefore, the decrease of Δ% to the resting values of the PEP/LVET ratio during recovery was greater in the sitting (22 to 25% in boys and 16 to 21% in girls) than in the supine position (9 to 15% in boys and 3 to 13% in girls) in all 3 age groups. In general, there were no sex and age group differences in the PEP/LVET ratio during recovery in the sitting and supine position except in the 10- to 11-year-old group of girls whose tachycardia during recovery were found in the sitting position.

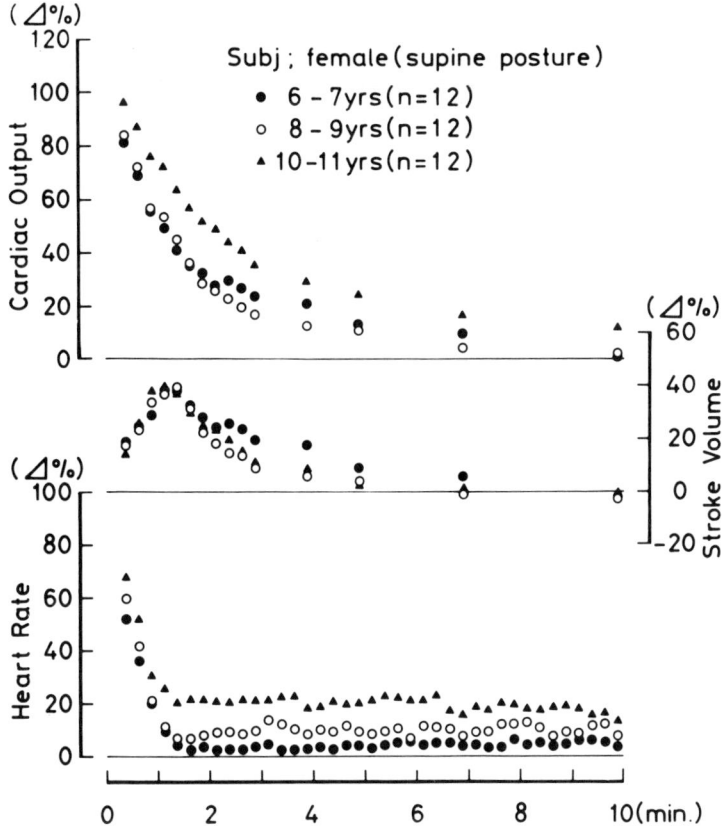

Figure 7—Percent changes in cardiac output, stroke volume, and heart rate during recovery compared to resting values in supine position of children aged 6-11 years (female).

Discussion

Stroke volume and stroke dimension during recovery from exercise have been investigated by Cumming (1972) and Stein, Michielli, Fox, and Krasnow (1978). However, they have studied the influence of supine bicycle exercise in patients, including children and healthy college students, on recovery of cardiac function. In the present study, the effects of 50 m sprint running resulting in a heart rate of 135 to 150 beats/min immediately after the exercise on cardiac function during recovery in healthy children aged 6- to 11-year-old were studied, and the influence of the sitting and supine positions on stroke capacity during recovery were investigated.

It was clearly observed in this study that transient increases in the mean stroke volume during recovery began at 15 s after the run and showed a peak value at average 65 s during recovery in 6- to 11-year-old healthy children of both sexes in the sitting and the supine position.

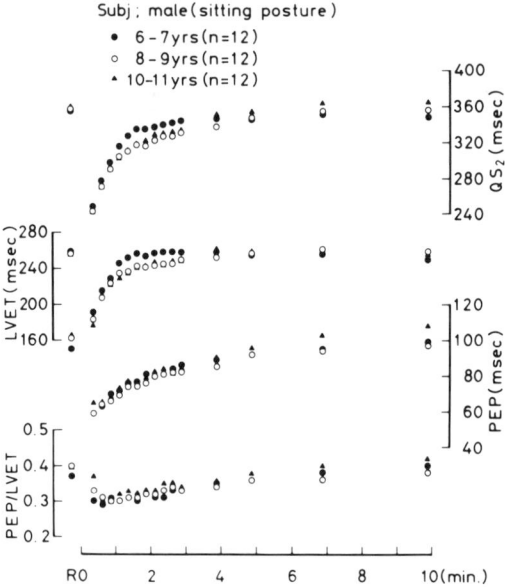

Figure 8—Changes in systolic time intervals at rest and recovery in sitting position of children aged 6-11 years (male).

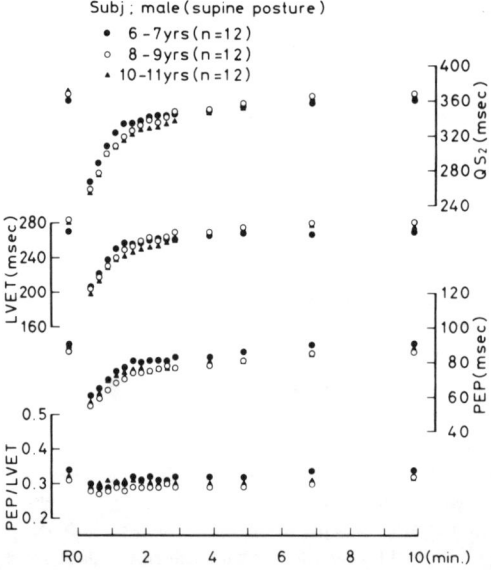

Figure 9—Changes in systolic time intervals at rest and recovery in supine position of children aged 6-11 years (male).

When the peak stroke volume during recovery was compared with values at rest, there was a significant increase in the Δ% of stroke volume by a mean value of 45 to 48% in the 6- to 7-year-old group and 31 to 35% in the 8- to 9- and 10- to 11-year-old group of both sexes in the sitting position. In the supine position the Δ% of stroke volume in all 3 age groups yielded almost the same values of 39 to 43% in both sexes.

A part of these results was consistent with the findings of Cumming (1972) and Stein, Michielli, Fox, and Krasnow (1978), whose investigations included supine bicycle exercise for a few minutes and recovery in the supine position. Stein et al. (1978) reported by using continuous echocardiographic recordings that there was a significant increase in end-diastolic and stroke dimensions increased by 35.1% (range 27 to 45%) in college students. Cumming (1972) also found by using a dilution method that the highest stroke volume occurred during the first 2 min of recovery and the percentages of stroke volumes were 27 to 29% higher during recovery of 15 to 120 s. In this study there was an equal number of peak stroke volumes in heart rates of 95 to 100 beats/min in all 3 age groups of both sexes, whereas Cummings' data showed higher values of 108 to 119 beats/min at the time of the peak stroke volume, because he required the subject to work against a heavy load, stimulating heart rates of 150 to 190 beats/min.

The increase in stroke volume during recovery from exercise might be due to the heart rate decreasing more rapidly than the cardiac output. Neurogenic factors which control for tachycardia at exercise are completely removed at the cessation of exercise so that the heart rate sharply decreases, whereas the cardiac output remains elevated and stimulated by humoral factors. It is said that stroke volume is dependent on venous return, myocardial contractility and peripheral resistance. The blood vessels in the active muscles remain dilated at the cessation of exercise while blood flow is no longer impaired by muscle contractions. Therefore, it might be assumed that these factors contribute to the elevated stroke volume by the fall in peripheral resistance and the increase in venous return. Stein, Michielli, Fox, and Krasnow (1978) suggested that the increased stroke dimension during recovery reflects a Frank-Starling mechanism which is unmasked in recovery because the heart rate appears to decrease faster than the metabolic demand and venous return. It was also postulated that enhanced myocardial contractility during recovery existed as indicated by the increased fractional shortening of the ventricular dimension.

Concerning the influence of position on the changes of stroke volume increase during recovery, it might be considered that the Δ% of stroke volume in the supine recovery was 3 to 12% greater in all 3 age groups of both sexes than the values in sitting recovery because venous return is unimpaired in the supine position. Moreover, a tendency of an increase in stroke volume during recovery in the sitting position was characterized much more in the 6- to 7-year-old group of both sexes (45 to 48%) than in the 8- to 9- and 10- to 11-year-old groups of both sexes (31 to 35%). Therefore, it might be suggested that the subjects in the 6- to 7-year-old age groups of both sexes might have had higher heart stroke capacities than the older aged children. On the other hand, the increase of stroke volume during recovery in the supine position showed higher consistency (39 to 43%) independent from age than the values in the sitting position. From these results, it might be postulated that an increase in stroke volume during recovery in the 8- to 9- and 10- to 11-year-old groups of both sexes were influenced greatly by hydrostatic factors associated with changing from sitting to supine position. The ratio of PEP/LVET reflected these hydrostatic changes of cardiac function; in the supine position this ratio during 15 to 30 s of recovery decreased by 15 to 18% and 22 to 24% in the 8- to 9- and 10- to 11-year-old groups of both sexes, respectively, compared with the values in the sitting position, whereas the 6- to 7-year-old groups showed no change in boys and 10% in girls. That is to say, in these older age groups of both sexes, cardiac contractility might be augumented by changing from the sitting to the supine position because venous return was unimpaired by removing hydrostatic pressure. Pigott, Spodick, Rectra, and Khan (1971) and McConahay, Martin, and Cheitlin (1972) also found that the ratio of PEP/LVET during recovery from supine exercise decreased in normal subjects, whereas this value increased in patients with cardiac failure. These consistent findings may be explained by a continued high level of venous return and enhancement of myocardial contractility during recovery in the supine position. The increase in stroke volume observed during recovery might have some application to development in aerobic work capacity and medical rehabilitation in children. Even in the 6- to 7-year-old groups of both sexes, the stroke capacities indicated superior function compared with the other older groups. Principally, it is reasonable to subject the heart to the repeated stimuli of high stroke volume by running exercise for development of heart stroke capacity in children, including 6- to 7-year-olds. Moreover, it might be suggested that to keep the supine position during recovery after exercise may have an advantage for enhancement of the heart's stroke capacity in children.

References

ASANO, K., & Hirakoba, K., (1984). Respiratory and circulatory adaptation during prolonged exercise in 10-to 12-year-old children and adults. *Children and Sport*. Springer Verlag. Berlin, Heidelberg, 119-128.

CUMMING, G.R. (1972). Stroke volume during recovery from supine bicycle exercise. *Journal of Applied Physiology*, **32**(5), 575-578.

DENNISTON, J.C., Maher, J.T., Reeves, J.T., Cruz, J.C., Cymerman, A., & Grover, R.F. (1976). Measurement of cardiac output by electrical impedance at rest and during exercise. *Journal of Applied Physiology*, **40**(1), 91-95.

KUBICEK, W.G., Karnegis, J.N., Patterson, R.P., Witsoe, D.A., & Mattson, R.H. (1966). Development and evaluation of an impedance cardiac output system. *Aerospace Medicine*, **37**, 1208-1212.

MCCONAHAY, D.R., Martin, C.M., & Cheitlin, M.D. (1972). Resting and exercise systolic time intervals. Correlations with ventricular performance in patients with coronary artery disease. *Circulation*, **45**, 592-601.

PIGOTT, V.M., Spodick,, D.H., Rectra, E.H., & Khan, A.H. (1971). Cardiocirculatory responses to exercise: Physiologic study by noninvasive techniques. *American Heart Journal*, **82**, 632-641.

REINDELL, H.L., Roskamm, H., & Gerschuler, W. (1962). Das Intervall-training (Interval training). Munchen: Fruh Morgen und Holzmann.

STEIN, R.A., Michielli, D., Fox, E.L., & Krasnow, N. (1978). Continuous ventricular dimensions in man during supine exercise and recovery—An echocardiographic study. *American Journal of Cardiology*, **41**, 655-660.

Children with Lung Disease and Exercise

Herman J. Neijens
Erasmus University, University Hospital, and
Sophia Children's Hospital, Rotterdam, The Netherlands

Children with lung diseases, as well as other chronic illnesses, often have a lower activity potential than healthy children. Various lung diseases may hamper exercise by different mechanisms. The causes of exercise limitation and the mechanisms involved in respiratory diseases will be discussed with special emphasis on exercise-induced bronchoconstriction. When patients complain about symptoms during or after physical activity, it is advisable to assess them objectively by exercise testing in order to analyze the limiting factors.

Respiratory Causes of Exercise Limitation

Breathlessness after exercise may be caused by one or more of the following disturbances in the respiratory system:

1. mechanical obstruction in the large or small airways—for example, obstructive lung disease;
2. low lung or chest wall compliance, as in restrictive lung disease;
3. alveolar hypoventilation, for example, abnormal control of ventilation or abnormally large physiological dead space; and
4. diseases of the lung parenchyma causing artero-venous shunting through hypoventilated lung, ventilation-perfusion abnormalities and diffusion disorders.

Patients who have difficulty exercising often avoid heavy work. This may lead to poor physical fitness which further diminishes the capacity to exercise.

Children with obstructive lung disease generally develop adequate cardiorespiratory adaptation to exercise. However, a great many of them develop a bronchoconstrictive reaction after a short period (5 to 8 min) of strenuous exercise. This is called exercise-induced bronchial obstruction (EIB) or exercise-induced asthma. In EIB arterial hyposaturation and CO_2 retention are either not present or not noticeable, even when airway obstruction is pronounced.

Bronchoconstriction after exercise can be quantified by lung function measurements which show a characteristic pattern after vigorous exercise in a susceptible person. During a 4- to 10-min period of exercise a small but detectable improvement in lung function (bronchodilatation) occurs. This is followed by a deterioration (bronchoconstriction) at the end of or shortly after the completion of the exercise period. The clinical and physiological abnormalities, regardless of severity, are usually most marked during the first 10 min after exercise and decrease over a period of 15 to 45 min.

Various lung function indices have been proposed to quantify the bronchial response. Generally the forced expiratory volume in 1 s (FEV_1) or peak flow rate is used as a measure of the degree of the bronchial response. The degree of EIB is usually expressed as the difference between the initial value and the lowest value after exercise as a percentage of the initial value.

Apart from an early reaction immediately after exercise, a delayed bronchial obstructive reaction has been observed recently (Kay & Lee, 1982) similar to that of antigen-induced bronchoconstriction. This late reaction occurs between 4 and 24 hr after the completion of exercise and seems to be correlated with release of the mediator neutrophil chemotactic factor of anaphylaxis (NCF).

Prolonged early reactions are also occasionally found. Delayed type reactions seem to be observed particularly in children. The observation that delayed type obstructive reactions may occur after exercise has practical clinical implications. It would, for instance, be important to appreciate that an apparent spontaneous exacerbation of asthma, especially at night, may be related to exercise undertaken several hours earlier.

Patients with restrictive lung disease easily develop dyspnea after exercise. At rest they usually have a small tidal volume, an increased respiratory rate and a high minute ventilation. With exercise, they increase their ventilation more than would be predicted by the augmentation in workload. The ventilation per minute will, therefore, be high for the work performed. The maximal ventilatory capacity is reached before they have exhausted their cardiovascular potential: the O_2-pulse (the quotient of O_2 uptake and pulse) tends to be relatively high. When they also have ventilation-perfusion abnormalities, arterial desaturation may occur. Repetition of the exercise test during 100% O_2 breathing provides additional information about the role of hypoxia.

Respiratory adaptation to exercise may be limited by abnormalities which affect the respiratory movements. These abnormalities can be located at different sites in the following pathway: the medulla oblongata, the neuromuscular system of the thorax, and the thoracic skeleton.

Centrally located disorders may be involved in Ondine's curse, which indicates a disturbance of the respiration regulation mainly occurring during sleep. Examples of neuromuscular disorders are poliomyelitis, myasthenia gravis, and muscular dystrophy. Skeletal diseases, such as kyphoscoliosis may limit chest movements and thus give rise to ventilatory restrictions. Children with cerebral palsy may have energy-wasting muscular spasticity and involuntary actions, which interfere with respiratory movements.

All these patients have a limited ability to increase their tidal volume, as is the case in restrictive lung diseases for different reasons. Increase in breathing rate, if possible, is the best way to increase their ventilation. Therefore, these patients are found to exercise with relative tachypnea. They have an increased risk of hypoxia.

In obesity, due to a marked increase in fat, the body is inappropriately large for the heart and lungs. In proportion to the degree of obesity, an increased O_2 uptake ($\dot{V}O_2$) is needed for any given degree of exercise. Various disorders may contribute to hypoventilation, such as a central cause, obstruction of the upper airways caused by adipose tissue, or muscular weakness. The ventilatory frequency and/or volume during exercise cannot be adapted to the requirements of the metabolic stress, resulting in a limited exercise tolerance. This will be obvious from the relatively low minute ventilation ($\dot{V}_E$) and possibly from hypercapnia, acidosis, and hypoxia.

Progressive abnormalities in the lung parenchyma, including tissue destruction and fibrosis, are usually present in children with cystic fibrosis (CF). These children have, besides other symptoms, decreased exercise tolerance along with their lung disease. The pathology in the lung causes alveolar hypoventilation, artero-venous shunting, and hypoxia. These conditions hamper the respiratory adjustment to an augmented workload. A progressively diminishing alveolar ventilation compared to the workload and an increase in artero-venous shunting through poorly or nonventilated parts of the lungs occurs. In this way the hypoxia may increase and may sometimes be associated with CO_2 retention. These patients tend to develop more acidosis than would be expected from exercise adaptation alone.

In a group of children with CF the arterial oxygen saturation was measured at the end of an exercise test. This was compared with the degree of lung disease, judged by a pulmonary function score. At rest these children had a saturation above 90%. After exercise a fall in arterial oxygen saturation occurred only in those who had advanced pulmonary disease.

In patients with diffusion defects, exercise easily results in hypoxia. Such patients have to be careful during strenuous exercise and should avoid exercise leading to marked arterial hyposaturation. A fall in saturation, but not a rise in PCO_2, can be decreased by oxygen administration during exercise. A consequence of arterial hyposaturation, if excessive and long standing, is often pulmonary hypertension, right ventricular hypertrophy, right arterial enlargement, and hence left ventricular dysfunction and arrhythmias. Repeated exercise by patients with hypoxia may promote these complications.

The Mechanisms of Exercise-Induced Bronchial Obstruction

In the last decade an increasing number of studies have appeared investigating the mechanism of EIB. The mechanism of EIB has long been obscure, but is now beginning to be elucidated. A number of factors are known now, although the precise interaction of these factors is not yet clear. The following variables may affect the response to exercise:

Amount of Metabolic Stress

Postexercise bronchial obstruction sharply increases with $\dot{V}O_2$. This relationship applies equally to an increase in exercise time or strength of exercise (Godfrey, 1974). Silverman and Anderson (1972) showed that increasing workloads not only increased bronchospasm but that a plateau was reached between 60 to 85% of the physical working capacity.

Type of Exercise

Differences in the bronchial response to exercise at the same workload have been reported in a group of asthmatic children by Anderson, Connolly, and Godfrey (1971).

Free-range running caused more bronchial obstruction than treadmill running. Cycling revealed a lower drop in lung function than running, while walking and swimming were even less effective in causing a postexercise fall. Sports such as swimming and kayaking, which primarily use the arms, are less likely to induce bronchial obstruction.

The differences in response to exercise were originally thought to be due to factors such as the use of different muscle groups. However, doubt about these explanations has been raised by several studies. Anderson, Silverman, König, and Godfrey (1975) have shown that cranking a bicycle ergometer with the arms can be as challenging as running, provided the oxygen consumption is comparable. Arm work produced a greater airway obstruction than leg work but was also accompanied by a greater metabolic load as judged by the heart rate (Strauss, Haynes, Ingram, & McFadden, 1977). If the load on the legs was increased, the differences between arm and leg exercise disappeared. The authors concluded that the workload and the mass of the exercising muscles determine the metabolic rate and thus the bronchial response. Similarly, running and cycling with equal metabolic load, defined by the oxygen consumption, revealed no differences in bronchial response to exercise (Miller, Davies, Cole, & Seaton, 1975).

It appears that metabolic load, assessed by the oxygen consumption, depends upon the muscle mass. This may explain to a great extent the variability in EIB between persons of different ages and sex and between different forms of exercise. Thus, it is most probable that the bronchial reaction after different forms of exercise is largely related to the metabolic load.

Physiology of Exercise

Heavy exercise is accompanied by hyperventilation, hypocapnia, and lactic acidosis (Godfrey, 1974; Wasserman, 1978). Formerly, these indices have been thought to play a role in exercise-induced bronchial obstruction, although no causal relationship could be observed between the degree of obstruction and hypocapnia, lactate acidosis, acidemia, or change in the arterial oxygen tension (Silverman, Anderson, & Walker, 1972). Various detailed studies have been performed which further deny such a relationship (Strauss, Ingram, & McFadden, 1977; Zeballos, Shturman-Ellstein, McNally, Hirsch, & Souhrada, 1978).

The Bronchial Mechanism and Reactivity

Bronchial reactivity is a characteristic which determines the response of the bronchi after a standardized stimulus. It varies between subjects and is related to the occurrence of symptoms. Bronchial reactivity is mostly quantified by the change in lung function parameters after the inhalation of histamine or metacholine.

The degree of bronchial obstruction after exercise and the reaction after inhaled histamine have been compared. Both reactions appeared to be related, indicating the more pronounced the bronchial reactivity the more bronchial obstruction usually develops after exercise (Neijens, Wesselius, & Kerrebijn, 1981). The association between the reactions after both stimuli suggests that the reaction after exercise is dependent upon some bronchial mechanism which is involved with nonspecific stimuli.

A number of factors are thought to be important for the bronchial mechanism, that is, the mucosa, the sympathetic and parasympathetic system, the mast cells, and the bronchial smooth muscles. In patients, these factors can most practically be assessed by the protective effects of pharmacological agents. In order to study the involvement of the airway sensory receptors, oropharyngeal anesthesia by a local anesthetic has been applied. Lidocaine per spray could not clearly inhibit bronchial obstruction after exercise (Fanta, Ingram, & McFadden, 1980). The impact of reflexes mediated by parasympathetic fibers has been examined by blocking studies using atropine. Atropine and related parasympathetic blocking agents could partially inhibit the bronchial obstruction after exercise. Thomson, Patel, and Kerr (1978) observed a marked protective effect in 8 of 13 patients. These findings were confirmed by Godfrey and König (1976), indicating that the parasympathetic system is at least partially involved in the generation of the bronchoconstriction.

The effect of cromoglycate, which is assumed to block mast cells, on the bronchial reaction due to exercise has been assessed in several studies, revealing a nearly complete inhibition of the bronchospasm in the majority of patients, but with little or no effect in the remaining ones (Silverman, Connolly, Balfour-Lynn, & Godfrey, 1972). Cromoglycate protects more patients than parasympatholytics (Thomson, Patel, & Kerr, 1978).

These results point to a protective role of cromoglycate, indicating that mediator release is probably important in the induction of bronchoconstriction after exercise. It must be stressed, however, that some doubt exists about its mode of action.

A role of mediator release from mast cells is further suggested by the following evidence. The occurrence of a refractory period after exercise suggests that a system is exhausted and mast-cell release seems the best candidate for it. James, Facian, and Sly (1976) repeated exercise-tests in asthmatic children at hourly intervals. They observed a progressively smaller bronchial response. The influence of previous exercise on exercise-induced bronchial obstruction was extensively studied by Edmunds, Tooley, and Godfrey (1978). The ability to induce the same amount of bronchial obstruction was mainly recovered within 2 hr and always fully within 4 hr. Thus, a refractory period of about 2 hr exists. These studies suggest a mast-cell depletion after exercise, while the mast cells need several hours to resynthesize mediators.

Kay and Lee (1982) were able to show that a mast-cell associated mediator, NCF, was released preceding the fall in lung function after exercise. The magnitude and kinetics of the reduction in FEV_1 and elevations in NCF were related, which strengthens the theory of mast-cell release in the generation of bronchial obstruction after exercise.

Although direct proof is lacking, these observations thus provide indirect evidence that mediator release from mast cells occurs and that they have a role in exercise-induced bronchoconstriction.

Several studies have shown that α-sympathetic blocking drugs (indoramine and thymoxamine) can partially inhibit bronchial obstruction after exercise (Patel & Kerr, 1976). Thus, the role of the α-sympathetic system in exercise-reactions is unclear, but may contribute to the obstructive reaction. The blocking capacity of β_2-sympathetic agonists in exercise-induced asthma is excellent in most patients when given by aerosol (Godfrey & Köning, 1976).

It may therefore be concluded that the stimulation of the β-sympathetic system is important in combating bronchoconstriction after exercise. The modulating effect of β-agonists may be directly on smooth muscle, mast-cell mediator release, or on a receptor site to mediator reactivity.

The effects of a β_2-sympathomimetic, a parasympatholytic, cromoglycate, and a placebo were compared in a group of asthmatic children under carefully standardized conditions (Neijens, Wesselius, & Kerrebijn, 1981). The results revealed that the β-sympathetic agonists are the most effective and parasympathetic antagonists the least effective. The effect of cromoglycate is intermediate, but variable among patients. In a further study, it was shown that the protective effects of the parasympathetic antagonist and those of the mast-cell stabilizer together were approximately equal to the degree of obstruction without protection. This suggests that the bronchospasm after exercise is brought about by a combination of the parasympathetic and the mast-cell system.

The Site of Airway Obstruction

Information about the localization of the obstruction, either in the large or in the small airway, may increase insight into the mechanism of the obstructive reaction.

Airflow obstruction in the more central—compared to the more peripheral—airways differ in density dependency using helium-oxygen mixtures. Studies using this technique have suggested that the predominant site of airway obstruction is located in the more central airways, whereas others have found the obstruction in the more peripheral airways. McFadden, Ingram, Haynes, and Wellman (1977) found that the subjects with predominately small airway response could be treated with cromoglycate, but not with parasympatholytics. In contrast, the patients who had their bronchial response in the large airway were more likely to be helped with the parasympatholytics. This suggests that chemical mediators affect the peripheral airways, which is in harmony with the relatively high density of mast cells at this location (Gold, Meijers, Dain, & Miller, 1977). The vagal nerves are not distributed in the peripheral bronchi, making more understandable the fact that obstruction in the central airway is mainly mediated via the parasympathetic system.

Neijens, Gargani, van Kralingen, Wezepoel, and Kerrebijn (1982) have measured the bronchial obstruction and site of narrowing after exercise in a group of children using helium-oxygen mixtures. In the majority of the patients the obstruction shortly after exercise (4 min) was maximal and located in the more peripheral airways. Later, 20 min after exercise, the obstruction decreased and moved to the more central airways. These results suggest that the bronchospasm seems to behave as a peristaltic wave. The site of maximal obstruction moves to the small or peripheral airways. Thereafter, the site of maximal obstruction moves back in the direction of the mouth towards the large or central airways while the overall degree of obstruction decreases.

Condition of Inhaled Air During Exercise

Several observations have highlighted the importance of the condition of the inhaled air in EIB. Weinstein, Anderson, Kvale, and Sweet (1976) studied the effect of humidification and found that exercise-induced bronchial obstruction was more severe when subjects breathed dry air compared to humidified air. This observation has been confirmed by Bar-Or, Neuman, and Dotan (1977) in a climatic chamber where a high relative humidity (90%) revealed a diminished bronchial response compared to a low relative humidity (25%). Strauss, McFadden, Ingram, Deal, and Jaeger (1978) compared temperature and humidity and their interaction with exercise-induced bronchial obstruction. Heating the air from room to body temperature had no clear effect on the bronchial response. When the humidity was increased, in combination with room temperature, the degree of bronchial obstruction diminished. The lung function changes could be completely prevented by fully saturated inhaled air at room temperature; and in patients with exercise-induced asthma when breathing with their mouths open, nasal breathing virtually abolished the postexercise bronchial obstruction. This may be explained by the humidifying and heating capacity of the nose (Shturman-Ellstein, Zeballos, Buckely, & Souhrada, 1978).

An excellent relationship was found between the condition of the inspired air, that is, the temperature and the humidity, and the degree of bronchoconstriction after exercise (McFadden & Ingram, 1979). Inspired air is known to be heated and humidified so that by the time it approaches the alveoli, it is fully saturated with water vapor at body temperature. Heat and water move from the mucosa to the incoming air as a function of temperature and vapor pressure gradients and the geometry of the exchanging surface. Heating occurs both by conduction and convection. During air warming, the capacity of air to hold water increases and humidification occurs by evaporation from the airway mucosa.

The net effect of the thermal exchanges on inspiration is mucosa cooling and drying. They depend not only upon the condition of inspired air and the intensity of ventilation, but also upon the time of exposure. High levels of ventilation with relatively cold air could surpass the warming and humidification capacity of the airways and challenge the deeper airways with cooling and drying. The decrease in temperature in the intrathoracic airways is confirmed by temperature measurements in the retrotracheal part of the esophagus, the magnitude being related to the minute ventilation and inversely to the inspired temperature and water content. Deal, McFadden, Ingram, and Jaeger (1979) found a mean temperature of 20°C in the trachea and of 27°C deep in the right lower lobe in normal subjects, inspiring air at $-17°C$ with a moderate hyperventilation. This indicates that very cold air is needed to drop the temperature of the intrathoracic airways without or with modest hyperventilation. However, during pronounced hyperventilation as in heavy exercise, less cold and dry environmental air may induce bronchial reactions. For the induction of an asthmatic response after exercise, Anderson et al. (1982) found the temperature of inhaled air during pronounced hyperventilation to be critical in the range of below 20°C and its water content below 30 mg $H_2O \cdot l^{-1}$.

Although no difference could be found in the degree of the temperature drop in asthmatics and normal subjects, those with hyperreactive airways are much more sensitive to airway cooling than normal subjects (Deal, McFadden, Ingram, Breslin, & Jaeger, 1980). In asthmatics, less cooling is required to induce obstruction as the disease worsens. The ability to induce bronchial obstruction by cooled air in normal subjects may come with an upper respiratory tract infection and later fade away.

The Effects of Airway Cooling

The mechanisms by which airway cooling produces bronchoconstriction is not yet known. A number of postulates about which system is sensitive to cooling have been put forward in the literature: cold-induced reflexes arising from the airways, release of mediators from mast cells, direct thermal effect on the airway's smooth muscle, and interconversion of β into α-sympathetic receptors.

Nearly 25 years ago, Wells, Walker, and Hickler (1960) found indications that the inhalation of cold air may induce reflex bronchoconstriction. Not only receptors inside the airways, but also those outside this system may generate reflex bronchoconstriction, as is shown by the following observations. Application of ice to the face of normal individuals and blowing cold air on the back of asthmatic patients (Josenhans, Melville, & Ulmer, 1969) cause bronchial obstruction. However, these bronchial effects are small and short lasting in comparison with cooling of the airways.

The role of the parasympathetic system in bronchoconstriction after cooling has been studied by blocking studies. Atropine, which blocks the parasympathetic fibers, causes some dose-dependent inhibition of the bronchial obstruction after voluntary eucapnic hyperventilation with cold air, whereby a higher dose is needed than for blockade of obstructive reactions after other triggers such as metacholine (Sheppard, Epstein, Holtzman, Nadel, & Boushey, 1982). However, another group of researchers (Griffin, Fung, Ingram, & McFadden, 1982) could not confirm these results and did not find any effect with atropine. Thus, the role of the parasympathetic system in cold air-induced bronchial obstruction is not yet established.

The role of mediator release from mast cells in obstructive reactions after airway cooling is assessed by studying the eventual occurrence of a refractory period or mediator release. Wilson, Barnes, Vickers, and Silverman (1982) found a refractory period in approximately 60% of the subjects after hyperventilation-induced bronchoconstriction. These investigators postulated that mast-cell release might be involved in respiratory heat exchange, besides other possible mechanisms like a parasympathetic reflex action. Cromoglycate was found to have a partial protective effect. Latimer, O'Byrne, Morris, Roberts, and Hargreave (1983) suggested that mast cells have some role in bronchoconstriction, stimulated by airway cooling. Nagakura, Lee, Denison, Newman-Tayler, and Kay (1983) tried to find direct evidence in the occurrence of mast cell release by the measurement of NCF-A, a mast-cell mediator. They found a peak of NCF-A after exercise with cold, dry air and not with warm, humid air. However, they found no rise in NCF-A after hyperventilation. These investigators concluded that mediator release from mast cells was related to the combined stimuli of respiratory heat loss and exercise and not after heat loss alone.

A change in receptor activity is a theoretical possibility by which cold air may change airway reactivity, based on animal studies (Kunos & Szentivanyi, 1968). The relevance under physiological conditions is unknown.

Sensitivity of bronchial smooth muscle to a decrease in temperature has been observed in vitro. Souhrada, Prestley, and Souhrada (1983) found that trachea strips from guinea pigs contracted after cooling in the range from 20 to 22°C, progressively. The Na^+K^+-ATPase enzyme of airway's smooth muscle, which is found to be increased in reactive bronchi, is sensitive to temperature changes. The eventual effect of cooling on the smooth-muscle contraction might be mediated by this enzyme (Souhrada & Souhrada, 1982). The degree of cold-induced contraction appeared to be dependent on the presence of histamine (Kolbeck, Chandhary, & Speir, 1983).

It will be clear that both the point where cooling and drying of the airways triggers the bronchoconstrictive mechanism and the components of the mechanism are far from resolved.

Differences Between Bronchial Reactions After Inhalation of Cold Air and Exercise

Although the respiratory heat loss is widely considered to be important in exercise-induced bronchial obstruction, differences between the bronchial reaction after cold air and exercise are reported. When patients inspired air, conditioned to body temperature and fully saturated with water vapor, bronchial obstruction after exercise was significantly reduced. However, half of the patients still had a weak obstruction following exercise which had induced no significant loss of heat or water (Anderson & Schaeffel, 1982). This indicates that also in the absence of respiratory heat loss, exercise can induce bronchial obstruction.

Hyperventilation of cold air does not seem to be associated with release of mediators like NCF, a phase of bronchodilatation and, in some patients, a refractory period. Thus, the role of the mast cells in exercise-induced bronchial obstruction is highly suggestive, in contrast to its role in bronchial obstruction after airway cooling. Parasympatholytic agents may block exercise-induced bronchoconstriction partially, while these agents are not clearly effective in reactions due to heat and water loss.

The Current Scheme of the Mechanism in EIB

Based upon present knowledge, the following scheme of exercise-induced bronchial obstruction can be constructed. Exercise produces respiratory heat loss, as well as another effect, probably mast-cell release. Respiratory heat loss induces bronchial obstruction, probably mediated by a direct effect upon the smooth muscles or other structures, that is, vascular or neurogenic responses. Activation of mediator release from mast cells in exercise reactions seems highly independent of cooling, but the trigger involved is unknown.

Godfrey and coworkers (Ben-Dov, Bar-Yiskay, & Godfrey, 1982) have proposed that a centrally located temperature-dependent area in the bronchi generates reflexes, whereas a more peripheral area induces mediator release. That the precise interaction of the various components differs among patients is highly probable.

The biological significance of the occurrence of bronchospasm in reaction to exercise or inhaled cold dry air may be protection of the lung against excessive heat and water loss. An increase in airway resistance will decrease ventilation and, hence, thermal demands. Why asthmatics respond more intensely than healthy individuals is a mystery and may represent the heightened airway reactivity of the disease. The part of the bronchial mechanism which is responsible for an exaggerated reaction is not known. Information about this regulation abnormality would be highly important in order to make it possible to prevent exercise-induced bronchial obstruction.

Practical Consequences

Exercise can benefit most children, including those with exercise-induced bronchoconstriction. One has to recognize children with other lung diseases or different disturbances by clinical examination and appropriate exercise tests because they may be at risk for serious complications. Physical education should be tailored to allow children of all physical conditions to reach their maximum potential.

The following action can be taken at this moment to combat exercise-induced bronchial obstruction. Based on the information of the respiratory heat exchange mechanism, the patient should try to respire through the nose. The gymnastic rooms should have an atmosphere with an optimal temperature and humidity.

An asthmatic patient should be advised to increase his or her speed gradually in order to run through an exercise-induced bronchial obstruction. A pronounced bronchial obstruction will not develop and a refractory situation is created in which intense exercise is permitted without generation of an obstructive response.

Asthmatics have a greater chance of success in certain sports than in others. Swimming, wrestling, sprinting, and team sports where running is of short duration are often well tolerated. Cold weather sports, however, are occasionally more difficult with which to cope for asthmatics than for healthy children. Downhill skiing can often be done very well. Activities with warm and moist air (swimming) are generally acceptable for asthmatics. Proper medication, such as cromoglycate or beta-sympathomimetics, taken prophylactically should allow most children with asthma to participate in nearly all sporting events.

References

ANDERSON, S.D., Conolly, N.M., & Godfrey, S. (1971). Comparison of bronchoconstriction induced by cycling and running. *Thorax,* **27,** 718-725.

ANDERSON, S.D., Silverman, M., König, P., & Godfrey, S. (1975). Exercise-induced asthma—A review. *British Journal of Diseases of the Chest,* **69,** 1-38.

ANDERSON, S.D., Schoeffel, R.E., Follet, R., Percy, C.P., Daviskas, E., & Kendall, M. (1982). Sensitivity to heat and water loss at rest and during exercise in asthmatic patients. *European Journal of Respiratory Diseases,* **63,** 459-471.

ANDERSON, S.D., & Schoeffel, R.E. (1982). Respiratory heat and water loss during exercise in patients with asthma. *European Journal of Respiratory Diseases,* **63,** 472-480.

BEN-DOV, I., Bar-Yishay, E., & Godfrey, S. (1982). Refractory period after exercise-induced asthma, unexplained by respiratory heat loss. *American Review of Respiratory Diseases,* **125,** 530-534.

BAR-OR, O., Neuman, I., & Dotan, R. (1977). Effects of dry and humid climates on exercise-induced asthma in children and preadolescents. *Journal of Allergy and Clinical Immunology,* **60,** 163-168.

DEAL, Jr., E.C., McFadden, Jr., E.R., Ingram, Jr., R.H., & Jaeger, J.J. (1979). Esophageal temperature during exercise in asthmatic and non-asthmatic subjects. *Journal of Applied Physiology,* **46,** 484-490.

DEAL, Jr., E.C., McFadden, Jr., E.R., Ingram, Jr., R.H., Breslin, F.J., & Jaeger, J.J. (1980). Airway responsiveness to cold air and hyperpnea in normal subjects and those with hay fever and asthma. *American Review of Respiratory Diseases,* **121,** 621-628.

EDMUNDS, A.T., Tooley, M., & Godfrey, S. (1978). The refractory period after exercise-induced asthma, its duration and relation to the severity of exercise. *American Review of Respiratory Diseases,* **177,** 247-254.

FANTA, C.H., Ingram, Jr., R.H., & McFadden, Jr., E.R. (1980). A reassessment of the effects of oropharyngeal anaesthesia in exercise-induced asthma. *American Review of Respiratory Diseases,* **122.** 381-386.

GODFREY, S. (1974). *Exercise testing in children.* London: Saunders Co. Ltd.

GODFREY, S., & König, P. (1976). Inhibition of exercise-induced asthma by different pharmacological pathways. *Thorax,* **31,** 137-143.

GOLD, W.M., Meijers, G.L., Dain, D.S., & Miller, R.L. (1977). Changes in airway mast cells and histamine. *Journal of Applied Physiology,* **43** 271-275.

GRIFFIN, M.P., Fung, K.F., Ingram, Jr., R.H., & McFadden, Jr., E.R. (1982). Dose-response effects of atropine on thermal stimulus-response relationship in asthma. *Journal of Applied Physiology,* **53,** 1576-1582.

JAMES, L., Faciane, J., & Sly, R.M. (1976). Effects of treadmill exercise on asthmatic children. *Journal of Allergy and Clinical Immunology,* **57,** 408-416.

JOSENHANS, W.T., Melville, G.H., & Ulmer, W.T. (1979). The effect of facial cold stimulation on airways conductance in healthy men. *Canadian Journal of Physiology and Pharmacology,* **47,** 453-457.

KAY, A.B., & Lee, T.H. (1982). Neutrophil chemotactic factor of anaphylaxis. *Journal of Allergy and Clinical Immunology,* **70,** 319-320.

KOLBECK, R.C., Chaudhary, R.A., & Speir, W.A. (1983). Effects of PGE_2, $PGF_2\backslash\backslash$, TXB_2 and histamine on tracheal smooth muscle response to thermal change. *American Review of Respiratory Diseases (abstract).*

KUNOS, G., & Sentivanyi, M. (1968). Evidence favouring the existence of a single adrenergic receptor. *Nature,* **217,** 1077-1078.

LATIMER, K.M., O'Byrne, P.M., Morris, M.M., Roberts, R., & Hargreave, F.E. (1983). Bronchoconstriction stimulated by airway cooling. Better protection with combined inhalation of terbutaline sulphate and cromolyn sodium than with either alone. *American Review of Respiratory Diseases,* **128,** 440-443.

McFADDEN, Jr., E.R., Ingram, Jr., R.H., Haynes, R.H., & Wellman, J. (1977). Predominant site of flow-limitation and mechanisms of post-exertional asthma. *Journal of Applied Physiology,* **42,** 746-742.

McFADDEN, Jr., E.R., & Ingram, Jr., R.H. (1979). Exercise-induced asthma, observations on the initiating stimulus. *New England Journal of Medicine,* **301,** 763-769.

MILLER, G.J., Davies, B.H., Cole, T.J., & Seaton, A. (1975). A comparison of the bronchial response to running and cycling in asthma using an improved definition of the response to work. *Thorax,* **30,** 306-311.

NAGAKURA, T., Lee, T.H., Denison, D.M., Newman-Tayler, A.J., & Kay, A.B. (in press). Neutrophil chemotactic factor in exercise- and hyperventilation-induced asthma. *Thorax.*

NEIJENS, H.J., Wesselius, T.R., & Kerrebijn, K.F. (1981). Exercise-induced bronchoconstriction as an expression of bronchial hyperreactivity: A study of its mechanisms in children. *Thorax,* **36,** 517-522.

NEIJENS, H.J., Gargani, G., van Kralingen, A., Weezepoel, H., & Kerrebijn, K.F. (1981). The site of maximal flow-limitation in exercise-induced bronchoconstriction. *Progress in Respiration Research,* **17,** 80-86.

PATEL, K.R., & Kerr, J.W. (1975). Alpha-receptor blocking drugs in bronchial asthma. *Lancet,* **i,** 348-349.

SHEPPARD, D., Epstein, J., Holtzman, J., Nadel, J.A., & Boushey, H.A. (1982). Dose-dependent inhibition of cold air-induced bronchoconstriction by atropine. *Journal of Applied Physiology,* **53,** 169-174.

SHTURMANN-ELLSTEIN, R., Zeballos, R.J., Buckely, J.M., & Souhrada, J.F. (1978). The beneficial effect of nasal breathing on exercise-induced bronchoconstriction. *American Review of Respiratory Diseases,* **118**, 65-73.

SILVERMAN, M., Anderson, S.D., & Walker, S.R. (1972). Metabolic changes preceding exercise-induced bronchoconstriction. *British Medical Journal,* **1**, 207-209.

SILVERMAN, M., Conolly, N.M., Balfour-Lynn, L., & Godfrey, S. (1972). Longterm trial of disodium cromoglycate and isoprenaline in children with asthma. *British Medical Journal,* **3**, 378-381.

SILVERMAN, S., & Anderson, S.D. (1972). Standardization of exercise-tests in asthmatic children. *Archives of Diseases in Childhood,* **47**, 882-889.

SOUHRADA, J.F., & Souhrada, M. (1983). Significance of the sodium pump for airway smooth muscle. *European Journal of Respiratory Diseases,* **64** (suppl.), 196-205.

SOUHRADA, J.F., Prestley, P., & Souhrada, M. (1983). Effects of quick cooling and warming on airway smooth muscle. *American Review of Respiratory Diseases,* **127**(4), 229. (abstract)

STRAUSS, R.H., Haynes, R.L., Ingram, Jr., R.H., & McFadden, Jr., E.R. (1977). Comparison of arm versus leg work in induction of acute episodes of asthma. *Journal of Applied Physiology,* **42**, 565-570.

STRAUSS, R.H., Ingram, Jr., R.H., & McFadden, Jr., E.R. (1977). A critical assessment of the role of circulating hydrogen ion and lactate in the production of exercise-induced asthma. *Journal of Clinical Investigation,* **60**, 658-664.

THOMSON, N.C., Patel, K.R., & Kerr, J.W. (1978). Sodium cromoglycate and ipratropium bromide in exercise-induced asthma. *Thorax,* **33**, 694-699.

WASSERMAN, K. (1978). Breathing during exercise. *New England Journal of Medicine,* **298**, 780-785.

WEINSTEIN, R.E., Anderson, J.A., Kvale, P., & Sweet, L.C. (1976). Effect of humidification on exercise-induced asthma. *Journal of Allergy and Clinical Immunology,* **57**, 250-251.

WELLS, R.E., Walker, J.E.C., & Hickler, R.B. (1960). Effects of cold air on respiratory airflow resistance in patients with respiratory disease. *New England Journal of Medicine,* **263**, 268-273.

WILSON, N.M., Barnes, P.J., Vickers, H., & Silverman, M. (1982). Hyperventilation-induced asthma; evidence for two mechanisms. *Thorax,* **37**, 657-662.

ZEBALLOS, R.J., Shturman-Ellstein, R., McNally, Jr., J.F., Hirsch, J.E., & Souhrada, J.F. (1978). The role of hyperventilation in exercise-induced bronchoconstriction. *American Review of Respiratory Diseases,* **118**, 877-884.

Exercise in Postoperative Tricuspid Atresia

Hans U. Wessel, Ronald L. Stout, and Milton H. Paul
The Children's Memorial Hospital, Chicago, Illinois, U.S.A.

It has been well established in human subjects that the time course of the $\dot{V}O_2$ in response to a step input of light to moderate work at a constant rate can be fitted to a single exponential such that

$$\Delta \dot{V}O_2(t) = \Delta \dot{V}O_2(ss)[1 - e^{-t/\tau}] \qquad (1)$$

where $\Delta \dot{V}O_2(t)$ is the $\dot{V}O_2$ increment at time t above baseline $\dot{V}O_2$, $\Delta \dot{V}O_2(ss)$ the steady-state increment, and τ the time constant of the exponential (Margaria, Mangila, Cuttica, & Cerretelli, 1965; Whipp, 1971).

In normal subjects, alveolar ventilation and cardiac output respond much faster to a step input of light to moderate work than $\dot{V}O_2$ (Cerretelli, Sikand, & Farhi, 1964). These rate differences suggest that neither cardiac output nor ventilation normally limit the $\dot{V}O_2$ on-response below the anaerobic threshold, and that under these conditions, τ of Equation 1 is independent of work rate (WR). However, heart disease could conceivably result in significant slowing of exercise $\dot{V}O_2$ kinetics. Therefore, exercise kinetics of ventilation ($\dot{V}_I$, $\dot{V}_E$), pulmonary gas exchange ($\dot{V}O_2$ and $\dot{V}CO_2$), and heart rate (HR) were studied in 14 patients with severely impaired right ventricular function. There were 10 males (mean age 15.6 years, range 6 to 21 years) and 4 females (mean age 17.3 years, range 13 to 19 years). Ten had tricuspid atresia and 4 others had functionally similar complex congenital cardiac defects. Ten had been surgically corrected by a Fontan procedure (Fontan & Baudet, 1971). Following this operation, systemic venous blood enters the pulmonary circulation either via a conduit from the right atrium to the main pulmonary artery or by two separate conduits from the superior vena cava to the right lung and from the inferior vena cava to the left lung.

Methods

Work Protocols

All work was done on a cycle ergometer (Quinton, Model 840), either nonsteady state work with 16.4 W increments of 60-s duration to the end of tolerance (11 studies), or steady state work of 4 min duration at rates varying from 0.27 to 1.33 W/Kg body weight (6 studies). Two patients performed both types of studies. The laboratory was maintained at 20°C and 40 to 50° relative humidity.

Measurements

Measurements began 3 min before and ended 4 min after exercise. Instantaneous heart rate (HR) was measured with a digital rate meter. Systemic blood pressure (BP) was measured intermittently at rest, during exercise, and at recovery with an automatic cuff system. A single lead bipolar ECG was monitored continuously.

Breath-by-breath (B-B) ventilation and pulmonary gas exchange were measured continuously with a computerized system (Wessel, Stout, & Paul, 1979). The patient breathes through a 42 ml deadspace, low-resistance, two-way valve. Inspiratory and expiratory flow rates are measured with separate pneumotachographs (Fleisch, #3), and fractional gas concentrations (O_2, CO_2, N_2, H_3, N_2O) are measured with a modified mass spectrometer (Perkin Elmer, Model 1140). The digitized data (200 samples/s/channel) are stored on disc for off-line analysis which yields permanent disc files of B-B and 1 min average data. The former characterize each breath in terms of gas flows, volumes, fractional concentrations, partial pressures, gas uptakes, rates of uptake, and respiratory timing events (50 variables). The latter contain 28 variables including HR and BP. To examine the HR response to a step input of work of 4 min duration, instantaneous HR and elapsed time at 5-s intervals were entered manually into separate disc files.

Data Analysis

Nonsteady State Work Protocol

Data analysis was based on 1-min average data. These were evaluated in terms of final WR (W/Kg), final $\dot{V}O_2$ (ml/min/Kg) and final HR. Final $\dot{V}O_2$ was related to the standards of Mocellin and Bastanier (1976) and final WR was expressed as percent of 3.4 W/Kg, the predicted average maximal work rate. Linear and exponential regressions were computed for regression of $\dot{V}_E$, $\dot{V}_A$, $\dot{V}O_2$, $\dot{V}CO_2$, and HR on WR and of $\dot{V}_E$, $\dot{V}_A$, and HR on $\dot{V}O_2$ and $\dot{V}CO_2$. Regression slopes were compared to standards developed in our laboratory from studies in 90 subjects (580 1-min averages) who were considered to have a normal ventilatory response to exercise as defined by a maximal end-tidal P_{CO_2} during submaximal exercise of $5.1 \leqslant P_{CO_2} \leqslant 5.5$ kPa.

Steady State Protocol

The time course of $\dot{V}O_2$, $\dot{V}CO_2$, $\dot{V}_I$, and the HR was evaluated by comparison with data obtained in 2 endurance-trained runners. Steady state increments represent the difference between the average of all breaths during the 4th min of exercise and the minute preceding exercise. All instantaneous B-B and HR values were expressed as a fraction of the steady state increment and plotted as a function of time. Time constant τ (see Equation 1) was estimated by superimposing a family of exponentials with τ varying from 30 to 90 s on the patient data.

Results

The maximal WR achieved was low in all patients (1.9 ± 0.4 W/Kg or 54 ± 13.5% of predicted). The final $\dot{V}O_2$ averaged only 20.7 ± 4.7 ml/min/Kg with a range from 11.1 to 25.1 ml/min/Kg or 24 to 56% of predicted maximal $\dot{V}O_2$.

Nonsteady State Work

In the tests with 16.4 W increments of 60 s duration, $\dot{V}O_2$ and $\dot{V}CO_2$ were uniformly low at all work rates even after normalization for body weight (W/Kg). In 9 of the 11 patients, the linear regression slope of $\dot{V}O_2$ and $\dot{V}CO_2$ on WR was > 3 S.E. below that of controls. Regression of ventilation ($\dot{V}_E$, $\dot{V}_E/Kg$, $\dot{V}_A$) on WR indicated an increased ventilatory response to exercise in 7 and a normal response in 4 patients. In the former group, $\dot{V}_E$ and $\dot{V}_A$ as a function of $\dot{V}O_2$ and $\dot{V}CO_2$, respectively, were markedly increased in all subjects, and end-tidal exercise PCO_2 was low (2.8 to 4.3 kPa). Ventilation relative to $\dot{V}O_2$ and $\dot{V}CO_2$ was also markedly increased in 3 of the 4 patients with normal ventilation relative to WR. There was only 1 patient with normal ventilation relative to both WR and gas exchange, and a normal end-tidal exercise PCO_2 (5.5 kPa).

Steady State Work

Of the 5 patients who completed work increments of 4-min duration (see Table 1), 3 had an increased and 2 a normal ventilatory response to exercise. In 4 of these pa-

Table 1

Time Constant τ of the Exponential Increase of Breath-by-Breath $\dot{V}O_2$, $\dot{V}CO_2$, $\dot{V}_I$, and of HR

# Subject	Age (Yrs)	Work Increment (W)	(W/Kg)	τ (s) $\dot{V}O_2$	$\dot{V}CO_2$	$\dot{V}_I$	HR
Moderate work							
1 runner	43	R- 98.0	1.63	30	45	50	< 30
2 runner	25	R- 89.8	1.50	30	45	45	< 30
3 TA	16	R- 65.4	0.99	30	40	45	< 30
4 TA	17	R- 65.4	1.32	30	40	35	< 30
	21	R- 65.4	1.33	40	65	75	35
5 TA	15	R- 49.0	0.82	30	35	40	< 30
6 TA	21	R- 16.3	0.27	40	50	55	—[a]
	21	16.3- 49.0	0.54	50	65	70	—[a]
Heavy work							
1 runner	43	98.0-196.1	1.63	50	50	60	50
7 TA	15	R- 81.7	1.33	50	45	60	50

Response to work increments of 4 min duration in endurance-trained runners and 5 tricuspid atresia (TA) patients.
R = rest.
[a]Absolute HR increase < 4 beats/min.

tients $\Delta\dot{V}CO_2(ss)$ was > 3 S.E. below the predicted value, and in 3 $_D\dot{V}O_2(ss)$ was low by the same criterion.

In all studies (see Table 1) the time course of $\dot{V}O_2$, $\dot{V}CO_2$, $\dot{V}_I$, and HR could be fitted to single exponentials (see Equation 1). For moderate WR increments below the anaerobic threshold, τ of $\dot{V}O_2(t)$ was 30 s in the 2 distance runners but also in 3 of the 5 tricuspid atresia (TA) patients. In each of these studies, work began from rest and τ of HR(t) was < 30 s (see Table 1 & Figure 1). In each study, τ of $\dot{V}CO_2(t)$ and $\dot{V}_I(t)$ was longer than the corresponding τ of $\dot{V}O_2(t)$, but the time constants for $\dot{V}CO_2(t)$ and $\dot{V}_I(t)$ were shorter in the tricuspid atresia (TA) patients than in the distance runners.

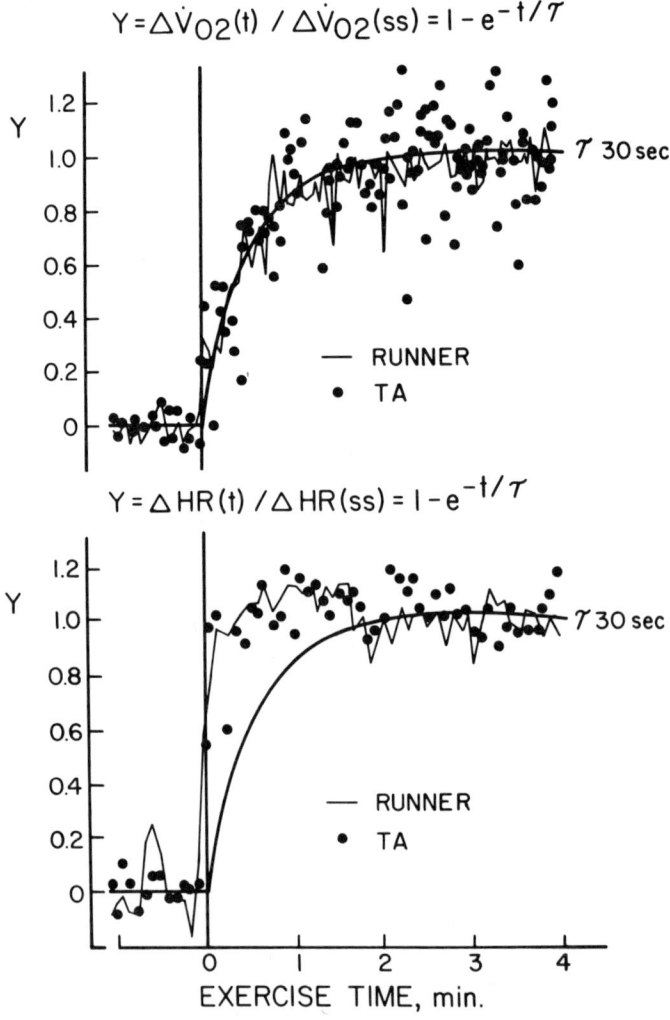

Figure 1—(a) Breath-by-breath $\dot{V}O_2$ response to step input of work at a constant rate (starting from rest) in an endurance-trained runner (89.9 W) and a patient with tricuspid atresia (TA, 49.0 W). Heavy line represents Equation 1 for τ of 30 s. (b) HR response during the same studies. Each data point represents instantaneous HR at 5 s intervals. See text.

Subject #4 (see Table 1) was studied twice at the same WR increment of 65.4 W, first at age 17 and again 4 years later. Note that τ of $\dot{V}O_2(t)$, $\dot{V}CO_2(t)$, and $\dot{V}_I(t)$ increased between the first and second study from 30, 40, and 35 s to 40, 65, and 75 s, respectively, while at the same time τ of the HR response increased from < 30 to 35 s. Similarly, for Subject #6, τ of $\dot{V}O_2(t)$ was 40 and 50 s for 2 WR increments, the first starting from rest and the second after 4 min of work at 16.3 W. In this patient the heart rate response to exercise was markedly reduced with steady increments of only 4 and 2 beats/min, respectively.

In one tricuspid atresia patient (Subject #7), a WR increment of 81.7 W represented heavy work above the anaerobic threshold. τ of $\dot{V}O_2(t)$ and HR(t) was 50 s, which was identical to the responses elicited in 1 of the distance runners (#1) for a WR increment from 98.0 to 196.1 W, which was also above the anaerobic threshold.

Discussion

There is general agreement that a step input of work elicits a monoexponential $\dot{V}O_2$ on-response as measured at the mouth. In human subjects, this response is task-specific (Cerretelli, Skindell, Pendergast, di Pampero, & Rennie, 1977) and has a time constant (τ) of approximately 45 s for upright leg work of moderate intensity. Although τ may be shortened by endurance training (Cerretelli, Pendergast, Panganelli, & Rennie, 1979), this effect appears to be independent of cardiovascular fitness since the cardiac output adjustments to exercise are normally considerably faster than the $\dot{V}O_2$ response. However, it has not been established if this response may be slowed by impaired cardiovascular fitness due to structural heart disease. Of subjects who are routinely exercised in our laboratory, tricuspid atresia (TA) patients represent the low end in a spectrum of cardiovascular fitness due to four factors: (a) an absent or diminutive right ventricle, (b) an often impaired HR response, (c) nonuniform distribution of pulmonary blood flow, and (d) lack of endurance training. Moreover, a reduced cardiac output response to recumbent leg exercise has been demonstrated in these patients (Shachar, Fuhrman, Wang, Lucas, & Lock, 1981). If slowing of the $\dot{V}O_2$ on-response due to reduced cardiovascular fitness occurs, it should be demonstrable in TA patients. Moreover, if such an effect exists, τ should be longer in TA patients than in endurance-trained subjects since this latter group represents the opposite end in the spectrum of cardiovascular fitness. For these reasons, the exercise kinetics of ventilation, gas exchange, and HR in TA patients were compared to endurance-trained distance runners.

In the TA patients, reduced cardiovascular fitness was manifested by reduced exercise tolerance, low final exercise $\dot{V}O_2$ of ≤ 25 ml/min/Kg, and low-anaerobic thresholds. The latter was reached at the first 16.4 W WR step in two patients who were incapable of any HR increase with exercise. The low $\dot{V}O_2$ relative to work rate found in all TA patients during the work test with small increments of short duration is consistent with a reduced cardiac output response. Equation 1 suggests that the linear regression slope of $\dot{V}O_2$ on WR is highly sensitive to an increase of τ if the WR increments are of short duration. In this study, these slopes averaged 0.19 ± 0.05 ml $\dot{V}O_2$/W and were significantly different ($p < .005$) from the slope of controls (0.27 ml $\dot{V}O_2$/W; SE 0.004; r = 0.938). Assuming a constant τ over the work rates tested and a normal $\Delta\dot{V}O_2(ss)$ of approximately 0.34 ml $\dot{V}O_2$/W, these slope differences translate into an increase of τ from approximately 40 s in controls to 80 s in TA patients. It is also apparent from Equation 1 that this change of τ could not measurably alter the slope of $\dot{V}O_2$ on WR for increments of 4 min duration or more. Both the low $\dot{V}O_2$ at all work rates and the low-anaerobic threshold in TA patients suggest that intramuscular O_2 delivery is inadequate to eliminate all anaerobic metabolites even at low-work rates. However, τ computed from $\Delta\dot{V}O_2(t)$ measured at the mouth is probably a considerable overestimate of τ for $\Delta\dot{V}O_2(t)$ of the working muscles since in TA patients the relative contribution of $\dot{V}O_2$ from venous and tissue O_2 stores to the overall $\dot{V}O_2$ of working muscles must be much greater than in normals.

The TA patients who completed WR increments of 4 min duration were considered the most active physically among the group. However, even these 5 patients had a reduced exercise tolerance, and none was able to complete a second 4-min increment of work at twice the WR shown in Table 1. Therefore, a longer τ of $\dot{V}O_2(t)$ than in the distance runners was expected. However, this was not the case. Even though the number of patients was small, the data suggest a similar pattern of $\dot{V}O_2$ kinetics in the TA patients and distance runners as WR is increased from moderate to heavy work. In both groups, $\dot{V}O_2$ and HR kinetics appeared to be closely linked, suggesting that the cardiac output response to a step input of work limits the speed of the $\dot{V}O_2$ on-response. At low-work rates below the anaerobic threshold, τ of $\dot{V}O_2(t)$ had a minimal value of approximately 30 s in all instances where the HR kinetics were extremely fast (see Figure 1 & Table 1). However, even at these low-work rates, τ of $\dot{V}O_2(t)$ increased when τ of HR(t) was either increased (see Table 1, Subject #4) or the absolute HR change was negligible (Subject #6). In the two studies at heavy work rates (Subjects #1, #7) $\dot{V}O_2$ and HR kinetics appeared similarly linked.

It was speculated from these data that in a given individual $\dot{V}O_2$ kinetics as measured at the mouth are independent of WR only over a narrow range which may, however, include all work rates below the anaerobic threshold as has been suggested by Whipp and Mahler (1980). As work rates are increased further, there is a progressive slowing of the cardiac output response. The $\dot{V}O_2$ kinetics of endurance-trained subjects differ from that of patients with compromised cardiac function (such as the TA patients in this study) only in that the sequence of changes occurs over a wider range of work rates. This suggests that $\dot{V}O_2$ kinetics may be independent of cardiovascular fitness only if WR is expressed as a percent of the WR which elicits maximal slowing of $\dot{V}O_2$ kinetics.

References

CERRETELLI, P., Pendergast, D., Paganelli, W.C., & Rennie, D.W. (1979). Effects of specific muscle training on VO_2 on-response and early blood lactate. *Journal of Applied Physiology: Respiratory, Environmental and Exercise Physiology, 47*, 761-769.

CERRETELLI, P., Sikand, R., & Farhi, L.E. (1964). Readjustments of cardiac output and gas exchange during onset of exercise and recovery. *Journal of Applied Physiology, 21*, 1345-1350.

CERRETELLI, P., Skindell, D., Pendergast, D.P., di Pampero, P.E., & Rennie, D.W. (1977). Oxygen uptake transients at the onset and offset of arm and leg work. *Respiration Physiology, 30*, 81-97.

FONTAN, F., & Baudet, E. (1971). Surgical repair of tricuspid atresia. *Thorax, 26*, 240-248.

MARGARIA, R., Mangila, F., Cuttica, F., & Cerretelli, P. (1965). The kinetics of oxygen consumption at the onset of muscular exercise in man. *Ergonomics, 8,* 49-54.

MOCELLIN, R., & Bastanier, C.K. (1976). Fur Frage Der Zuverlässigkeit der W_{170} als Mass der körperlichen Leistungsfähigkeit bei der Beurteilung von Kindern mit Herzkrankheiten. *European Journal of Pediatrics,* **122**, 223-239.

SHACHAR, G.B., Fuhrman, B.P., Wang, Y., Lucas, R.U., & Lock, J.F. (1981). Rest and exercise hemodynamics after Fontan procedure. *American Journal of Cardiology,* **47**(2), 432 (abstract).

WESSEL, H.U., Stout, R.L., & Paul, M.H. (1979). Minicomputer based system for breath-by-breath analysis of ventilation and pulmonary exchange. In J.R. Lox & P.G. Hugenholz (Eds.), *Proceedings of the 5th Annual Conference of Computers in Cardiology.* New York: IEEE Computer Society.

WHIPP, B.J. (1971). The rate constant for the kinetics of oxygen uptake during light exercise. *Journal of Applied Physiology,* **30**, 261-263.

WHIPP, B.J., & Mahler, M. (1980). Dynamics of pulmonary gas exchange during exercise. In J.B. West (Ed.). *Pulmonary gas exchange, Vol. II, Organism and environment.* New York: Academic Press.

Spiroergometric Criteria of Patients With Idiopathic Scoliosis: A Long-Term Study

Hans Stoboy and Bärbel Speierer-Kharazi
Orthopädische Klinik und Poliklinik der Freien Universität,
Berlin, Federal Republic of Germany

The most important consequence of major scoliotic chest deformity is cardiopulmonary insufficiency (Bergofsky, 1979). Lung volumes and capacities, especially vital capacity (FVC), are the best and most highly investigated parameters of decreased pulmonary function. Reduced vital capacity is negatively correlated with the Cobb angle (Meister, 1980). Maximum voluntary ventilation (MVV) may be decreased from 50 to 80% (Meister, 1980; Ogliati, Levine, Smith, Briscoe, & King, 1982; Stoboy, 1978; Westgate & Moe, 1969).

These changes are mainly due to pulmonary restriction. The aim of Harrington rod surgery is to maintain respiratory function at presurgical values (Bergofsky, 1979; Meister, 1980; Scheier, 1967). Bergofsky (1979) states that a critical Cobb angle of 70° and more increases the risk of respiratory failure and facilitates the development of pulmonary hypertension. Nilsonne and Lundgreen (1968) found a mean expectancy of 46.4 years in untreated scoliotic patients. Haber, Kummer, Lukschitsch, and Derda (1982) investigated lung function and spiroergometric parameters in untreated young patients with idiopathic scoliosis, applying factor analyses to their data. They found no cause-and-effect relationship between the degree of scoliosis and the results obtained with pulmonary function and spiroergometric tests. Reduced aerobic capacity is not due to scoliosis but to sedentary life habits. The latter leads to impairment of respiration, circulation, and aerobic metabolism.

Kafer (1975) observed that correction of scoliosis fails to yield long-term functional improvement. Shneerson and Edgar (1979) point out that no information is available concerning the long term effect upon respiratory function after spinal fusion.

Lindh and Bjure (1975), who assessed lung volumes and capacities over a period of 3 years, found significant increases in static volumes. In a follow-up study extending over a period of 4 to 5 years, Meister (1980) noted a significant improvement in volumes and capacities, accompanied by an increase of $P_A O_2$.

The aim of this investigation was to measure spirometric and ergometric parameters over a period of 5 years with special reference to values obtained for patients with moderate and severe scoliosis and to investigate the changes in these values in both groups.

Material and Methods

Patients with idiopathic scoliosis (m = 62) between 10 and 21 years of age underwent Harrington rod surgery and spinal fusion. Patients were divided into two groups according to the severity of the impairment. Group A consisted of subjects with Cobb angle <70° (39 to 68°), n = 47; Group B >70° (70 to 102°), n = 15. After surgery, median angles were 27° and 45°, respectively. Four weeks prior to surgery, the patients underwent endurance training and spinal mobilization therapy. All of them remained under clinical observation for a period of 14 months. A strict regimen of casts and braces was maintained including breathing therapy as well as strength and endurance training (Stoboy, 1978).

Standard spirographic investigations were carried out at the time of admission and at annual intervals following surgery. Spiroergometric values were assessed on a bicycle at 0.5, 1.0 W/kg and at maximum work loads. Drop-out rate was extremely high, mainly due to changes of residence, influence of an overprotective family or physicians, and at times, to disinterest. In the fifth year after surgery, Group A consisted of 11 and Group B of 7 patients.

Statistical calculations were performed using the Wilcoxon-paired nonparametric test and the Mann-Whitney U-test for unpaired observations.

Results

The physical characteristics of the patients (noncorrected values) are shown in Tables 1 and 2. Changes of height, weight, body-surface, and Cobb angle (lateral deviation of the spine) are provided in detail.

Table 1

Physical Characteristics of the Patients (noncorrected values)

Total	0		2 Years	
	<70	>70	<70	>70
Body Height (cm)				
N	47	15	35**	15*
$\overline{X}$	161.0	156.0	168.0	161.0
$P_{25} - P_{75}$	153.0 - 168.0	150.0 - 162.0	165.0 - 174.0	160.0 - 169.0
Body Weight (kg)				
N	43	15	35**	15*
$\overline{X}$	51.0	46.0	55.0	55.0
$P_{25} - P_{75}$	43.0 - 55.0	36.0 - 53.0	50.0 - 64.0	52.0 - 60.0
Body Surface (m²)				
N	43	15	35**	15*
$\overline{X}$	1.51	1.40	1.64	1.57
$P_{25} - P_{75}$	1.39 - 1.60	1.25 - 1.56	1.52 - 1.73	1.50 - 1.63

*P = .01 ≤.05
**P = .001 ≤.01

Table 2

Physical Characteristics of the Patients (noncorrected values)

	< Cobb Total			Total
	<70°	>70°		<70° - >70°
Preop.				
N	46	15		
X	52.0	85.0	Preop.	P <.0001
$P_{25} - P_{75}$	46.0 - 60.0	73.0 - 94.0		
Postop.				
N	41***	15***		
X	27.0	45.0	Postop.	P <.0001
$P_{25} - P_{75}$	22.5 - 34.5	40.0 - 55.0		

***P <.0001

In both groups, vital capacity (FVC) increased significantly during the period between admission and the second year of observation ($p \leq .05$ and $\leq .01$), respectively. Thereafter, values remained approximately constant until the end of the 5-year observation period (see Figure 1). In Group A, FVC was definitely larger than in Group B at admission as well as after 2 years. Values ranged from approximately 60% to 80% of reference values (normal range of values).

FEV_1 expressed in % FVC, fluctuated between 75% and 84% of normal values during the period of observation. Maximum voluntary ventilation (MVV) was significantly and continually enhanced until the fifth year ($p \leq .001$ and $\leq .05$), respectively (see Figure 2). After the second year, MVV was significantly larger in Group A ($p \leq .05$). Values were approximately 40 to 50% less than reference values at time of admission, and the 5-year values were only 10% less than the reference values.

Maximum work load (W) increased continually in Group A (see Figure 3), from 120 to 160 W ($p \leq .005$). In Group B, the increase took place until the second year ($p \leq .05$) from 115.5 to 140 W ($p \leq .005$). However, there were no statistically significant differences between the two groups.

At the time of admission, heart rates (HR) at rest were considerably above normal (102 to 105/min). Decreases were noted only in Group A. First and final values were definitely smaller in Group A (87/min, $p \leq .05$) than in Group B ($p \leq .05$).

In Group A, maximum HR remained constant at 186/min. In Group B it increased slightly at first, then markedly to 198/min, the last values for Group A were significantly smaller than those in Group B ($p \leq .01$).

In Group A, minute volume of ventilation ($\dot{V}$) at rest decreased from 11 l min^{-1} to 9 l min^{-1} ($p \leq .05$). In Group B, a decline was followed by a moderate increase. Final values were distinctly smaller than at the time of admission ($p \leq .05$).

In Group A, rates of respiration at rest (BF) decreased continually from 21 to 14/min ($p \leq .001$). In Group B, no significant changes were observed.

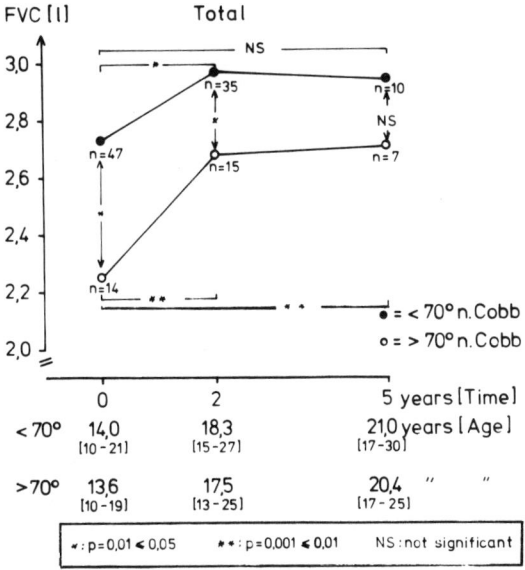

Figure 1—Changes of FVC in Groups A and B during the observation period (O = admission; Total = Totality of patients under investigation).

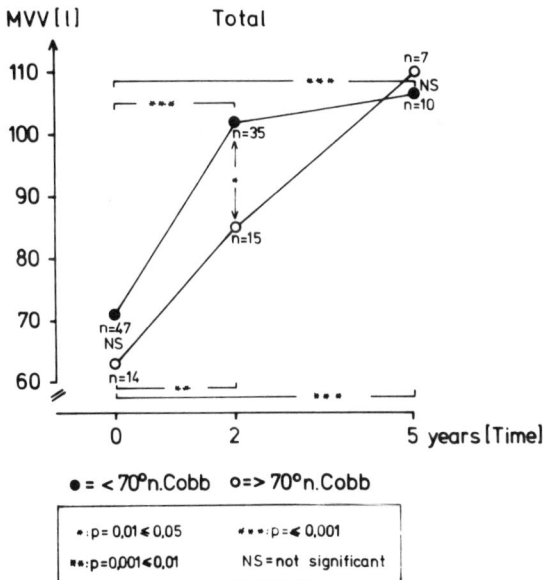

Figure 2—Changes of maximal voluntary ventilation during the period of observation.

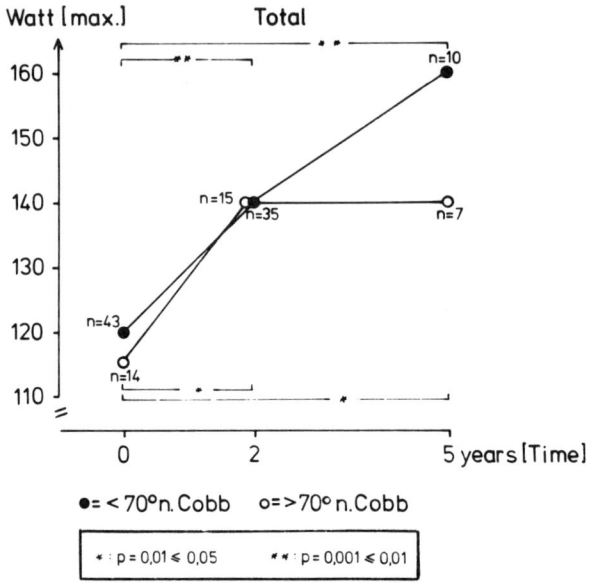

Figure 3—Changes of maximum work load during the observation period.

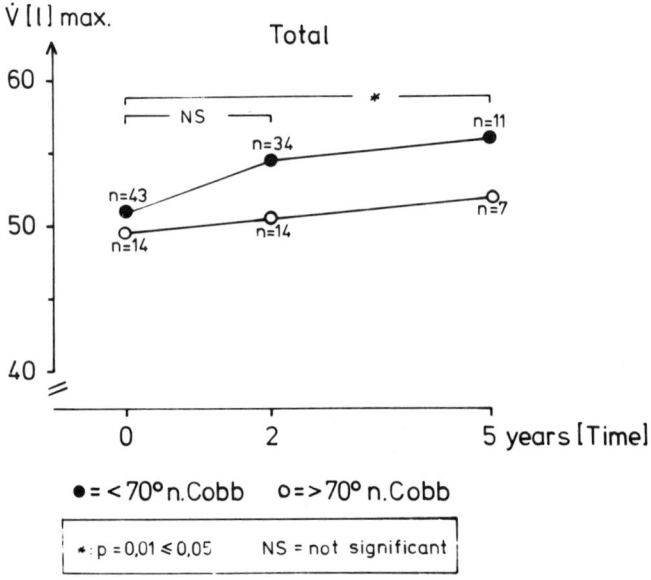

Figure 4—Changes of minute volume of ventilation during the observation period.

In Group A, the minute volume of respiration during maximum work load ($\dot{V}$ max) increased significantly from 51 to 56 l min^{-1} ($p \leq .05$), (see Figure 4). In Group B, no significant changes occurred. Minimal and maximal values (V) were approximately 40% and 30% below reference values, respectively.

Breathing frequencies at maximum work load (BF max) did not change significantly (39 & 36/min).

Maximum O_2-uptake ($\dot{V}O_2$ max) increased significantly in Group A ($\cong$ 1600 to 2100 ml•min^{-1}), (see Figure 5). In Group B enhancements of approximately 300 ml were noted until the second year. No statistically different values between the two groups were obtained. Maximal and minimal values were approximately 40 to 30% less than reference (normal) values.

In Group A, $\dot{V}O_2$ max•min^{-1}/m$_2$ body surface was significantly enhanced until the end of the second year (1100 to 1200 ml•min^{-1}/m$_2$), thereafter, values remained unchanged. In Group B, $\dot{V}O_2$ max•min^{-1}/m$_2$ values fluctuated. There were no statistically significant differences between Groups A and B.

In Group A, maximum O_2-pulse values increased (see Figure 6) until the end of the second year from 9 to 10.8 ($p\leq.05$). In Group B, values remained nearly constant ($\approx$ 8.5).

In Group A, O_2-pulse values were larger at the end of the fifth year ($p\leq.05$). Smallest and highest values were approximately 50 and 40% less, respectively, than those of the normal reference sample.

In both groups, ventilatory equivalent measurements ($\dot{V}_EO_2$) at rest declined until the end of the second year, by 8.5 and 6, respectively ($p\leq.01$ and $\leq.05$). Minimal $\dot{V}_EO_2$ values at maximum work load declined significantly in both groups by 4 and 5 ($p\leq.005$ and $\leq.05$), respectively. A small increase was noted after the end of the second year continuing until the end of the fifth year (see Figure 7). In Group A, final values still remained below admission values ($p\leq.05$). No significant differences were

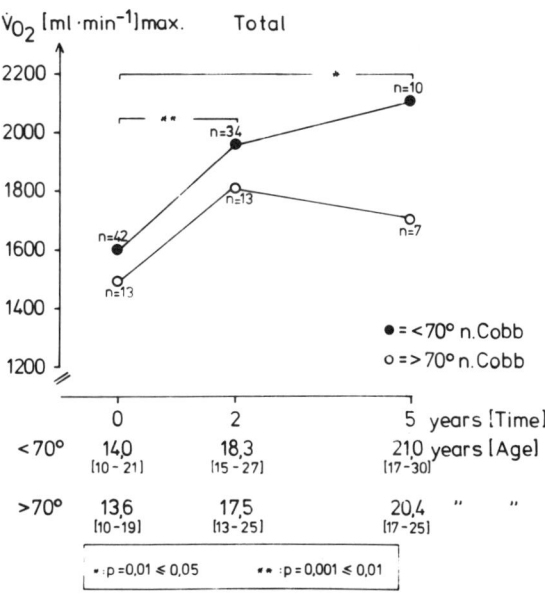

Figure 5—Changes of maximal O_2 uptake during the period of observation.

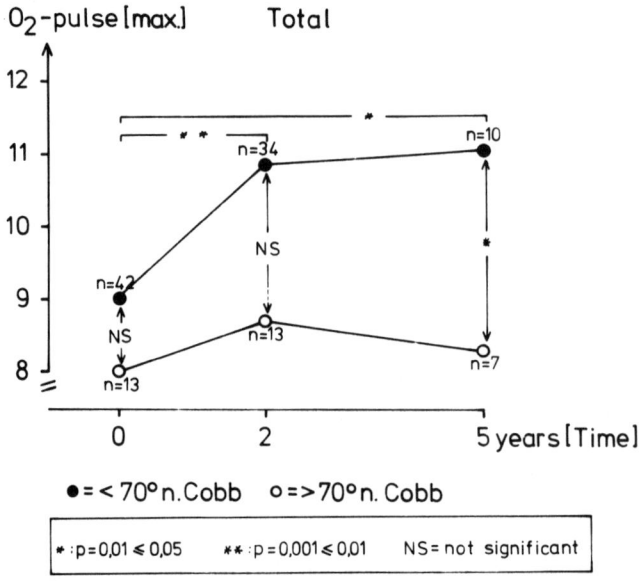

Figure 6—Changes of maximal O_2 pulse during the period of observation.

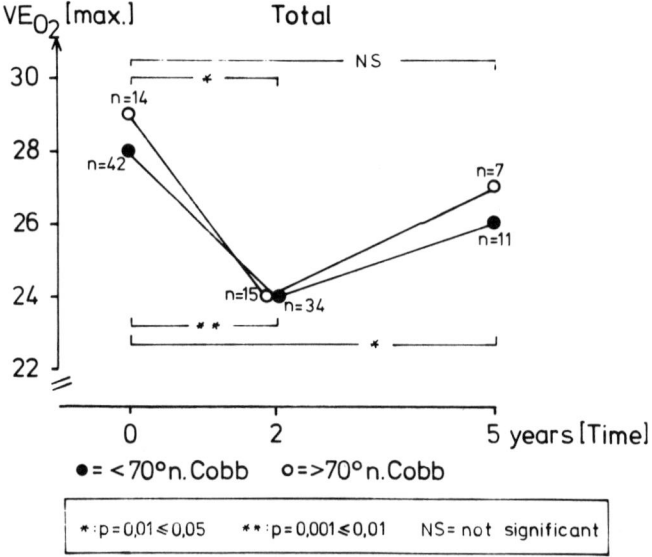

Figure 7—Changes of minimal ventilatory equivalent at maximum work load.

found between the two groups. Smallest and largest values lagged behind the normal reference values by 40 to 50%.

Discussion

Due to the fact that in the present study, larger numbers of patients were examined, FVC and FEV_1 values showed a more marked trend than had previously been obtained (Stoboy, 1978). These findings correspond to those reported by Meznik, Koller, and Kummer (1972); Lindh and Bjure (1975); and Meister (1980). The FEV_1/FVC ratios were within normal ranges.

MVV values which at the time of admission were definitely low, rose markedly and ascended toward normal ranges. By contrast, Shneerson and Edgar (1979) and Shneerson (1980) found MVV values within normal ranges. They were not enhanced after spinal fusion. The differences may have been due to the small sample (n = 10), to the short time of observation (17 to 23 months) and to the different rehabilitative regime in previous researches. According to Bergofsky (1979), dyspnea or hyperventilation is a leading symptom in scoliosis resulting in a breathing pattern distinguished by small tidal volumes and high-breathing frequencies (Meister, 1980).

In scoliotic patients, work expenditure with breathing is extremely high. Values vary with the square or tidal volume (Bergofsky 1979). At admission $\dot{V}$ and BF at rest were far above reference values. $\dot{V}_E O_2$ revealed a distinct uneconomical ventilation pattern. These findings corresponded to the increased work expenditure with respiration and the diminished alveolar ventilation. The pattern of breathing was advanced with respect to energy production, even though total ventilation had to be incremented (Meister, 1980).

In Group A, BF, $\dot{V}_E O_2$, and HR at rest decreased until the end of the second year, an observation suggesting improved alveolar ventilation and enhanced cardiac function.

In Group A, HR at maximum work load corresponded to reference values. In Group B, values increased during the entire observation period. Shneerson (1980) referred to this observation as "true exercise tachycardia." In contrast to Shneerson's interpretation these findings were not explained by increases in body weight. In this sample, body weights remained fairly constant between the end of the second year until the end of the fifth year.

In Group A, V max, $\dot{V}O_2$ max, $\dot{V}O_2$ max•min^{-1} and O_2 pulse values rose until the second year corresponding to the end of bodily growth. In Group A, BF max decreased at the same time. However, $\dot{V}_E O_2$ decreased in both groups until the second year, indicating more efficient respiration during exercise. Uneven distribution of ventilation during exercise appears to be less responsible for the deficit of alveolar-arterial O_2 transfer than at rest (Haab, Chinet, & Micheli, 1971).

Meister (1980) reported during rehabilitation 4 to 5 years following spinal correction a rise of PA_{O_2} (approximately 4 mm Hg) during rest as well as during exercise. PA_{CO_2} remained nearly constant in this study. Thus, aleveolar-arterial O_2-pressure gradient was reduced. Shannon, Riseborough, Valenca, and Kazemi (1961) demonstrated an improved ventilation perfusion ratio following surgical correction of scoliosis. The treatment exerts a favorable effect upon PA_{O_2} and efficiency of respiration (Meister, 1980).

In 19 patients in the current study, PA_{O_2} rose from 75 to 77 mm Hg until the second year. After that, maximum work load values had increased to 93 to 96 mm Hg.

Conclusion

During a longitudinal study extending over 5 years, most parameters under investigation (FVC, MVV, BF, $\dot{V}_E O_2$, HR, $\dot{V}$ max, $\dot{V}O_2$ max, and O_2 pulse) showed significant improvements in patients with moderate scoliosis. A constant improvement was evident until the end of the second year following surgery (Lindh & Bjure, 1975; Meister, 1980). In interpreting the above findings, consideration must be given to the fact that in the present sample of patients, the second year corresponded to the end of bodily growth.

In patients with severe scoliosis, most parameters remained at preoperative levels with the exception of FVC and $\dot{V}_E O_2$. Combined surgical and exercise treatment yielded improvement of uneven distribution, enhanced maximum work load, or prevented deterioration in physical exercise capacity (Shneerson & Edgar, 1979). In this context, it should be noted that in untreated subjects, distinct progression of scoliosis occurs during bodily growth (Meister, 1980).

Correction of scoliosis ought to be performed at moderate Cobb angles, preferably at an early age. Prognosis is definitely superior if the Cobb angle does not exceed the critical limit of 70°.

Endurance exercises improve alveolar ventilation shown by changes in $V_E O_2$ and PA_{O_2}. Long-term endurance training ought to be applied to all scoliotic patients if possible.

References

BERGOFSKY, E.H. (1979). Respiratory failure in disorders of thoracic cage. *American Review of Respiratory Diseases*, **119**, 643.

BJURE, I., Grimby, G., & Nachemson, A. (1969). The effect of physical training in girls with idiopathic scoliosis. *Acta Orthopedica Scandinavica*, **40**, 325.

HAAB, P., Chinet, A., & Micheli, J.L. (1971). Model analysis of apparent steady state pulmonary diffusing capacity at exercise. In *Pulmonary diffusing capacity at exercise*, Bern: Huber.

HABER, P., Kummer, F., Lukschitsch, G., Derda, W. (1982). Die Beziehung von Deformationsgrad und Lungenfunktionseinschränkung bei Skoliosepatienten (Relation between degree of deformation and decreased lung function in scoliosis). *Respiration*, **43**, 241.

KAFER, E.R. (1975). Idiopathic scoliosis. Mechanical properties of the respiratory system and the ventilatory response to carbon dioxide. *Journal of Clinical Investigation*, **55**, 1153.

LINDH, M., & Bjure, J. (1975). Lung volumes in scoliosis before and after correction by the Harrington instrumentation method. *Acta Orthopedica Scandinavica*, **46**, 934.

MEISTER, R. (1980). Atemfunktion und Lungenkreislauf bei thorakaler Skoliose (Breathing function and circulation in scoliosis). *Bücherei des Pneumologen*, **5**. Stuttgart: Thieme.

MEZNIK, F., Koller, H., & Kummer, F. (1972). Die Entwicklung der Lungenfunktion nach Skolioseoperationen (Development of lung function after surgical correction of scoliosis). *Z. Orthop.*, **110**, 542.

NILSONNE, U., & Lundgren, K.-D. (1968). Long-term prognosis in idopathic scoliosis. *Acta Orthopedica Scandinavica*, **39**, 456.

OGLIATI, R., Levine, D., Smith, J.P., Briscoe, W.A., & King, Th.K.C. (1982). Diffusing capacity in idiopathic scoliosis and its interpretation regarding alveolar development. *American Review of Respiratory Diseases*, **120**, 229.

SCHEIER, H. (1967). *Prognose und Behandlung der Skoliose (Prognosis and treatment of scoliosis)*. Stuttgart: Thieme.

SHANNON, D.C., Riseborough, E.Y., Valenca, L.M., & Kazemi, H. (1970). The distribution of abnormal lung function in scoliosis. *Journal of Bone and Joint Surgery*, **52A**, 131.

SHNEERSON, J.M., Edgar, M.A. (1979). Cardiac and respiratory function before and after spinal fusion in adolescent idiopathic scoliosis. *Thorax*, **34**, 658.

SHNEERSON, J.M. (1980). Cardiac and respiratory responses to exercise in adolescent idiopathic scoliosis. *Thorax*, **35**, 347.

STOBOY, H., Speierer, B., & Schick, A. (1977). Spirometric parameters during rehabilitation of patients with idiopathic scoliosis. In St. Kovacić (Ed.), *Scoliosis and Kyphosis*. Zagreb: Medicinska Naklada.

STOBOY, H. (1978). Pulmonary function and spiroergometric criteria in scoliotic patients before and after Harrington rod surgery and physical exercise. In E. Jokl (Ed.), *Medicine and sport*, **11**. Basel: Karger.

WESTGATE, H.K., & Moc, J.H. (1969). Pulmonary function in kyphoscoliosis before and after correction by the Harrington instrumentation method. *Journal of Bone and Joint Surgery*, **61A**, 935.

Anaerobic Threshold in Children

Milos Mácek and Jan Vávra
Laboratory for Physical Fitness Research, Faculty of Pediatrics
Prague, Czechoslovakia

Anaerobic threshold (At) has been defined as the level of physical work load beyond which the energy demands of muscle work reach a level where the products of anaerobic metabolism cannot be sufficiently removed by aerobic pathways. (Wasserman, Whipp, Koyal, & Beaver, 1973.) This level is indicated by the increased production of lactic acid (LA) creating an increase in blood concentration levels and incidental manifestation of metabolic acidosis. Anaerobic threshold has been intensively studied by using various invasive or noninvasive indicators during increasing work load. Most studies have been done using adults, in particular athletes, in order to obtain some information on specific changes due to sport participation or training effects. Yet hardly any definite conclusions can be drawn concerning either the significance of AT (examination in various sport activities) or the correlation among various indicators and their reliability for AT determination.

There is a lack of existing information on anaerobic threshold in children and its significance. It is generally accepted that the LA production is lower during exercise in these younger age groups. (Eriksson & Koch, 1973; Godfrey, Davies, Wozniak, & Barnes, 1971; Mácek & Vávra, 1971; Reybrouck, Weymans, Ghesquiere, Van Gerven, & Stinjns, 1983.) The hypothetical explanations for this statement fluctuate between the incapacity of young organisms to realease anaerobic energy and the lack of need for this metabolic pathway. The main purpose of this study was to obtain more information on the reliability of AT estimation in young populations of both sexes by using various indicators.

Methods

The study was conducted with a group of 47 boys and 52 girls between the ages of 6 and 14 years without any previous history of cardiopulmonary disease from a school in the center of Prague. The weight and height of all children under study were within 2 SD of the average population values. None of the subjects had taken part in an organized sport activity.

Children rode a bicycle ergometer for 4 successive days, 5 minutes each day without any warm-up. On the first day, the load was 1 W/kg body weight (bw), the second day, 2 W/kg bw, the third day, 2.5 W/kg bw, and the 4th day 3 W/kg bw. The highest work load (i.e., 3 W/kg bw) could not be fulfilled by all children, particularly the girls. In the girls' group, this work-load was completed by only 70% of the girls.

The expired air was collected into a system of Douglas bags in the last 2 min of exercise. Its volume was determined by a Tissot spirometer, and the gas content analyzed on a Scholander apparatus. The blood was sampled in the third min after cessation of work from the brachial vein, and the LA values were estimated by the enzymatic method using the Boehringer tests.

Results

All children were divided in four weight groups regardless of age, that is, 20 to 29 kg (A), 30 to 39 kg (B), 40 to 49 kg (C), and 50 to 59 kg (D). The average values of the blood Δ LA, of the minute ventilation (V_E) per kg bw, and of the ventilatory equivalent for oxygen—V_E/VO_2 were calculated for each of the weight groups of both sexes and were plotted against the work load in W/kg bw.

The blood levels of Δ LA in boys (see Figure 1) indicate that a steeper increase begins between 2 and 2.5 W/kg bw in all weight groups. In girls, the exponential increase in the LA curve was more pronounced in the lowest weight group, at a work load of 2.5 W, whereas in higher weight groups this abrupt change was less noticeable. The minute ventilation in boys (see Figure 2) increased linearly with increasing work load up to the load of 2 W/kg bw, in all weight groups, but at higher work loads the slopes of these curves were noticeably steeper. In girls, the increase in minute ventilation (see Figure 3) with increasing work load was practically linear up to the highest work load, with much less distinct changes in shape.

The ventilatory equivalent for oxygen (see Figure 4) decreased up to a load of 2 W/kg bw, which it increased in all boys' weight groups. In girls, these curves reached

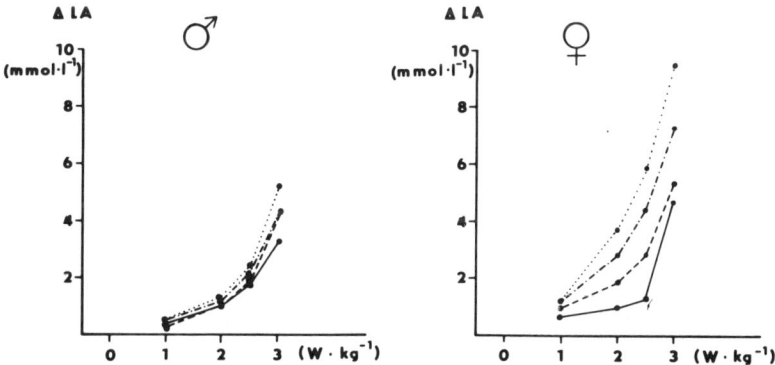

Figure 1—The increase of lactic acid for various work loads in boys and girls. The weight groups A: 20-29 kg ⎯⎯⎯⎯⎯ ; B: 30-39 kg ⎯⎯⎯⎯ ; C: 40-49 kg -•-•-•- ; D: 50-59 kg ....

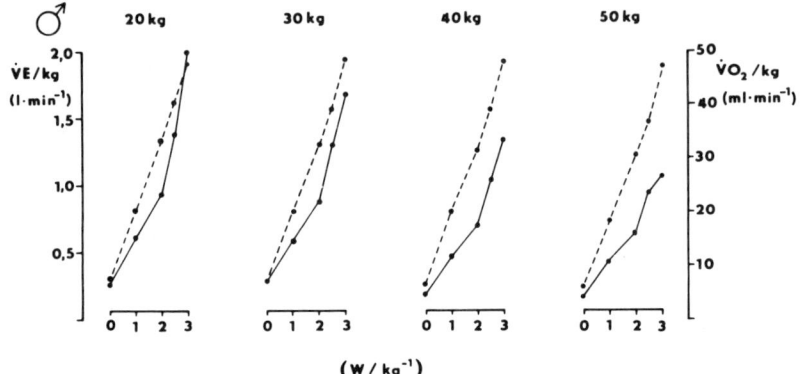

Figure 2—The minute ventilation per kg bw (V_E/kg ——————) and the oxygen uptake per kg bw. ($\dot{V}O_2$/kg --------) in various weight groups for the boys.

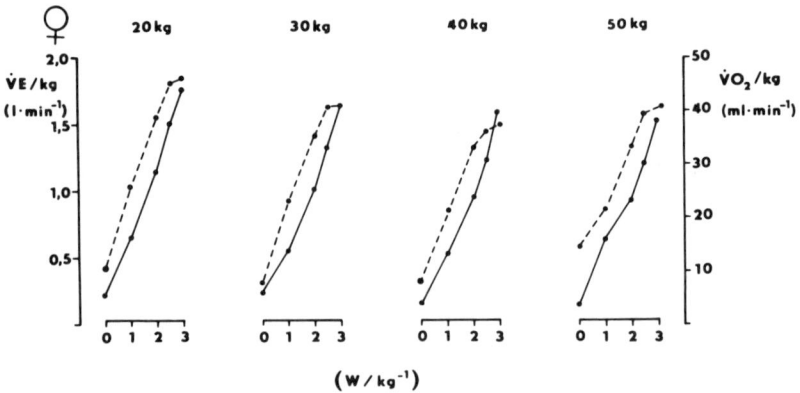

Figure 3—The minute ventilation per kg bw (V_E/kg ——————) and the oxygen uptake per kg bw ($\dot{V}O_2$/kg --------) in various weight groups of girls plotted against work load.

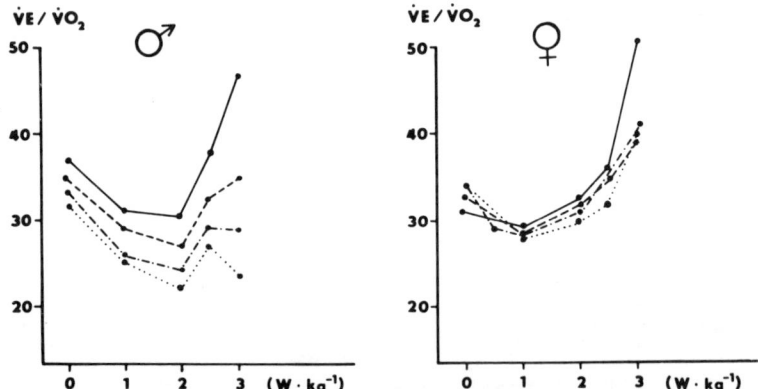

Figure 4—The ventilatory equivalent for oxygen in various work loads in various weight groups of boys and girls. (Same legend for groups as in Figures 1, 2, and 3.)

their lowest point at the workload of 1 W/kg bw in all weight groups. At higher work loads the slopes of these are reversed, the increase being less distinct between 1 and 2 W/kg bw, but later the steeper slopes are obvious.

Discussion

The AT is usually determined by various arrangements of progressive exercise tests on a bicycle ergometer or on a treadmill in a single test session. In this study, the estimation of AT was created from work-loads of increasing intensities on 4 days. Each day only one exercise test was conducted. The interval between any two measurements never exceeded a maximum of 3 days. In this experimental arrangement, the response of organism seems to be more linked with the given load, whereas in progressive exercise tests, the obtained values may be distorted, mainly in LA, because these values can be influenced by a time delay between muscle production and blood level equilibrium.

The results of the present study suggest that the anaerobic threshold can be found in boys by using various methods, such as the LA, the minute ventilation, and the ventilatory equivalent for oxygen curves. All these curves show a distinct changes in slope namely at the work-load of 2 W/kg bw with a very good agreement among all three indicators.

Nevertheless, the AT estimation in girls is more difficult or quite impossible. Which is the valid value for the minute ventilation curve when the increase is practically linear from rest to the highest applied load? From the LA curve, the anaerobic threshold could be detected in the lowest weight group only, with a work-load at an intensity of 2 to 2.5 W/kg bw. For higher weight groups, the AT detection is questionable. the AT estimation from the ventilatory equivalent for oxygen curve in girls suggests its level is at the work-load of 1 W/kg bw or between 1 and 2 W/kg bw. Thus, some discrepancies in AT estimation were apparent in girls when using different indicators. The most reliable method of those used was the estimation of AT from the ventilatory equivalent.

References

ERIKSSON, B.O., & Koch, G. (1973). Effect of physical training on hemodynamic response during submaximal and maximal exercise in 11-13 years old boys. *Acta Physiologica Scandinavia*, **87**, 27-39.

GODFREY, S., Davies, C.T.M., Woznial, E., & Barnes, C.A. (1971). Cardiorespiratory response to exercise in normal children. *Clinical Science*, **40**, 419-431.

MÁČEK, M, Vávra, J. (1971). Cardiopulmonary and metabolic changes during exercise in children 6-14 years old. *Journal of Applied Physiology*, **30**, 202-204.

REYBROUCK, T., Weymans, M., Ghesquiere, D., Van Gerven, D., & Stinjns, H. (1982). Ventilatory threshold during treadmill exercise in kindergarten children. *European Journal of Applied Physiology*, **50**, 79-86.

WASSERMAN, K., Whipp, B., Koyal, N.S., & Beaver, W.L. (1973). Anaerobic threshold and respiratory gas exchange during exercise. *Journal of Applied Physiology*, **35**, 236-243.

Influence of Age and Sex on the Ventilatory Anaerobic Threshold in Children

Maria Weymans, Tony Reybrouck, Hugo Stijns, and Jacqueline Knops
University of Leuven, Belgium

In adults, the exercise intensity at which a nonlinear increase in pulmonary ventilation ($\dot{V}_E$) and derived variables occurs with increasing oxygen uptake is considered to be a ventilatory (anaerobic) threshold (VAT), which is an indirect indicator for the onset of metabolic acidosis (Wasserman, Whipp, Koyal, & Beaver, 1973).

Similarly, in healthy children a VAT has been shown during exercise (Reybrouck, Weymans, Ghesquiere, Van Gerven, & Stijns, 1982) or could be deduced from published data (Eriksson & Koch, 1973; Godfrey, 1981; Lange-Andersen, Seliger, Rutenfranz, & Messel, 1974; Máček & Vávra, 1969). The VAT has also been shown both in adults (Wasserman & Whipp, 1975) and children (Reybrouck, Weymans, Ghesquiere, Van Gerven, & Stijns, 1982) to represent an index of physical performance capacity.

The purpose of the present study was to investigate the influence of age and sex on the VAT during graded exercise in children.

Methods

A group of 52 children, aged 6, 11, and 14 years, performed a graded maximal exercise test on a treadmill. Some anthropometrical characteristics are given in Table 1.

The speed of the treadmill was set at 4.8 km/hr for children younger than 6 years of age and 5.6 km/hr for children above 6 years of age (Chandramouli, Ehmke, & Lauer, 1975). The inclination of the treadmill was increased by 2% every minute until exhaustion. After a rest period of half an hour, a supramaximal exercise test at an inclination which corresponded to a predicted heart rate of 220 beats•min^{-1} was performed for 3 min.

Respiratory variables were measured by the open-circuit method. Expired air was collected every minute in Douglas bags. The volume was determined by a dry gas meter and the concentrations of O_2 and CO_2 were analyzed by electronic gas analyzers.

Heart rate (HR) was calculated from the ECG. The VAT was determined as the starting point of the nonlinear change in $\dot{V}_E$ with increasing $\dot{V}O_2$ (Wasserman, Whipp, Koyal,

Table 1

Anthropometrical Characteristics of the Children

Variables	Boys			Girls		
Age (years)	6	11	14	6	11	14
Height (cm)	120.2	145.2	164.9	118.5	143.6	162.4
	±4.4	±4.3	±3.8	±4.3	±12.9	±6.2
Weight (kg)	21.2	35.6	51.1	21.2	34.9	50.8
	±2.1	±4.1	±8.8	±2.1	±4.5	±6.1
Number of subjects	7	9	10	5	7	14

Note. The data represent mean and standard deviation of the mean.

& Beaver, 1973). This breakpoint of the $\dot{V}_E$ was checked by referring to the exercise intensity at which (a) the $\dot{V}CO_2$ began to increase nonlinearly, (b) a systematic increase of the ventilatory equivalent for O_2 ($\dot{V}_E/\dot{V}O_2$), without a concomitant increase in the ventilatory equivalent for CO_2 ($\dot{V}_E/\dot{V}CO_2$), (c) a progressive increase of the O_2 concentration in the mixed air (F_EO_2), and (d) an excess rise of the respiratory gas exchange ratio (R) occurred (Caiozzo et al., 1982; Davis, Frank, Whipp, & Wasserman, 1979; Reybrouck, Heigenhauser, & Faulkner, 1975; Reybrouck, Weymans, Ghesquiere, Van Gerven, & Stijns, 1982).

Results

In boys, aged 6, 11, and 14 years, the VAT averaged 32.28 ± 5.14 ml $O_2 \cdot min^{-1} \cdot kg^{-1}$. In the girls, this VAT was reached at a significantly ($p < .0001$) lower $\dot{V}O_2$ of 26.56 ± 3.87 ml $O_2 \cdot min^{-1} \cdot kg^{-1}$. When expressed as a percentage of $\dot{V}O_2$max, this VAT was reached at 66.0 ± 10.5 and 66.4 ± 7.5%, respectively, in boys and girls and no sex difference ($p > .05$) existed.

$\dot{V}O_2$max was significantly lower in girls (40.14 ± 5.35 ml $O_2 \cdot min^{-1} \cdot kg^{-1}$) than in boys (49.85 ± 6.03 ml $O_2 \cdot min^{-1} \cdot kg^{-1}$). The VAT expressed in ml $O_2 \cdot min^{-1} \cdot kg^{-1}$ or as a percentage of $\dot{V}O_2$max was reached at a significantly lower ($p < .05$) value or percentage of $\dot{V}O_2$max in the 14-year-old children compared to the 11- and 16-year-olds. However, no age differences were found for $\dot{V}O_2$max (Table 2). No interaction ($p > .05$) of sex and age could be detected for the VAT (ml $O_2 \cdot min^{-1} \cdot kg^{-1}$ or as a % of $\dot{V}O_2$max) and $\dot{V}O_2$max (see Figure 1).

Discussion

In girls, the VAT was observed at a significantly lower $\dot{V}O_2$ (ml $O_2 \cdot min^{-1} \cdot kg^{-1}$) than in boys, which is in agreement with the observations of Máček and Vávra (1969),

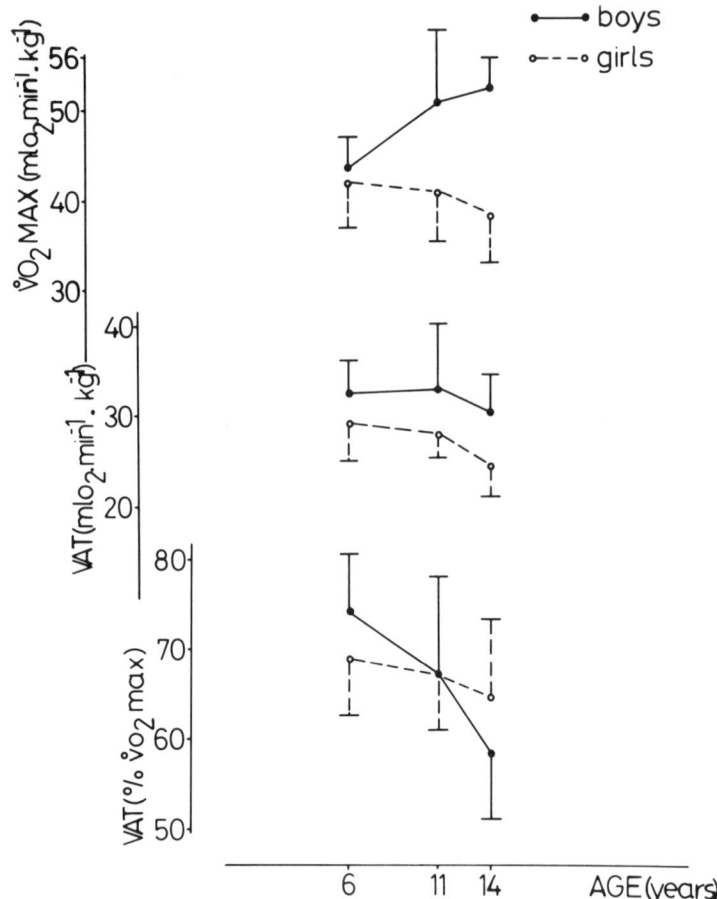

Figure 1—Influence of sex and age on the ventilatory anaerobic threshold both expressed in ml $O_2 \cdot min^{-1} \cdot kg^{-1}$ and as a percentage of $\dot{V}O_2max$, and the maximal aerobic capacity expressed in ml $O_2 \cdot min^{-1} \cdot kg^{-1}$.

who found that anaerobiosis starts at a lower work intensity in girls compared to boys. The significant difference for the VAT, expressed both in ml $O_2 \cdot min^{-1} \cdot kg^{-1}$ or as a percentage of $\dot{V}O_2max$, between the 6- and 11-year-olds compared to the 14-year-old children can be explained by the growth spurt, which starts at an average age of 12 and 14 years in girls and boys, respectively (Tanner, Whitehouse, & Takaishi, 1966).

The capacity to perform anaerobic metabolism can be assessed by expressing the VAT as a percentage of the $\dot{V}O_2max$. In boys the maximal aerobic power increases from age 6 to 14 years, which is in agreement with the observations of Åstrand (1952), Lange-Andersen, Seliger, Rutenfranz, and Messel (1974), Davies, Barnes, and Godfrey (1972), and their VAT expressed as ml $O_2 \cdot min^{-1} \cdot kg^{-1}$ drops over the same age span. In girls, on the other hand, this VAT (ml $O_2 \cdot min^{-1} \cdot kg^{-1}$) drops at a greater rate than the $\dot{V}O_2max$ from age 6 to 14 years (see Figure 1). From this combined effect

Table 2

Influence of Age on the Ventilatory Anaerobic Threshold and Maximal Aerobic Capacity

Variables	Age (Years) 6	11	14
VAT (ml $O_2 \cdot min^{-1} \cdot kg^{-1}$)	31.36 ± 4.28	31.28 ± 5.99	27.21 ± 4.68
VAT (% $\dot{V}O_2max$)	72.33 ± 6.43	67.44 ± 8.76	62.29 ± 8.68
$\dot{V}O_2max$ (ml $O_2 \cdot min^{-1} \cdot kg^{-1}$)	43.32 ± 3.96	47.29 ± 7.97	44.30 ± 8.33

Note. The data represent mean and standard deviation of the mean.
|_____| : represents subsets from a TUKEY test.

of changes in $\dot{V}O_2max$ (ml $O_2 \cdot min^{-1} \cdot kg^{-1}$) and VAT (ml $O_2 \cdot min^{-1} \cdot kg^{-1}$) with increasing age, it is obvious that the VAT, when expressed as a percentage of $\dot{V}O_2max$, decreases with age without any sex difference.

The higher capacity to perform lactacid anaerobic metabolism with increasing age has also been shown by Åstrand (1952), who found higher maximal blood lactate concentrations after exercise, and Davies, Barnes, and Godfrey (1972) who showed that the maximal anaerobic capacity, as measured by the Margaria stair climbing test, increases with age and is independent of sex in children.

A higher lactacid anaerobic capacity with increasing age in children can be explained by their enzymatic profile. In the older children lower concentrations of the oxidative enzyme succinic dehydrogenase and also higher concentrations of the glycolytic enzyme phosphofructokinase have been found compared to the youngest children (Eriksson, 1972; Eriksson & Saltin, 1974).

In conclusion, the higher percentage of $\dot{V}O_2max$ at which this nonlinear increase in ventilation starts in the youngest children compared to the older ones suggests that the lactacid anaerobic capacity increases with age and is independent of sex in children.

References

ÅSTRAND, P. (1952). *Experimental studies of physical working capacity in relation to sex and age.* Copenhagen: Ejnar Munksgaard.

CAIOZZO, V., Davis, J., Ellis, J., Azus, J., Vandagriff, R., Prietto, C., & McMaster, W. (1982). A comparison of gas exchange indices used to detect the anaerobic threshold. *Journal of Applied Physiology,* **53,** 1184-1189.

CHANDRAMOULI, B., Ehmke, D., & Lauer, R. (1975). Exercise induced elektrocardiographic changes in children with congenital aortic stenosis. *Journal of Pediatrics,* **87,** 725-730.

DAVIES, C., Barnes, C., & Godfrey, S. (1972). Body composition and maximal exercise performance in children. *Human Biology,* **44**, 195-214.

DAVIS, J., Frank, M., Whipp, B., & Wasserman, K. (1979). Anaerobic threshold alterations caused by endurance training in middle-age men. *Journal of Applied Physiology,* **41**, 544-550.

ERIKSSON, B. (1972). Physical training, oxygen supply and muscle metabolism in 11-13 year old boys. *Acta Physiologica Scandinavica,* **384**(suppl), 1-48.

ERIKSSON, B., & Koch, G. (1973). Effect of physical training on hemodynamic response during submaximal and maximal exercise in 11-13 year old boys. *Acta Physiologica Scandinavica,* **87**, 27-39.

ERIKSSON, B., & Saltin, B. (1974). Muscle metabolism during exercise in boys aged 11 to 16 years compared to adults. *Acta Paediatrica Belgica,* **28**(suppl), 257-265.

GODFREY, S. (1981). The growth and development of the cardiopulmonary responses to exercise. In J. Davies & J. Dobbing (Eds.), *Scientific Foundations of Pediatrics*, pp. 450-460. London: Heinemann Medical Books.

LANGE-ANDERSEN, K., Seliger, V., Rutenfranz, J., & Messel, S. (1974). Physical performance capacity in children in Norway, Part III. Respiratory responses to graded exercise loadings—Population parameters in a rural community. *European Journal of Applied Physiology,* **33**, 265-274.

MÁČEK, M., & Vávra, J. (1969). Aerobic and anaerobic metabolism during exercise in childhood. *Malatti Cardiovasculari,* **10**, 409-420.

REYBROUCK, T., Heigenhauser, G., & Faulkner, J. (1975). Limitations to maximum oxygen uptake in arm, leg and combined arm-leg ergometry. *Journal of Applied Physiology,* **38**, 744-779.

REYBROUCK, T., Weymans, M., Ghesquiere, J., Van Gerven, D., & Stijns, H. (1982). Ventilatory threshold in kindergarten children during treadmill exercise. *European Journal of Applied Physiology,* **50**, 79-86.

TANNER, J., Whitehouse, R., & Takaishi, M. (1966). Standards from birth to maturity for height, weight, height velocity and weight velocity; British children. *Archives of Disease in Childhood,* **41**, 454-471.

WASSERMAN, K., Whipp, B., Koyal, S., & Beaver, W. (1973). Anaerobic threshold and respiratory gas exchange during exercise. *Journal of Applied Physiology,* **35**, 236-243.

WASSERMAN, K., & Whipp, B. (1975). Exercise physiology in health and disease. *American Review of Respiratory Disease,* **112**, 219-249.

Development of Anaerobic Capacity in Early and Late Maturing Boys

Donald H. Paterson and David A. Cunningham
University of Western Ontario
London, Ontario, Canada

Anaerobic Capacity and Maturation

Boys of different onset of maturation (early or late) may show markedly different responses to exercise. At comparable chronological ages, earlier maturers have greater size and strength and show distinct performance advantages (Malina, 1980). The purposes of the present study were to compare anaerobic capacity (AnC) of young boys of different maturative groups (a) at given chronological ages (from 11 to 15 years) to observe possible performance advantages with early (or late) maturation, and (b) at given stages of growth (indicated by peak height velocity, PHV) to observe, theoretically, whether development of AnC differs. Early- and late-maturing boys were identified by skeletal age.

Previous investigators have suggested that AnC may be developed in conjunction with sexual development, and, hence, early maturers would show a performance advantage throughout pubescence over boys of similar chronological age but late to mature. Eriksson, Karlsson, and Saltin (1971) suggested that "sexual maturation has a role" in development of anaerobic energy in light of an "almost significant correlation" between muscle lactate (La) following maximal exercise and testicular volume in 12- and 13-year-old boys. Wirth, Trager, Schede, Mayer, Diehm, Reisch, and Weicker (1978) have associated an increased blood La beyond age of puberty with increased insulin concentrations during exercise indicating, perhaps, an enhanced glycogen synthesis in the muscle (Hermansen, 1980).

Methods

Nineteen subjects completed an annual battery of tests over 5 years (mean age 10.8 to 14.9 years). Included was the performance of a treadmill run designed specifically to estimate AnC. The boys were a subgroup of the sample of a longitudinal investigation of growth and physiological characteristics of active children (Cunningham, Paterson, Blimkie, & Donner, 1984).

All boys performed habituation tests in the fall of their entry year and their annual tests occurred in the spring. Tests were performed in a laboratory with temperatures 20 to 23 °C. Body weight and height were recorded and subcutaneous fat thickness was measured at 12 sites using Harpenden calipers. A computer plot of height vs. age for each subject was fitted by a polynomial curve (Akima, 1970) and the point of greatest slope, or instantaneous change in height defined as the age of PHV. Hand–wrist x-rays were taken in the year of entry and final year of study for each boy. Skeletal age was determined by a radiologist according to methods of Greulich and Pyle (1959). Boys were grouped into earlier and later maturing groups using the skeletal age measures. Early maturers were those with skeletal age in advance of chronological age at both determinations. In late maturers, skeletal age was less than chronological age. The age at PHV was used to confirm these groupings; that is, age of PHV in early maturers was in advance of the group average (12.9 ± 1.2 years), and age of PHV in late maturers was later than the group average.

The AnC test was a treadmill run at 20% grade as designed by Cunningham and Faulkner (1969) to maximally stress the capacity of the anaerobic energy system. Speed was adjusted for the boys to 130 m•min^{-1} in 10- and 11-year-olds, 160 m•min^{-1} in 12- and 13-year-olds, and 190 m•min^{-1} for the 14- and 15-year-olds. Performance times could not, therefore, be compared across ages, but only within ages. AnC was determined from measurements of postexercise blood lactate and O_2 debt. Blood samples were drawn from the finger tip at 5 minutes postexercise and lactate concentrations determined using an enzymatic analysis (Hohorst, 1965). The O_2 debt was calculated from the recovery oxygen consumption less the preexercise oxygen consumption. A 5-min determination of oxygen consumption was made with the subject seated prior to the treadmill test. The postexercise oxygen consumption was measured over a 15-min period. To obtain these measurements of $\dot{V}O_2$, subjects breathed through a Koegel valve (dead space 64 ml); inspired ventilation was recorded from a dry gas meter, and expired gases collected in a spirometer or meteorological balloons for subsequent analysis using a paramagnetic O_2 analyzer and infrared CO_2 analyzer.

Descriptive variables and data for O_2 debt in liters and ml•kg^{-1}, La, and performance time at each chronological age were compared (in the early- and late-maturing groups) by independent t-tests. Data of each individual were also expressed at yearly intervals from the age of PHV using the polynomial curve (Akima, 1970) to derive data at -2, -1, 0, +1 and +2 years from age of PHV. Early and late maturers were compared using independent t-tests at each stage of growth.

Results

Physical characteristics of the 19 subjects from ages 10.9 through 14.9 years, and the subgroups of 6 early maturers and 7 late maturers are given in Table 1. Throughout the age span, early maturers were significantly taller (by 8 to 12 cm) than late maturers, and heavier (by 4 to 7 kg) although the weight differences were not significant. Skinfold measures were not different between these subgroups. The early- and late-maturing groups were significantly different in skeletal age, the factor used to define group membership. In early maturers, skeletal age was 0.9 and 0.8 years in advance of chronological age for the determinations made at ages 10.5 and 14.5 years, respectively; in late maturers, the skeletal ages were 1.1 and 0.9 years behind the chronological

Table 1

Physical Characteristics of the Total Sample (n=19) and Early (n=6) and Late (n=7) Maturers

Variable	Group	Test 1	Test 2	Test 3	Test 4	Test 5
Age (yrs)	Early	10.8±0.4	11.9±0.4	12.9±0.4	13.9±0.4	14.9±0.4
	Late	10.9±0.3	12.0±0.3	13.0±0.3	14.0±0.3	14.9±0.3
	Total Sample	10.9±0.3	12.0±0.3	12.9±0.3	13.9±0.3	14.9±0.3
Height (cm)	Early	145.3±2.6	153.4±5.2	161.6±6.5	169.3±6.3	174.0±4.1
	Late	137.8±4.9*	144.8±5.2*	151.2±6.0*	160.2±7.6*	165.9±7.4*
	Total Sample	142.9±5.6	151.3±7.4	158.6±8.6	166.7±8.5	171.6±7.5
Weight (kg)	Early	36.1±2.3	41.3±3.9	48.1±6.6	55.2±7.7	60.6±6.3
	Late	32.8±3.3	36.3±3.8	40.9±4.5	47.9±6.3	54.7±7.9
	Total Sample	36.4±4.8	41.1±6.2	46.9±7.7	54.4±8.7	60.4±9.0
Skinfolds (mm)	Early	82.7±18.5	97.5±25.4	98.8±25.7	92.2±23.8	94.4±28.3
	Late	84.4±18.0	88.1±28.1	90.9±42.3	84.5±29.9	102.7±37.7
	Total Sample	96.2±35.5	100.4±33.5	99.8±37.9	97.3±48.0	106.6±53.2

Values are means ± S.D.
*Significant difference between early and late maturers, (p<0.05).

age. In early maturers, PHV averaged 12.0 ± 1.1 years and in late maturers, 13.8 ± 0.6 years.

Performance times on the AnC test ranged from means of 80 to 100s through ages 10.9 to 13.9 years. At age 14.9 years, the performance time averaged 52 s. Performance times comparing the two groups at each age showed no significant differences (see Figure 1). O_2 debt in liters and ml·kg^{-1}, and La at each chronological age for early and late maturers, as well as the total group are shown in Figures 2, A, B, and C. For the total group, O_2 debt in liters increased 171% from age 10.8 to 14.9 years, and 64% when weight gain (O_2 debt, ml·kg^{-1}) was considered. The increase in La, also a measure in which size was at least partially factored out, was 38%. O_2 debt in liters was generally larger (nonsignificant) in early maturers (see Figure 2A), but in ml·kg^{-1} early and late maturers were similar (Figure 2B). Lactic acid was also similar in the two groups (Figure 2C).

Data were also aligned relative to age of PHV (Figures 3A, B, C). At a given stage of growth, early maturers were approximately 2 years younger; however, height (within 2 cm) and weight (within 3 kg) were very similar in the two groups. O_2 debt in liters, nevertheless, was slightly larger in late maturers (see Figure 3A), and O_2 debt in ml·kg^{-1} (see Figure 3B) and La (see Figure 3C) were consistently larger in late maturers. In light of the large standard deviation on each of these AnC measures and

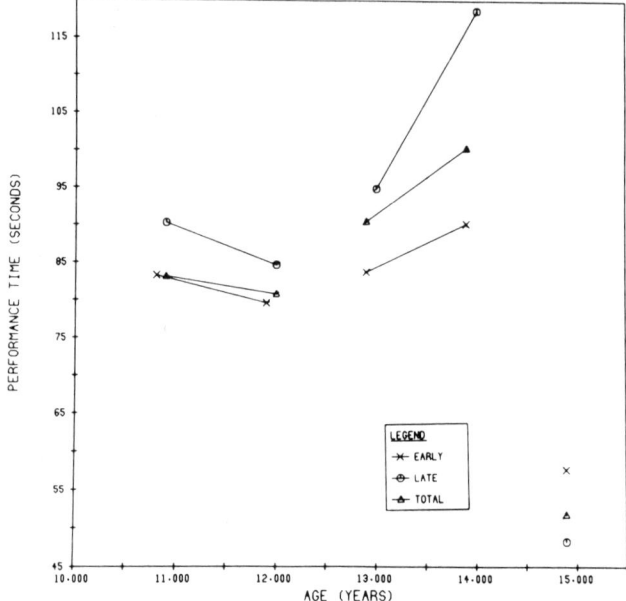

Figure 1—Chronological age and performance times (seconds) on the anaerobic treadmill test in early- and late-maturing boys.

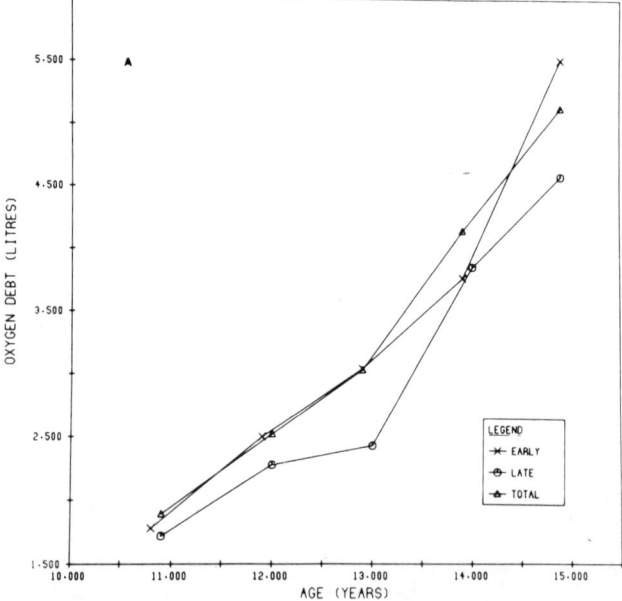

Figure 2A, 2B, 2C—Chronological age and AnC measured as: (A) O_2 debt in liters; (B) O_2 debt in $ml \cdot kg^{-1}$, and (C) La in $mmol \cdot l^{-1}$ in early- and late-maturing boys.

ANAEROBIC CAPACITY AND MATURATION

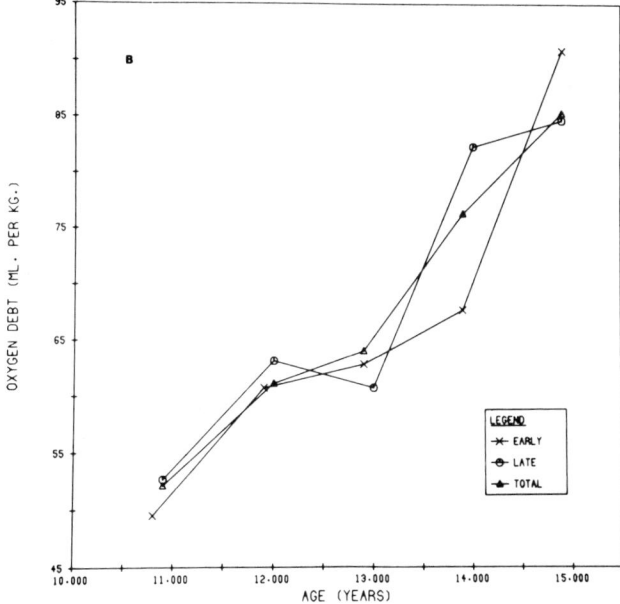

Figure 2B.

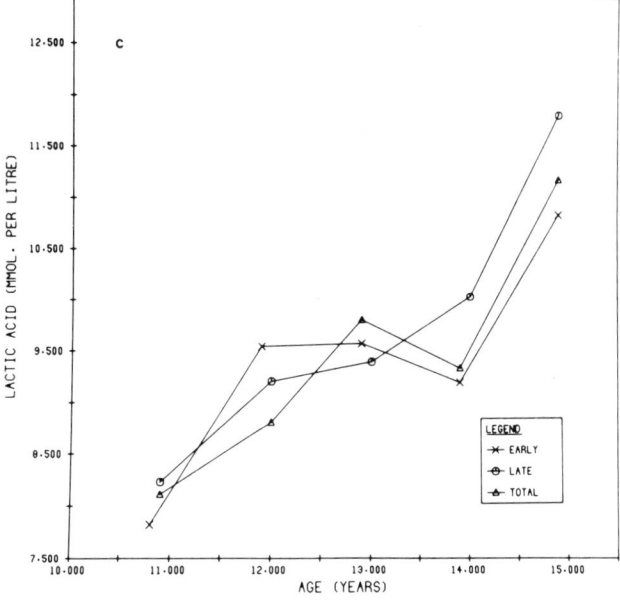

Figure 2C.

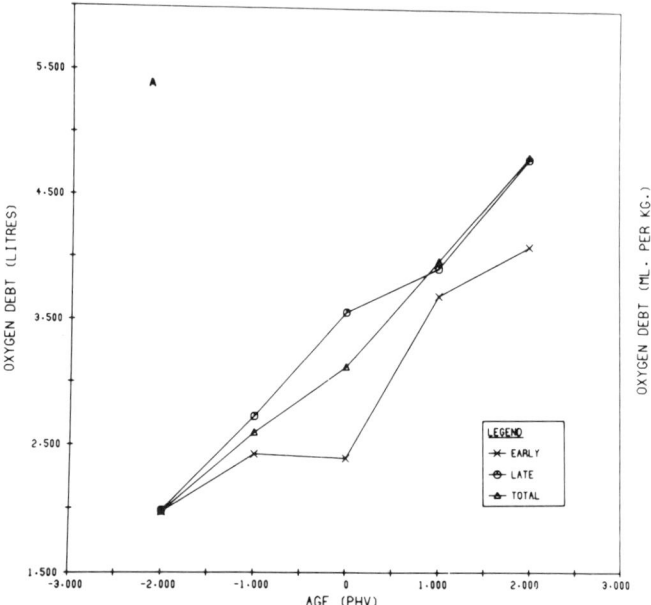

Figure 3A, 3B, 3C—Age of peak height velocity and AnC measured as: (A) O_2 debt in liters, (B) O_2 debt in ml·kg^{-1}, and (C) La in mmol·l^{-1} in early- and late-maturing boys.
(Sample size at -2, -1, 0, +1, +2 years was in early maturers, 3, 4, 6, 6, 4 and for late maturers 7, 7, 7, 6, 5).

the relatively small group sizes, differences between groups were not statistically significant with exception of a higher La in the late maturers at PHV +2 years. Performance times could not be realigned individually to age of PHV due to the differences in running speeds on the test across the age span. Nevertheless, late maturers at age 13.9 years ran for 119 s at 20% grade and 160 or 190 m·min^{-1}, while early maturers at age 12.0 years performed at 20% grade and slower speed (130 or 160 m·min^{-1}) for only 80 s. Thus, performance appeared substantially better in late maturers when examined at similar stages of maturation (PHV age).

In the total group, the largest AnC changes occurred following age of PHV. Increases in O_2 debt (1 and ml·kg^{-1}) from 0 to +1 and +1 to +2 years were the only significant year-to-year increments (see Figure 3A, B). The largest La increment, between +1 and +2 years, was not significant (see Figure 3C). In the subgroups, early maturers showed their greatest increases for each of the measures (O_2 debt, 1, ml·kg^{-1}, and La) in the year following PHV, while late maturers showed increases in all three measures prior to PHV, with a second spurt from +1 to +2 years (see Figure 3A, B, C).

Discussion

The 19 boys in the present study were taller (3 to 5 cm) and heavier (1 to 3 kg) at each age compared to the 81 boys in the parent longitudinal study (Cunningham

ANAEROBIC CAPACITY AND MATURATION

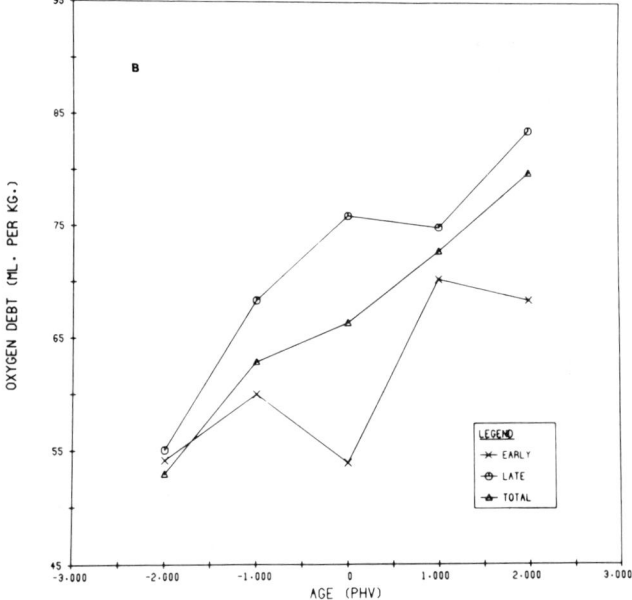

Figure 3B.

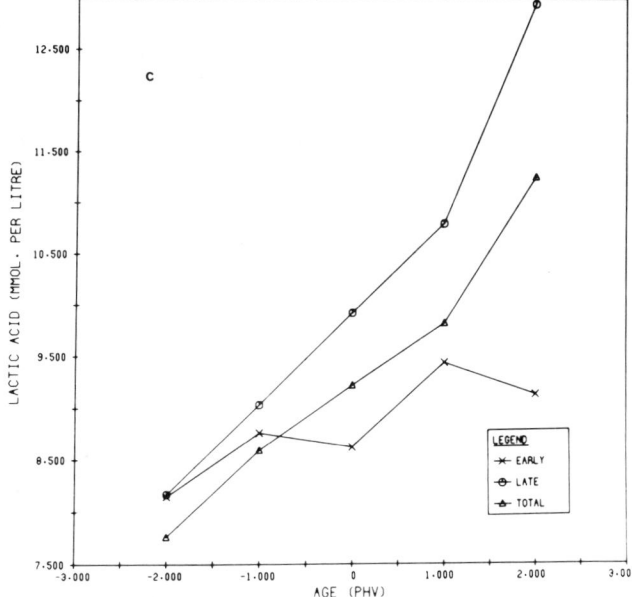

Figure 3C.

& Paterson, unpublished). In the present study, early maturers were bigger boys than late maturers. The size differences between early and late groups were not as large as in the sample of 81 boys, in which early and late maturers represented only 17% and 15% of the sample, respectively. In this sample of 19 the definition of earlier and later maturers was less stringent with 32% (6/19) and 37% (7/19) included in these groups, respectively.

The treadmill AnC test was evaluated previously in children aged 10 and 15 years (Paterson, Cunningham, & Bonk, 1980). Subjects duplicated their performance times on a test-retest ($r > .76$) and O_2 debt measures were reliable ($r > .76$) and reproducible, with no significant difference between the two trials. Postexercise La showed poorer reliability ($r > .53$) with the usual wide intraindividual variability, but group means were reproducible.

The possibility of a growth dependent development of AnC was investigated in the present study with expression of data relative to age of PHV. It was recognized that measurements of height only once per year could not conclusively define age of PHV in an individual and had an accuracy of ± 6 months. Nevertheless, alignment of AnC measures to coincide with this approximation of each individual's greatest growth period allowed examination as to whether the AnC increases paralleled the growth spurt. A greatly improved AnC in conjunction with the pubertal growth spurt was expected on the basis of the reports of Eriksson, Karlsson, and Saltin (1971) and Wirth et al. (1978). Year-to-year increments in AnC (either O_2 debt or La) were not accentuated in relation to the period of greatest growth (Paterson, Cunningham, & Bumstead, 1981). Further, although the AnC for the total group showed the largest increments following PHV age, there was not a consistent increase of AnC in both the early- and late-maturing groups at the same stage of growth.

A larger AnC in early maturers at ages following their age of PHV was expected compared to late maturers. As well as the data in children which suggested a larger AnC following puberty (Eriksson, Karlsson, and Saltin 1971; Wirth et al., 1978), studies in the rat have demonstrated that testosterone (a) influences the maturation of glycolytic potential of skeletal muscle (Beitner, Nordenberg, & Cohen, 1979); (b) is critical in the maturative development of the muscle lactate dehydrogenase isozyme pattern (Dux, Dux, Mazarean, & Guba, 1979); (c) is critical in the development of phosphorylase activity (Krotkiewski, Krol, & Karlsson, 1980); and (d) alters morphometric properties (Dux, Dux, & Guba, 1982). Nevertheless, there were no differences between the early- and late-maturing groups contrary to the expectation that AnC might develop in association with growth and growth-related factors. In fact, at each chronological age, including ages in which the early maturers had passed PHV age but late maturers had not, the measures of AnC were not significantly greater in the larger early maturers. There were also no differences in performance of the two groups on the anaerobic capacity task. These findings of similarity of AnC in early and late maturers at a given age are different from the findings of a larger VO_2 max in early maturers when absolute values ($l \cdot min^{-1}$) were considered and greater values in late maturers when weight was included in the expression of VO_2 max ($ml \cdot kg^{-1} \cdot min^{-1}$) in the study of Cunningham, Paterson and Blimkie (1984).

In early- and late-maturing boys, not only is the chronological age of peak growth different, but there are also differences between the groups in the process and rate of maturation (Malina, 1980). The process of development of AnC with maturation in boys classified in early- or late-maturing groups could be compared, therefore, only when the individual data (and thus averaged group results) were aligned to common growth stages (approximating prePHV, during PHV, or after PHV). At these common stages of growth, the size (height, weight) was similar in the two groups despite the two-year difference in chronological age. Alignment of the AnC data to PHV ages revealed larger differences between early and late groups than found when the groups were compared at given chronological ages. The late maturers tended generally toward larger values for O_2 debt in liters and when corrected to body size, and a significantly greater La at +2 years relative to PHV age. The late maturers at given chronological ages also showed superior running performances. These data suggest that late maturers are progressing towards a superior AnC and performance at mature adult levels when differential growth effects on early and late maturers are completed.

To conclude, the growth of AnC appeared unrelated to the growth spurt or the occurrence of maturative or pubertal events. AnC was not different in early compared to late maturers at any age from 11 to 15 years. Late maturers may, in fact, show a greater AnC beyond the age of 15 years.

References

AKIMA, H. (1970). A new method of interpretation and smooth curve fitting based on local procedures. *Journal of Comparative Mathematics,* **17,** 589-602.

BEITNER, R., Nordenberg, J., & Cohen, T.J. (1979). Correlation between the levels of glucose—1,6 -biphosphate and the activities of phosphofructokinase, phosphoglucomutase, and hexokinase in skeletal and heart muscle from rats of different ages. *International Journal of Biochemistry,* **10,** 603-608.

CUNNINGHAM, D.A. & Faulkner, J.A. (1969). The effect of training on aerobic and anaerobic metabolism during a short exhaustive run. *Medicine and Science in Sports and Exercise,* **1,** 65-69.

CUNNINGHAM, D.A. & Paterson, D.H. (Unpublished). Development of aerobic capacity in early and late maturing boys. A longitudinal study.

CUNNINGHAM, D.A. Paterson, D.H., & Blimkie, C.J.R. (1984). The development of the cardiorespiratory system with growth and physical activity. In R.A. Boileau (Ed.), *Advances in Pediatric Sport Sciences* (pp. 85-116). Champaign, IL: Human Kinetics.

CUNNINGHAM, D.A., Paterson, D.H., Blimkie, C.J., & Donner, A.P. (1984). Development of cardiorespiratory function in circumpubertal boys: A longitudinal study. *Journal of Applied Physiology: Respiratory, Environmental and Exercise Physiology,* **56,** 302-307.

DUX, L., Dux, E., & Guba, F. (1982). Further data on the anaerobic dependency of the skeletal musculature. The effect of prepubertal castration on the structural development of the skeletal muscles. *Hormone Metabolism Research,* **14,** 191-194.

DUX, L., Dux, E., Mazarean, H., & Guba, F. (1979). A non-neural regulatory effect on the metabolic differentiation of the skeletal muscle. Effect of castration and testosterone administration on the skeletal muscles of the rat. *Comparative Biochemistry and Physiology,* **64A,** 177-183.

ERIKSSON, B.O., Karlsson, J., & Saltin, B. (1971). Muscle metabolites during exercise in pubertal boys. *Acta Paediatrica Scandinavica Supplement,* **217,** 57-63.

GREULICH, W.W., & S.J. Pyle. (1959). *Radiographic atlas of skeletal development of the hand and wrist* (2nd ed.). Stanford: Stanford University Press.

HERMANSEN, L., Resynthesis of muscle glycogen stores during recovery from prolonged exercise in non-diabetic and diabetic subjects. *Acta Paediatrica Scandinavica Supplement,* **283**, 33-38.

HOHORST, H.J. (1965). L-(+) lactate determination with lactic dehydrogenase and DPN. In H.A. Bergmeyer (Ed.), *Methods of enzymatic analysis* (2nd ed.). New York: Academic Press.

KROTKIEWSKI, M., Krol, J.G., & Karlsson, J. (1980) Effects of castration and testosterone substitution on body composition and muscle metabolism in rats. *Acta Physiologica Scandinavica,* **109**, 233-237.

MALINA, R.M. (1980). Physical activity, growth and functional capacity. In F.E. Johnson, A.F. Roche, & C. Susanne (Eds.), *Human physical growth and maturation. Methodologies and factors* (pp. 161-175). New York: Plenum Press.

PATERSON, D.H., Cunningham, D.A., & Bonk, J.M. (1980). Anaerobic capacity of athletic males aged 10, 15 and 21 years. *International Symposium: Growth and Development of the Child.* Trois-Rivères, Quebec.

PATERSON, D.H., Cunningham, D.A., & Bumstead, L.A. (1981). Development of anaerobic capacity in boys aged 11 to 15 years. *Canadian Journal of Applied Sports Sciences,* **6**, 134.

WIRTH, A., Trager, E., Schede, K., Mayer, D., Diehm, K., Reisch, K., & Weicker, H. (1978). Cardiopulmonary adjustment and metabolic response to maximal and submaximal physical exercise of boys and girls at different stages of maturity. *European Journal of Applied Physiology and Occupational Physiology,* **39**, 229-240.

The Optimization of Endurance Training in Adolescent Middle-Distance Runners

Georgine Gaisl and Hubert König
University Graz, Austria

The behavior of lactate has proved to be a sensitive parameter and a highly reproducible one for the definition of the aerobic and anaerobic work capacity of athletes (Aghemo, Ceretelli, Margaria, & Sassi, 1963). The results found from the examinations in the field or in the laboratory have been reported to be related to running speed or to training heart rate and can so be used for the individual regulation of top and adolescent athletes in endurance sports (Föhrenbach, Hollmann, & Mader, 1981).

During this research project field lactate examinations were carried out among others in long- and middle-distance runners. For this article, only the results of the middle-distance runners who were not over 18.2 years of age at the first examination were evaluated.

The schedule of the examinations was in accordance with the following periods of the training year: preparation period 1—competition period for cross-crountry and indoor track; preparation period 2 and competition period.

At the beginning of preparation period 1, there was an examination on the treadmill with the determination of the anaerobic threshold and the maximal performance work capacity. The lactate tests were carried out at the beginning and at the end of preparation period 1 and at the end of preparation period 2. This article deals with only a comparison of the first two examinations.

Subjects and Methods

The first lactate-test (T_1) was carried out in early November 1982, the 2nd (T_2) 3½ months later, in the middle of February 1983. At the first test, the runners were 14.7 to 18.2 years old ($X=17$, $SD=1.20$). Five runners were members of the best Austrian junior team; the other 5 belonged to the best Styrian runners of their age.

The data recording form for the field test is shown in Table 1. The athletes run three times either 2400 m or 2800 m with increased speed on a 400 m running track. After a break of 20 min, a 400 m run is completed with maximal speed. Heart rate is measured by hand (apex beat) before the start and after the end of each run and is, in addition, partly controlled by a telemeter or with the help of a heart rate monitor.

Table 1

Field-Lactate Test
Aerobic Test: 3 × 2,800 m
Anaerobic Test: 1 × 400 m

	Time Planned min/km	Time Reached min	m/s	HR	Lactate mmol/l
At rest					1.55
1. Run	3:45	10:18	4.53	156	2.32
2. Run	3:30	9:30	4.91	180	3.74
3. Run	3:15	8:50	5.28	192	7.43
20 min interval					2.47
400 m		53.5			10.87
3 min					14.60
6 min					14.30
10 min					13.14
20 min					7.90
30 min					5.32

Blood samples were taken from the earlobes and analyzed immediately by means of a lactate analyzer (Roche 640) at the following times: At rest, after each run, 20 min after the 3rd run, and during the 3rd, 6th, 10th, 20th and 30th minute of recovery after the 400 m run. From the graphically presented measured values (Figure 1), the running speed and heart rate at the anaerobic threshold (AT) were determined. The AT is, in accordance with Keul, Kindermann, and Simon (1978), fixed at a lactate value of 4 mmol/l.

Results and Discussion

Table 2 contains the results of the first field test (T_1), which are compared to the results of the second examination (T_2).

The times of runs 1, 2 and 3 were not compared because for technical reasons on the first test, a distance of 2400 m was run while in the second test, the distance was 2800 m. For the determination of the anaerobic threshold, it is the running speed which is critical and not the length of the run. In order to standardize the running speed in the 3 runs, the current work capacity at AT was used. This was done at T_1 by subjective evaluation by the coach and by the athlete, including the results of the previous examination on the treadmill, at T_2 by means of the performance in the previous training period. The running speed was fixed so that a lactate value of 2 to 2.5 mmol/l was expected in the first run, a value slightly less than AT in the second run, and a value higher than AT in the third run. With the help of a course table, the regularity of the running speed was checked and respective information was given to the runner.

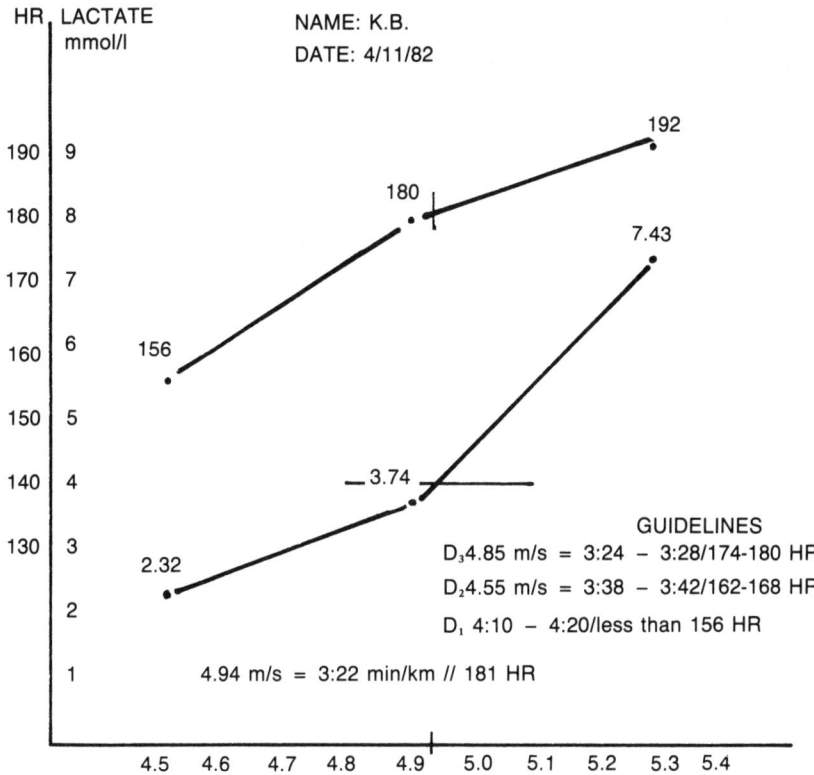

Figure 1—Graphic presentation of field–lactate test. Facsimile of original data form.

Table 2 shows that satisfying this criterion was no problem for the runner. From the determined heart rate and running speed at AT, definite recommendations for the realization of different kinds of endurance training were worked out for each runner individually. A comparison of the running speed at AT during T_1 with the running speed during T_2 showed a distinct improvement. The increase of the middle-running speed at AT was 0.27 m/s—from 4.41 to 4.68 m/s, corresponding to an improvement of 6.12%. Similar improvement was found in running speed at AT under the same type of conditions in cross-country skiers. Members of the best Austrian cross-country skiing team improved 6.15% after a training of 3½ months in preparation period–(Franz & Gaisl, in press). According to the improvement of the variables at AT, the guiding principles related to the recommended running speed and heart rate for different kinds of endurance training were established. In Table 3, the definitions of these training forms are constructed from practice: D_3 for an intensive endurance training, T_2 for extensive training and D_1 for regenerative endurance training. In order to make instruction more understandable for the athlete, the running speed was converted from m/s into a so-called "kilometer-average"—that is to say, how fast a kilometer should be run.

Table 2

Field-Lactate Test—Part 1

Determination of the anaerobic threshold

Variables		Units	1 Test Mean	SD	2 Test Mean	SD
Lactate at rest		(mmol/l)	1.19	0.21	1.15	0.26
1. run:	Speed	(m/s)	4.01	0.33	4.38	0.26
	Heart rate	(b/min)	163.2	12.26	166.2	12.35
	Lactate	(mmol/l)	2.44	0.76	2.32	0.98
2. run:	Speed	(m/s)	4.32	0.43	4.65	.29
	Heart rate	(b/min)	179.4	11.82	184.0	7.12
	Lactate	(mmol/l)	3.17	0.96	3.95	1.70
3. run:	Speed	(m/s)	4.60	0.45	4.92	0.30
	Heart rate	(b/min)	194.4	10.28	195.6	9.47
	Lactate	(mmol/l)	5.78	2.01	6.82	1.83
	Lactate 20th min of recovery		2.45	1.13	3.17	1.32
Anaerobic threshold:	Speed	(m/s)	4.41	0.42	4.68	0.24
	Speed	(min/km)	3:48.7	22.7	3:34.3	10.0
	Heart rate	(b/min)	185.4	11.15	181.7	10.94

Table 4 illustrates the second part of the field test, which provides information about the present anaerobic state of performance. The athlete had to run 400 m using maximal effort. The criteria for the judgment were the lactate-value attained related to the 400 m running time and the speed of the reduction of lactate. During preparation period 1, the athletes practiced exclusively under aerobic conditions. Thus, in this part of the examination, the change of the anerobic work capacity was examined.

After the 400 m run the heart rate at T_1 was measured by hand and in 6 athletes at the same time registered telemetrically. The comparison of the measured values showed that the number of errors of the measurement by hand was relatively high because of the high heart-rate, as opposed to the relatively low number of errors in the first part of the test. Moreover, the measured heart rates after the 400 m run offer no suggestions for training. Therefore, no more heart rates were measured after the 400 m run during the second test.

Conclusion

The determination of the lactate concentration in the blood as an expression of the anaerobic part of energy metabolism allows the differentiation of top-performance capacity and endurance performance capacity. This differentiation is very important for endurance kinds of sport. The knowledge of the variables of AT is also important for

Table 3

Field-Lactate Test

Guiding principles for the training practice
(Mean (min) and Standard Deviation (s) given)

Variables	Units	1 Test		2 Test	
D_3 Speed	(min/km)	3:50.5	- 3:55.1	3:38.1	- 3:42.5
		21.79	22.12	11.93	11.97
Heart rate	(b/min)	177.0	183.0	175.8	181.6
		10.3	10.3	11.33	11.15
D_2 Speed	(min/km)	4:05.3	4:10.4	3.54.3	3:58.7
		22.14	23.65	14.61	14.61
Heart rate	(b/min)	167.4	173.4	168.0	172.8
		9.14	9.14	10.95	9.30
D_1 Speed	(min/km)	4:33.0	- 3:52.0	4:19.0	- 4:31.0
		20.58	24.40	11.01	8.76
Heart rate	(b/min)	159.6		162.2	
		6.45		7.86	

D_3 = intensive endurance training
D_2 = extensive endurance training
D_1 = regenerative endurance training

Table 4

Field-Lactate Test—Part 2
Determination of the Anaerobic State of Performance

Variables	Units	1 Test Mean	SD	2 Test Mean	SD
400	(s)	58.26	3.29	58.4	3.08
Lactate	(mmol/l)	8.59	2.49	7.00	1.98
Lactate	3rd min of recovery	12.49	1.43	11.67	1.71
Lactate	6th min of recovery	13.26	1.76	11.90	1.64
Lactate	10th min of recovery	12.41	2.02	11.38	1.54
Lactate	20th min of recovery	9.45	2.44	7.81	1.58
Lactate	30th min of recovery	6.43	2.51	5.66	1.63

purposes of practical training because an optimal intensity stimulus can be expected for the improvement of the aerobic capacity during endurance training in this zone

(Heck, Liesen, & Mader, 1976). Repeated examinations in the laboratory and in the sports field must be conducted because a change of the heart rate at AT is to be expected with the continuance of training. The movements, the working muscles and the achieved intensities in the laboratory and in the field test must largely correspond (Berg, Dickhuth, & Keul, 1981). Only then can it be assumed that endurance training with a load intensity at AT is optimal and that it leads to the greatest possible effect with the least training effort; that is to say, to the most distinct development of general endurance (Gaisl, König, Pessenhofer, & Schwaberger, 1980). For the determination of the optimal training intensity, repeated field tests are of great importance.

Acknowledgments

This study was supported by Grant no. 4619 from the Austrian Research Council (Fonds zur Förderung der wissenschaftlichen Forschung).

References

FÖHRENBACH, R., Mader, A., & Hollmann, W. (1981). Umfang und Intensität im Dauerlauftraining von Mittelstreckenläuferinnen des DLV und Maβnahmen zur individuellen Trainings— und Wettkampfoptimierung (Extent and intensity of the endurance training of female middle-distance runners of the DLV and measure for the individual optimization of training and competition). *Leistungssport,* **11**, 458-472.

FRANZ, W., & Gaisl, G. (in press). Felduntersuchungen bei den Skilangläufern in der Vorbereitungsperiode (Field-examinations in cross country skiers during the preparation period). *Leistungssport.*

GAISL, G., König, H., Pessenhofer, H., & Schwaberger, G. (1980). Die Trainingsoptimierung im Mittel- und Langstreckenlauf mit Hilfe der Bestimmung des aerob-anaeroben Schwellenbereiches (Optimization of training in medium- and long-distance running, aided by determination of the aerobic and anaerobic threshold zones). *Deutsche Zeitschrift für Sportmedizin,* **31**, 131-140.

KEUL, J., Dickhuth, H.H., & Berg, A. (1981). Allgemeine und sportartspezifische Leistungsdiagnostik im Hochleistungssport (General and discipline—specific diagnosis of performance in top performance sport). *Leistungssport,* **11**, 382-398.

KEUL, J., Kindermann, W., & Simon, G. (1978). Die aerobe und anerobe Kapazität als Grundlage für die Leistungsdiagnostik (The aerobic and anaerobic capacity as a basis for diagnostic achievement). *Leistungssport,* **8**, 22-32.

KINDERMANN, W., Simon, G., & Keul, J. (1978). Dauertraining-Ermittlung der optimalen Trainingsherzfrequenz und Leistungsfähigkeit (Endurance training—determination of optimal training heart frequency and working capacity). *Leistungssport,* **8**, 34-39.

MADER, A., Liesen, H. & Heck, H. (1976). Zur Beurteilung der sportartspezifischen Ausdauerleistungsfähigkeit im Labor (For the estimation of the discipline specific endurance work capacity in the lab). *Sportarzt,* **27**, 80-88, 109-112.

MARGARIA, R., Cerretelli, P., Aghemo, P., & Sassi, G. (1963). Energy cost of running. *Journal of Applied Physiology,* **18**, 367-371.

Effects of Supplemental Physical Activity on Body Composition, Aerobic and Anaerobic Power in 13-Year-Old Boys

Anthony J. Sargeant, Patricia Dolan, and Adrian Thorne
Polytechnic of North London
London, England

An interesting question is how much of an effect physical education programs might reasonably be expected to have upon the short-term physical fitness of children (Duquet & Gregoire, 1978; Kemper et al., 1978; Rutenfranz & Singer, 1980).

In an attempt to provide some insight into this question, the effects of supplementing the normal school physical education program with additional periods specifically devoted to fitness training were studied.

Methods

A sample of 13-year-old boys (n=28) attending a secondary school in North London were studied over an 8-week period during the fall term (September to December). The school authorities, parents, and boys, gave their informed consent for participation in the study. The children were divided into a control and a training group. Both groups followed the normal curriculum, nominally consisting of 150 min of sports activities per week, but the training group had two additional periods amounting to a further 150 min each week. These periods were specifically devoted to fitness training. The content of the supplementary periods was designed to include a balanced mixture of short-term power and endurance training as well as some weight training.

Maximum oxygen uptake was directly determined using standard techniques as previously described by Sargeant, Dolan, and Thorne (1983).

Short-term (anaerobic) power was assessed using the isokinetic cycle ergometer developed and described by Sargeant, Hoinville, and Young (1981). The data reported here are maximal peak power (PPmax), that is, the power generated at the instant of maximal peak force, measured at a pedaling speed of 108 rev/min. PPmax is expressed as the sum of both legs. For further discussion of these techniques, readers are referred to Sargeant et al. (1981).

Lean body mass was estimated from the sum of four skinfolds (Durnin & Rahaman, 1967). Leg muscle (plus bone) volumes were estimated by anthropometry (Sargeant & Davies, 1977).

Results

At the start of the study there were no significant differences in age, height, weight, lean body mass, or leg (muscle plus bone) volume, although it might be noted that members of the training group were slightly taller and heavier than the control group (see Table 1). Following the 8-week period of study, both groups were taller and heavier than at the start ($p<.001$). The control group showed an increase in lean body mass which was proportional (2.5%; $p<.01$) to the overall increase in body size, whereas in the training group there was an increase in lean body mass of nearly twice that level (+4.8%; $p<.001$). The increases in lean body mass were associated with larger leg muscle volumes. For example, in the control group, upper leg muscle (plus bone) volume increased, although not significantly, by 3%, while the training group showed a much more dramatic and highly significant increase of 9.7% ($p<.01$). It is only in this last physical characteristic that there was a significant difference between the groups at the end of the study period ($p<.05$).

Maximum oxygen uptake was not significantly different between the groups before training but there was a slightly higher absolute value for the training group, reflecting the tendency for this group to be somewhat larger and heavier than the controls. This difference was largely accounted for when standardized for body weight (see Table 2). During the study period the $\dot{V}O_2$ max of the training group increased in direct proportion to body size. Hence when expressed in relation to body weight, there was no change from the initial value of 53 ml/kg/min. In marked contrast, the control group showed a significant decrease of 6% in absolute terms, and this difference was exacerbated when account was taken of the growth-related increase in body weight so that there was a 9% reduction in $\dot{V}O_2$ max when expressed in ml/kg/min ($p<.01$). As a consequence of the deterioration in the control group, there was a significant difference

Table 1

Physical Characteristics of Subjects

Mean (SD) data for age, height, weight, lean body mass (LBM), leg muscle plus bone volume (LV), and upper leg muscle plus bone volume (ULV)

		Age (yrs)	Height (cm)	Weight (kg)	LBM (kg)	LV (l)	ULV (l)
Control (n = 13)	Before	13.6(0.27)	158.3(8.5)	48.9(6.1)	40.6(5.1)	5.11(0.87)	3.38(0.66)
	After	13.8(0.27)	159.8(8.7)	50.0(6.2)	41.6(5.3)	5.24(0.82)	3.48(0.58)
	% Change	+1.1%***	+0.9%***	+2.2%**	+2.5%**	+2.5%	+3%
Training (n = 15)	Before	13.7(0.28)	164.8(10.6)	52.5(9.7)	43.7(7.1)	5.78(1.07)	3.82(0.75)
	After	13.8(0.28)	166.6(11)	54.1(9.8)	45.8(7.5)	6.24(1.23)	4.19(0.85)±
	% Change	+1.1%***	+1.1%***	+3%***	+4.8%***	+8%***	+9.7%**

Significance: Between groups, ± $p<.05$
Significance: Within groups, * $p<.05$; ** $p<.01$; *** $p<.001$

Table 2

Maximum Oxygen Uptake

Mean (SD) of directly measured maximal oxygen uptake
in absolute terms (1/min) and standardized for body weight (ml/kg/min)

	Control Group (n=8)		Training Group (n=8)	
	1/min	ml/kg/min	1/min	ml/kg/min
Before	2.41(0.39)	50(6)	2.67(0.33)	53(8)
After	2.27(0.35)	45(3)	2.73(0.29)	53(8)
% Change	-6%*	-10%**	+2%	0%

Significance as for Table 1.

($p<.05$) between the groups at the end of the study in absolute values of $\dot{V}O_2$ max and when standardized for body weight.

Maximum peak power output (PPmax) was slightly, though not significantly, greater in the training group compared to the control. This difference again reflects the slight size difference between the groups. Hence, when expressed in terms of body weight, PPmax was almost identical for the two groups: 30.9 and 31.2 W/kg for the control and training groups, respectively (see Table 3). During the study, the control group increased their PPmax from 1522 to 1578 W (3.7%; $p<.05$), but because this was associated with a concomitant increase in body size, there was no significant change in the PPmax expressed as W/kg body weight. The training group showed a larger increase from 1622 to 1760 W (8.5%: p<01). Thus, when expressed in terms of body weight, there was a 4.5% increase in PPmax from 31.2 to 32.6 W/kg, although this change did not reach conventional levels of significance.

Table 3

Maximum Peak Power (2-Legs)

Mean (SD) data for maximal peak (anaerobic) power
given in absolute terms (W) and standardized
for body weight (W/kg)

	Control Group (n=11)		Training Group (n=15)	
	W	W/kg	W	W/kg
Before	1522(292)	30.9(3.6)	1622(298)	31.2(5.2)
After	1578(342)	31.3(4.8)	1760(312)	31.2(5.2)
%Change	+3.7%*	+1.2%	+8.5%**	+4.5%

Significance as for Table 1.

Discussion

The normal curriculum followed by the children in this study consisted of 150 min of sports-related activities per week, which included only a relatively small proportion of time devoted specifically to elements of fitness training. In contrast, the supplementary periods were devoted entirely to fitness training organized on a group basis, using standard gymnasium equipment and activities. These included interval sprints, 4-min pursuit races, and weight training. Clearly some caution should be exercised in attempting to extrapolate the results of the present study to other situations.

It should also be noted that the study was carried out during the fall term between September and December, immediately following the long summer vacation. It seemed reasonable to assume that for boys of this age, the habitual physical activity level was much higher during the summer vacation than on return to school, when most of the time was spent in sedentary classroom-based activities. At the same time, there was an additional factor, which was the effect of shorter daylight hours which progressively curtailed outdoor activities during this period.

In the light of these observations, it is perhaps not surprising that the normal physical education curriculum of only 150 min/week fails to compensate for the enforced overall reduction in habitual physical activity, and that as a consequence, the control group showed a significant deterioration in maximum oxygen uptake from 50 to 45 ml/kg/min (-10%; $p<.05$). Even with the two-period supplement, the training group only managed to maintain maximum oxygen uptake at the initial value of 53 ml/kg/min and did not improve it.

In contrast short-term (anaerobic) power output, presented here as maximal peak power (PPmax), increased significantly in both groups. In the control group, this increase was 3.7% ($p.<.05$) which can be seen as an accurate reflection and consequence of physical growth over the experimental period. Total body weight increased by 2.2% and upper leg muscle mass increased by 3% (see Table 1). The training group also showed an increase in PPmax expressed in absolute terms, from 1622 to 1760 W. Although this mean change of 8.5% was over twice that of the control group, it was associated with a similarly large increase in upper leg muscle volume (+9.7%: $p<.01$).

In conclusion, when considered in terms of maximum oxygen uptake, it may be directly or indirectly possible to at least compensate for the enforced reduction in habitual physical activity on returning to school after the summer vacation by supplementing the normal school physical education program. It also appears that changes in maximal short-term power were closely related to the size of the active muscles in these groups and that it is possible to increase this by means of a training program occupying relatively little time. This may be in contrast to the time needed to sustain or increase maximum oxygen uptake.

References

DUQUET, W., & Gregoire, D. (1978). Work capacity, strength, and body measurements of adolescent boys in a special sports program compared to normal boys: initial comparison. In J. Borms & M. Hebbelinck (Eds.), *Pediatric work physiology* (pp. 167-172). Basel: Karger.

DURNIN, J.V.G.A., & Rahaman, M.M. (1967). The assessment of the amount of fat in the human body from measurements of skinfold thickness. *British Journal of Nutrition,* **21**, 681-689.

KEMPER. H.C.G., Verschuur, R. Ras, K.G.A., Snel, J., Splinter, P.G., & Tavecchio, L.W.C. (1978). Investigation into the effects of two extra physical education lessons per week during one school year upon the physical development of 12- and 13-year-old boys. In J. Borms & M. Hebbelinck (Eds.), *Pediatric work physiology* (pp. 159-166). Basel: Karger.

RUTENFRANZ, J. & Singer, R. (1980). The influence of sport activity on the development of physical performance capacities of 15-17-year-old boys. In K. Berg, & B.O. Eriksson (Eds.), *Children and Exercise IX* (pp. 160-165). Baltimore: University Park Press.

SARGEANT, A.J. & Davies, C.T.M. (1977). Limb volume composition and maximum aerobic power output in relation to habitual 'preference' in young male subjects. *Annals of Human Biology*, **4**, 49-55.

SARGEANT, A.J., Dolan, P. & Thorne, A. (in press). Isokinetic measurement of maximal leg force and anaerobic power output in children. In *Children and Exercise X*. Berlin: Springer-Verlag.

SARGEANT, A.J., Hoinville, E., & Young, A. (1981). Maximum leg force and power output during short-term dynamic exercise. *Journal of Applied Physiology: Respiratory, Environmental, Exercise Physiology*, **51** (5), 1175-1182.

Treadmill Endurance Times, Blood Lactate, and Exercise Blood Pressures in Normal Children

Gordon R. Cumming, Laverne Hastman, and Joy McCort
The Children's Hospital of Winnipeg and The University of Manitoba
Winnipeg, Manitoba, Canada

Normal values for the Bruce treadmill protocol using as test subjects children sent for cardiac evaluation for what proved to be innocent heart murmurs have been reported previously (Cumming, Everatt, & Hastman, 1978) and have been compared to normal values obtained in volunteers from the school system (Cumming & Hnatiuk, 1980). It has also been emphasized that when patients are to be compared to normal subjects all subjects should be exercised in the same laboratory over the same time period (Cumming, 1978). Data for normal children exercised over the last 4 years have been calculated and compared to the normal values obtained over the 3 preceding years. The new normal values were higher. This was attributed to the greater experience of the laboratory in knowing how to get close to maximal efforts from the children tested in a clinical situation. In addition to presenting new norms for the Bruce treadmill protocol in children, data on exercise blood pressure and postexercise lactic acid are presented in this article.

Subjects

All subjects were referred to cardiology because of heart murmurs. All had normal electrocardiograms at rest, normal heart size and sounds, and normal pulses and blood pressures. M-mode echocardiography was carried out in 78% of the subjects and showed normal dimensions and structures. The heart was considered clinically normal in all subjects. All but 6 of 788 exercise tests done consecutively on normal children in the laboratory from 1978 to 1981 were included in the analysis. These 6 children were excluded because the technicians subjectively felt that their efforts were well short of maximal. The remaining 782 subjects were arbitrarily divided into 6 age groups by sex. Their anthropometric data are given in Table 1.

Methods

The Bruce protocol (Bruce, Kusumi, & Hosmer, 1973) was followed on a programmed treadmill. The belt speed and the grade indicator were calibrated at regular intervals.

Table 1
Anthropometric Data

Age Group	Boys				Girls			
	Number of Subjects (m)	Mean Age (years)	Height (cm)	Weight (kg)	Number of Subjects (m)	Mean Age (years)	Height (cm)	Weight (kg)
4-5	107	4.6 ± 0.5	109.3 ± 5.6	19.5 ± 2.7	95	4.6 ± 0.5	107.4 ± 5.7	18.3 ± 2.8
6-7	72	6.5 ± .05	119.4 ± 6.3	23.2 ± 4.4	71	6.3 ± 4.9	118.0 ± 5.9	22.1 ± 3.3
8-9	66	8.4 ± 0.5	130.8 ± 7.6	29.4 ± 4.8	37	8.5 ± 0.5	128.1 ± 8.9	27.3 ± 5.6
10-12	83	11.0 ± 0.8	146.6 ± 8.6	39.9 ± 8.5	65	10.9 ± 0.8	144.7 ± 9.3	38.7 ± 7.9
13-15	58	13.9 ± 0.9	162.2 ± 9.2	53.7 ± 11.2	66	14.1 ± 0.7	160.8 ± 6.5	54.3 ± 12.3
16-20	43	17.2 ± 1.4	170.8 ± 6.8	66.8 ± 11.9	19	17.4 ± 1.4	159.3 ± 9.7	56.5 ± 11.5

ECG lead CM5 was monitored during the test. Children were encouraged to continue until they seemed to be nearly exhausted. Hanging on to the guard rails was prohibited. Some children under 6 years were allowed to hang on to one finger of the technician for light support and encouragement.

Two minutes after cessation of the exercise, 2.0 ml of venous blood was obtained without stasis from an anticubital vein, placed in a chilled tube containing 14 mg of dried potassium oxalate and 17.5 mg of sodium fluoride and kept on ice, and later centrifuged and frozen for lactate estimation using an enzymatic method adapted to autoanalyzer technology (Westgard, Lahmeyer, & Birnbaum, 1972). Blood pressure was measured by sphygmomanometry at rest, during exercise for Stages 1 to 3, and within 30 s of stopping exercise with the subject sitting in a chair, and after 2 and 5 min of recovery. Phase 5 was used for diastolic pressure, but if this went below 50 mm Hg during recovery from exercise, Phase 4 (muffling) was used if a distinct end point was noted.

Results

The mean endurance time results along with the centile values are given in Table 2 for the previous (Cumming, Everatt, & Hastman, 1978) and the current normal subjects. Period 1 study involved 167 boys and 160 girls tested from 1975 to 1977; the current Period 2 study included 429 boys and 353 girls tested form 1978 to 1981. Comparing Period 1 to Period 2, boys aged 4 to 5 years showed an increase in mean endurance time of 1.1 min (11%; $p<.05$), and the 10th centile level increased from 8.1 to 9.5 min (17%). Girls aged 4 to 5 years showed an increase in mean endurance time of 1.5 min (16%; $p<.05$), and the 10th centile level increased from 7.0 to 9.5 min (21%). Girls aged 6 to 7 years showed an increase in mean endurance time of 1.1 min (10%; $p<.05$), and the 10th centile level increased from 9.5 to 11 min (16%).

While the changes in the mean times for the 8- to 12-year-old girls were of small magnitude, the 10th centile values for Period 2 subjects were higher by over 10%. For the remaining girls groups, the differences in mean values were smaller than 5%, as were the 10th centile values. The major differences in these normal values collected at different times were in the mean values and the 10th centile values for age groups 4 to 5 and 6 to 7 for both boys and girls, and the 10th centile levels in the 10- to 12-year-old boys. At the upper end of the scale the times for the most fit children (the 90th centile) did not differ from one study period to the other.

The age trends in treadmill endurance with the Bruce protocol were similar to those in our previous studies (Cumming, Everatt, & Hastman, 1978). For boys there was an increase in mean endurance time from 11.5 min at ages 4 to 5, to 14.3 min at ages 16 to 20 years. Even so, the top 25% of the 4- to 5-year-old boys were able to last longer than the bottom 20% of the 13- to 20-year-old boys. The mean endurance times for the girls peaked at age 6 to 7 years, was essentially stable to age 12 years, and then decreased. The 4- to 7-year-old girls had mean values within a half minute of boys of the same age. The top 25% of the 10- to 20-year-old girls were able to do more work than the bottom 15% of boys in the comparative age groups.

Our earlier studies provided values for $\dot{V}O_2$ max for children in relation to their treadmill endurance times (Cumming, Everatt, & Hastman, 1978). For 8- to 12-year-old girls 12.0 min corresponds to a $\dot{V}O_2$ max of about 44 ml·kg^{-1}min^{-1}, and for boys 14.0

Table 2

Centiles and Mean Values for Treadmill Endurance Times

Age Groups (years)	Number of Subjects P1	Number of Subjects P2	Centiles 10 P1	Centiles 10 P2	Centiles 25 P1	Centiles 25 P2	Centiles 50 P1	Centiles 50 P2	Centiles 75 P1	Centiles 75 P2	Centiles 90 P1	Centiles 90 P2	Endurance Time (min) Mean ± Standard Deviation P1[a]	Endurance Time (min) Mean ± Standard Deviation P2
Males
4– 5	40	107	8.1	9.5	9.0	10.5	10.0	11.5	12.0	12.5	13.3	13.5	10.4 ± 1.9	11.5 ± 1.5*
6– 7	28	72	9.7	10.8	10.0	12.0	12.0	12.5	12.3	13.0	13.5	14.0	11.8 ± 1.6	12.5 ± 1.2
8– 9	30	66	9.6	12.0	10.5	12.5	12.4	13.0	13.7	13.5	16.2	15.0	12.6 ± 2.3	13.2 ± 1.4
10–12	31	83	9.9	11.0	12.0	13.0	12.5	13.5	14.0	14.0	15.4	15.5	12.7 ± 1.9	13.5 ± 1.7
13–15	26	58	11.2	12.0	13.0	12.9	14.3	13.8	16.0	14.9	16.1	15.5	14.1 ± 1.7	13.8 ± 1.4
16–20	12	43	11.3	10.5	12.1	13.0	13.8	14.3	14.5	15.8	15.8	17.5	13.5 ± 1.4	14.3 ± 2.3
Females
4– 5	36	95	7.0	9.5	8.0	10.0	9.0	11.0	11.2	12.0	12.3	12.5	9.5 ± 1.8	11.0 ± 1.4*
6– 7	34	71	9.5	11.9	9.6	11.5	11.4	12.3	13.0	13.0	13.0	13.5	11.2 ± 1.5	12.3 ± 1.2*
8– 9	26	37	9.9	10.5	10.5	11.0	11.0	12.1	13.0	13.0	14.2	13.5	11.8 ± 1.6	12.2 ± 1.1
10–12	28	65	10.5	10.5	11.3	11.0	12.0	12.1	13.0	13.0	14.6	13.6	12.3 ± 1.4	12.1 ± 1.3
13–15	24	66	9.4	9.0	10.0	10.0	11.5	11.1	12.0	12.0	13.0	13.0	11.1 ± 1.3	11.1 ± 1.7
16–20	12	19	8.1	9.2	10.0	10.3	10.5	11.1	12.0	12.3	12.4	15.0	10.7 ± 1.4	11.6 ± 1.7

[a]P1 = Period 1, P2 = Period 2
*$p<.05$

min corresponds to a $\dot{V}O_2$ max of about 55 ml·kg⁻¹min⁻¹. The aerobic fitness of these children with innocent heart murmurs would seem to be about the same as has been reported for other groups of normal children (Rutenfranz, Lange-Andersen, Seliger, & Maseroni, 1982; Shephard, Allen, & Bor-Or, 1968), better than some (Eriksson, 1972; Matsui, Miayshita, & Miura, 1970), and below some (Åstrand, 1972; Kemper & Verscheur, 1980; Rode & Shephard, 1973; Wilmore & Sigerseth, 1967).

Comparing Period 1 to Period 2, the mean maximal heart rates (see Table 3) increased for all age groups but the significant changes were for the 4- to 5- and 6- to 7-year-old age groups for both sexes and the 16- to 20-year-old age group for the girls. In the entire population of new normals, only 5% of the subjects had maximal heart rates less than 190 beats/min. Using the mean minus 2 standard deviations as the lower limit for normal maximal heart rates, these values ranged from 177 to 192 beats/min for boys and 182 to 187 beats/min for girls in the various age groups.

The submaximal heart rates during Stage III (see Table 4) were high (163 to 194 beats/min) considering that most subjects continued to exercise 3 or more minutes after this recording. The mean heart rates for Stage III showed no consistent differences between Period 1 and Period 2.

The mean lactate values are given in Table 5, and ranged from 8.1 to 13.7 mmol·L⁻¹ for males and 8.4 to 11.5 mmol·L⁻¹ for girls. Mean values showed a steady increase in the boys with age with a greater increase after age 15. The mean values for the girls were minimally higher than for the boys for all age groups except after age 15 years. Using minus 2 standard deviations from the mean as the lowest level for normal for the subjects, values were as low as 2.9 for 4- to 5-year-old boys, 5.0 for the 13- to 15-year-old boys.

However, only 13% of subjects under age 12 had lactate values below 6.0 mmol·L⁻¹. Only 3 subjects (0.5%) under age 12 had both lactate below 6.0 mmol·L⁻¹ and maximal heart rate below 190 beats·min⁻¹; only 2 subjects (1%) age 12 and over had both lactate below 8.0 mmol·L⁻¹ and maximal heart rate below 190 beats·min⁻¹.

The blood pressure values are given in Table 6. The highest systolic values were recorded immediately after exercise and showed a gradual increase with age. The normal range was wide. The values tended to be higher after the age of 9 years in the

Table 3

Maximal Heart Rates

	Males		Females	
Age	Period 1	Period 2	Period 1	Period 2
4- 5	200 ± 9	205 ± 10*	199 ± 10	206 ± 10*
6- 7	201 ± 7	206 ± 7*	206 ± 4	207 ± 10
8- 9	200 ± 6	204 ± 8	202 ± 9	206 ± 9
10-12	199 ± 7	203 ± 7	204 ± 8	205 ± 8
13-15	198 ± 6	201 ± 12	196 ± 6	200 ± 9
16-20	201 ± 6	201 ± 10	193 ± 5	200 ± 8

*Increase Period 2, $p \leq .05$

Table 4

Heart Rates at the End of Stage III of the Treadmill Protocol (Beats·min⁻¹)

Age	Males		Females	
	Period 1	Period 2	Period 1	Period 2
4- 5	189 ± 13	189 ± 14	195 ± 14	194 ± 15
6- 7	188 ± 12	188 ± 11	196 ± 6	188 ± 15
8- 9	177 ± 12	178 ± 16	180 ± 13	187 ± 14
10-12	174 ± 13	173 ± 15	188 ± 11	187 ± 13
13-15	163 ± 14	169 ± 17	180 ± 16	187 ± 14
16-20	174 ± 12	163 ± 19	186 ± 9	180 ± 18

(No significant differences)

Table 5

Post Exercise Serum Lactate (mmol·L⁻¹)

Age	n	Males Mean	n	Females Mean
4- 5	61	8.1 ± 2.6[a]	48	8.4 ± 2.3
6- 7	58	8.9 ± 2.7	60	9.4 ± 2.3
8- 9	60	9.0 ± 2.8	34	10.5 ± 3.1
10-12	71	9.5 ± 2.5	58	10.7 ± 2.7
13-15	56	10.8 ± 2.9	54	11.5 ± 3.2
16-20	39	13.7 ± 3.4	16	11.5 ± 2.8

[a]mean plus standard deviation

boys. The 95% confidence limits for systolic blood pressure recorded within 20 or 30 s of stopping exercise in 13- to 15-year-old boys ranged from 116 to 200 mm Hg. This very large range of normal values makes the measurement of blood pressure of limited values except in specific situations such as patients with myocardial disease, aortic stenosis, or coarctation of the aorta. Other studies have found similarly wide ranges for blood pressure values during exercise in children (Riopel, Taylor, & Hohn, 1979).

Discussion

The longer endurance times of subjects in Period 2 could be explained by postulating higher levels of fitness. If this were the case, submaximal heart rates for a given exercise load should have been lower, but they were not. One of the major determinants

Table 6
Blood Pressures—1981 Normals

Age	m	Rest Syst.	Rest Diast.	Stage 1 Syst.	Stage 1 Diast.	Stage 2 Syst.	Stage 2 Diast.	Stage 3 Syst.	Stage 3 Diast.	Early Recovery Syst.	Early Recovery Diast.	Recovery 2'R Syst.	Recovery 2'R Diast.	Recovery 5'R Syst.	Recovery 5'R Diast.
Males															
4- 5	107	98± 9	59±10	109±11	64± 9	117±11	66± 8	125± 5	76± 8	127±13	68±11	113±14	63±10	102±12	59± 8
6- 7	72	101±11	58± 9	115±14	65± 9	123±12	66±11	130±14	71±12	133±14	70±14	119±15	64±12	106±12	60±12
8- 9	66	105±11	64±12	117±12	66±10	126±12	69±10	131±12	73±10	140±12	73±15	124±13	65±12	112±12	62±10
10-12	83	106±10	65±10	121±13	70± 8	129±13	69±10	135±13	71±10	146±15	73±12	129±12	67±11	113±10	62± 9
13-15	58	113±14	65±10	130±17	69±10	140±17	69± 9	151±18	70±11	158±21	68±12	143±19	61±10	121±15	61±10
16-20	43	121±16	70±12	135±17	73±10	145±19	73±10	156±17	75±12	163±19	75±13	149±19	64±11	125±16	61±10
Females															
4- 5	95	96± 8	56± 9	105±10	61± 8	112±91	65± 8	118± 7	73± 8	126±14	65±13	112±12	60±10	100±11	56± 9
6- 7	71	98± 9	60± 9	110±12	64± 9	119±12	67± 9	127±12	73±10	132±17	70±16	117±14	63±11	104±12	58±10
8- 9	37	100±10	60±11	115±12	66±10	124±12	67±11	130±12	70±12	136±14	71±13	122±11	66±10	108± 9	59±11
10-12	65	108±14	64±11	122±16	65±11	131±15	67± 9	140±17	69±10	144±16	67±13	129±15	60±12	113±14	56± 9
13-15	66	108±13	66±11	123±16	70±10	133±16	71±10	144±17	75±10	146±21	72±15	122±18	67±12	177±18	62±11
16-20	19	109± 9	67±11	125±13	69±11	136±16	70±12	140±15	72±13	144±21	74±13	135±17	63±11	199±13	59± 9

Syst. = systolic mm Hg
Diast. = diastolic mm Hg

of treadmill endurance is body weight with heavier and fatter subjects not surprisingly having reduced endurance times (Cumming & Hnatiuk, 1980). Since there were no significant differences in the mean height/weight ratios for subjects studied in Periods 1 and 2; this tended to exclude body build as a possible explanation for the differences in endurance. It is likely that the longer endurance times for the Group 2 subjects were due to the technicians knowing what to expect from the children, thus setting definite minimal goals, and encouraging the subjects to reach these goals. At the time of obtaining the Period 1 values, there were no published standards for children for the Bruce protocol.

At present all 4- and 5-year-olds are encouraged to at least perform 1 min at Stage IV, and the technologists try to have children persevere until this level of performance is reached. All boys over 7 years of age were encouraged to do at least a minute of Stage V of the protocol. The termination of the test was most commonly a mutual agreement between the exercise technician and the children: The children claimed severe fatigue and a desire to stop, while the technician urged them to finish just another 30 or 100 s, the end point most commonly decided by arbitration.

The experience and tenacity of the technician is of paramount importance. After leaving the exercise room, the subjects were routinely asked if they could have run a little longer, and while some pleaded absolute exhaustion, most indicated they could have continued for another 30 s. Another factor likely contributing to the higher values for the lower centiles of endurance was the larger number of subjects studied in Period 2.

The finding of a significant increase in some of the mean endurance times and an increase in the lower limits for endurance times in a second study performed in the same laboratory with the same direction and philosophy points out two fundamental principles. First, each laboratory needs to establish its own normal values for exercise capacity; and second, all tests should be carried out continuously over the same time period in the same laboratory when different groups of subjects (i.e., cardiac patients vs. normals) are to be compared.

The lactate values in this study confirm earlier work from this laboratory (Cumming, Hastman, McCort, & McCollough, 1980). While the younger children had slightly lower values for mean post exercise lactate, most of the lactate values in prepubertal children in the present study were higher than have been reported (Åstrand, 1952; Eriksson, 1972). The current values in postpubertal children were about the same as those reported (Åstrand, 1952). While methodological differences cannot be completely excluded as an explanation for the higher lactates in our younger children, the most likely explanation is that our children were encouraged to work harder and utilized more of their anaerobic reserves than the children in the other studies. If methodological factors were responsible for the differences, the lactate results for the postpubertal children should have been higher than previously reported, but they are in the same range.

The maximal heart rates reported for children vary. Most investigators have not been able to reproduce the very high rates reported by Åstrand (1952). The maximal rates in Åstrand's study were obtained by auscultation, and at rates above 200 in a moving subject, the changes for error were perhaps greater. Our large experience suggests that mean maximal heart rates of less than 200 beats/min in young children performing treadmill exercise (as in the study of Riopel, Taylor, & Hohn, 1979) likely indicate that the exercise was terminated well before the point of severe fatigue, and such tests should not be regarded as maximal.

The blood pressure of normal children during exercise shows wide fluctuations as it also does for normal adults (Bruce, DeRouen, & Hossack, 1980). Our maximal pressures are lower than those reported by others for children, and lower than what we have obtained with bicycle exercise. In part this is because pressure measurements were not taken when the children started to run during Stage 4 of the Bruce test so that pressure was not measured during near-maximal work. Pressures obtained during Stage III of the protocol are below those found at peak exercise, and pressures obtained 20 to 30 s after stopping the exercise are also lower than those obtained during maximal exercise. It is difficult to know how reliable indirect pressure measurements are when the subject is straining with near-maximal effort.

We found that our previous mean values for endurance time were about 10% below mean values obtained with volunteers in the schools (Cumming & Hnatiuk, 1980). The new clinic mean values were within 5% of the school values in 7 of the 10 age and sex groups, and equalled or slightly exceeded the school mean values in 4 of the 10 sex and age groups.

Previous clinic lower limits (the 10th centile) for endurance time were as much as 25% below the school values. The new clinic values were equal or slightly above the school 10th centile values for age groups 6 to 7 and 8 to 9 but were about a minute lower for the older age groups, and 1.9 min lower for the 13- to 15-year-old girls. These differences are likely because less active children or less fit children were referred for evaluation in the clinic series, while many children not keen on exercise were eliminated from the school series because of the need to have a voluntary selection system.

When has a child produced an effort that can be accepted as near maximal? Previous studies have shown that less than 50% of children reach a plateau in oxygen intake as work load is increased (Åstrand, 1952; Cumming & Friesen, 1967), and that this physiological end point is not reproducible in children (Cunningham, Van Watershoot, & Patterson, 1977). Many of the children in this current study might have stayed another 1 or even 2 min longer on the treadmill and these may have been the children with peak lactates below 6.0 mmol•L^{-1}. The choice of criteria for maximal remains arbitrary. These studies did not involve air collection apparatus which we have found reduces exercise time by about 30 s in children age 9 and older, and by more in younger children.

By selecting serum lactates of under 6 mmol•L^{-1} for prepubertal children and under 8 mmol.L^{-1} for postpubertal children as indicating less than a maximal effort, 13% of our test subjects were in this category. By arbitrarily selecting a maximal heart rate of less than 190 beats.min^{-1} as indicating less than a maximal effort, 5% of children fell into this category. When both the lactate and the heart rate 190 criteria were applied, only 0.75% of children in this study would be categorized as possibly not giving a near-maximal effort. While these criteria are arbitrary, they are suggested as practical guidelines that a near-maximal effort has been made.

One purpose of this report is to show what can be achieved by children exercising in a clinical laboratory where exercise testing is a routine part of patient workup on a daily basis. Our values for maximal heart rate and postexercise lactate exceed the values published for many clinical laboratories and even most research studies where special attention can be given to motivation.

For clinical purposes we have arbitrarily taken the 10th centile endurance time as the lower limit of normal, as we feel that children unable to complete this amount of work should be classified as below normal in fitness. These lower limits of fitness, based on the Bruce protocol, for children are summarized in Table 7 with a minimal

Table 7

Lower Limits of "Normal" (1982) Bruce Treadmill Protocol

Age Group	Boys	Girls
4- 5	0.5 min stage IV	0.5 min stage IV
6- 7	2.0 min stage IV	2.0 min stage IV
8- 9	finish stage IV	1.5 min stage IV
10-12	finish stage IV	1.5 min stage IV
13-15	finish stage IV	finish stage III
16-20	1.5 min stage IV	finish stage III

Based on 10th centile values with minimal rounding off.

rounding off of less than 20 s. Values for boys and girls are the same for ages 4 to 7 years and values for boys are constant from ages 8 to 15 years (being able to finish Stage IV). Girls up to 12 years should be able to get halfway through Stage IV, and older girls should at least finish Stage III.

References

ÅSTRAND, P.O. (1952). *Experimental studies of physical working capacity in relaxation to sex and age*. Copenhagen: Munksgaard.

BRUCE, R.A., Kusumi, F., & Hosmer, D. (1973). Maximal oxygen intake and momographic assessment of functional aerobic impairment in cardiovascular disease. *American Heart Journal*, **85**, 546-562.

BRUCE, R.A., DeRouen, T.A., & Hossack, K. (1980). Value of maximal exercise tests in risk assessment of primary coronary heart disease events in healthy men. *American Journal of Cardiology*, **46**, 371-378.

CUMMING, G.R. (1978). Maximal exercise capacity of children with heart defects. *American Journal of Cardiology*, **42**, 613-619.

CUMMING, G.R., Everatt, D., & Hastman, L. (1978). Bruce treadmill test in children: Normal values in a clinical population. *American Journal of Cardiology*, **41**, 69-75.

CUMMING, G.R., & Friesen, W. (1967). Bicycle ergometer measurement of maximal oxygen uptake in children. *Canadian Journal of Physiology Pharmacology*, **45**, 937-946.

CUMMING, G.R., Hastman, L., McCort, J., & McCullough, S. (1980). High serum lactates do occur in young children after maximal work. *International Journal of Sports Medicine*, **1**, 66-69.

CUMMING, G.R., & Hnatiuk, A. (1980). Establishment of normal values for exercise capacity in a hospital clinic. In K. Berg & B.O. Eriksson (Eds.), *Children and exercise IX* (pp. 79-91). Baltimore: University Park Press.

CUNNINGHAM, D.A., Van Watershoot, P.M., & Patterson, D.H. (1977). Reliability and reproducibility of maximal oxygen uptake in children. *Medicine and Science in Sports*, **9**, 104-108.

ERIKSSON, B.O. (1972). Physical training, oxygen supply and muscle metabolism in 11-13 year old boys. *Acta Physiology Scandinavica,* Suppl. 384.

KEMPER, H.C.G., & Verscheur, R. (1980). Measurement of aerobic power on teenagers. In K. Berg & B.O. Eriksson (Eds.) *Children and exercise* **IX** (pp. 55-63). Baltimore: University Park Press.

MATSUI, H., Mayashita, M., Miura, M., et al. (1970). Aerobic work capacity of Japanese people. *Research Journal of Physical Education,* **14,** 137-142.

RIOPEL, D.A., Taylor, A.B., & Hohn, A.R. (1979). Blood pressure, heart rate, pressure rate product, and electrocardiographic changes in healthy children during treadmill exercise. *American Journal of Cardiology,* **44,** 697-704.

RODE, A., & Shephard, R.J. (1973). Growth, development and fitness of the Canadian Eskimo. *Medicine and Science in Sports,* **5,** 160-169.

RUTENFRANZ, J., Lange-Andersen, K., Seliger, V., & Maseroni, R. (1982). Health standards in terms of exercise fitness of school children in urban and rural areas in various European countries. *Ann. Clin. Res.* Suppl. 34 (pp.33-36).

SHEPHARD, R.J., Allen, C. & Bar-Or, O. (1968). The working capacity of Toronto school children. *Canadian Medical Association Journal,* **100,** 560-566.

WESTGARD, J.O., Lahmeyer, B.L., & Birnbaum, M.C. (1972). Use of the DuPont "automatic clinical analyzer" in direct determination of lactic acid in plasma stabilized with sodium fluoride. *Clin. Chem.,* **18,** 1334-1338.

WILMORE, J.H., & Sigerseth, P.O. (1967). Physical work capacity of young girls 7-13 years of age. *Journal of Applied Physiology,* **22,** 923-928.

Reference Values for Aerobic Power of Healthy 4- to 18-Year-Old Dutch Children: Preliminary Results

Wim H.M. Saris
University of Limburg, Maastricht, The Netherlands

Annemieke M. Noordeloos, Bini E.M. Ringnalda, Martin A. Van't Hof, and Rob A. Binkhorst
University of Nijmegen, Nijmegen, The Netherlands

Comparative data of areobic power are generally considered to be indispensable in applied research areas like clinical sports and occupational health care. However, most data are based on selected groups of children with respect to age and population (for instance, school or sports club). This was the impetus for beginning an investigation with a randomly selected group of healthy children. Currently, about half of the target group of children has been studied, and the results of these tests are reported here. Furthermore, it will be possible to compare these data with those gathered 15 years ago in The Netherlands (Bink & Wafelbakker, 1968), as well as the data collected in Czechoslovakia, also based on a randomly selected sample of the population (Seliger & Bartinek, 1976). Comparative data are also available from Sweden (Åstrand, 1952) and from the U.S.A. (Robinson, 1938), which were gathered 30 and 40 years ago, respectively, so it will be possible to evaluate the degree to which this aspect of the PPC of children has changed.

Methods

This cross-sectional study was performed in the city of Nijmegen (population 150,000). A random selection was made from the total census of people who were 4, 6, 8, 10, 12, 14, 16, and 18 years of age, plus or minus 2 weeks on the day of the experiment.

The goal and design of the experiment was explained in a letter to the parents and to the children above the age of 10 years. If no answer was received within 2 weeks, a second letter was sent asking for permission or requesting the reasons for refusal.

After the first 3 experimental months, and following the second letter, about 15% still had not responded. Cooperation was then requested by telephone and house calls were made (see Table 1). In this way, it was possible to determine whether there was

Table 1

Response and Participation of the Total Group of Children Requested by Letter for Permission to Participate in the Study (see text for further explanation)

	Total Addresses	Moved	Negative Response Letter	Negative Response Call/Visit	Positive Response Letter	Positive Response Call/Visit	Not Healthy	Refusal During Test
Total	294	16	66	24	154	11	17	6
				(90)		(165)		
%	100	5		31		56	6	2

a correlation between a low PPC and a refusal to participate. The reasons for refusal were noted for the group which was personally approached. Table 1 gives a summary of the response and the participation.

Information concerning the height and weight of the child was requested but if this was not known, they were measured. There was no age or sex effect on the participation rate except for the youngest age group. Mental retardation, physical handicaps, fractures, and asthma were some of the reasons why 17 children were removed from the sample. These are identified in Table 1 as "not healthy."

A general medical examination was performed during the first visit to the laboratory. Anthropometric measurements were made: height and weight, the thickness of 4 skinfolds (triceps, biceps, subscapular and crista iliaca) measured with a Holtain caliper, and the percentage fat calculated according to the Durnin and Womersley method (1974). Furthermore, the subjects practiced walking on the treadmill for 5 min at different speeds and gradients and the procedure for the maximal test was discussed.

The maximal exercise test on the treadmill was performed during the second visit to the laboratory during the morning hours. The measurements were made in an air conditioned room at a temperature of 18° C. The scheme developed by Bruce, Blackman, Jones, and Strait (1963) was used as a test protocol. The expired air was collected in Douglas bags. The collected volume of expired air was measured with a Tissot-spirometer, and the gas analyses were performed with a paramagnetic O_2 analyzer (Servomex, Taylor, England) and an infrared CO_2 analyzer (Uras, Hartmann, & Braun, Federal Republic of Germany). Heart rate was calculated from the continuous E.C.G. recording with a one/channel E.C.G. apparatus (Cardiostat, Siemens, Federal Republic of Germany).

A blood sample was taken from the fingertip during the 3rd min of the recovery phase in order to determine the lactate concentration with the Boehringer-Mannheim enzymatic method (Federal Republic of Germany).

The criteria for reaching maximal exercise were the leveling off of the heart rate despite an increasing workload during the test, and the appearance of an extreme forced ventilation. Subsequently, data were excluded from the results for children with a maximal heart rate lower than the mean max. HR minus two times the standard deviation, as given by Åstrand (1952) for the corresponding age. Data of children with a maximal respiratory exchange ratio (R) lower than 1.1 were also excluded. The R-limit for the 4-year-olds was set at 1.0 because most of the children did not reach the 1.1 R-level. In total, data were excluded for 35 children equally spread over the age groups and both sexes.

Results

The means and SDs for the different anthropometric measurements for boys and girls of the different ages are shown in Table 2. The boys as well as the girls were representative samples compared to the Dutch standard growth tables.

An evaluation of body composition is desirable for making comparisons with earlier studies. However, only the average weight of each age group was reported by Bink and Wafelbakker (1968) so that, although these values were comparable to the present data on the weight of boys, no definite statement can be made with respect to body composition. Furthermore, no skinfolds were measured in the study of Robinson (1938) and Åstrand (1952). A comparison is therefore only possible on the basis of the Quetelet index (QI = weight [kg]; height [m]. Keys, Aravanis, and Blackburn (1972) and others have shown that the QI correlates well with the percentage of fat. It can be seen in Figures 1A and 1B, with the exception of the 18-year-olds in the study by Seliger and

Table 2

Anthropometric Data (Mean ± SD) of Boys and Girls of Different Age Groups

	Age (years)	n	Height (cm)	Weight (kg)	Sum of 4 Skinfolds (mm)	Body Fat (%)
Boys	4	3	105.3 ± 2.5	18.1 ± 1.0	30.1 ± 7.2	12.6 ± 2.8
	6	7	119.6 ± 4.7	22.7 ± 3.6	23.6 ± 6.1	9.6 ± 3.2
	8	7	130.0 ± 5.3	27.6 ± 3.6	23.2 ± 5.4	9.6 ± 2.5
	10	9	140.7 ± 6.8	33.4 ± 3.5	30.8 ± 5.1	12.0 ± 5.4
	12	6	146.8 ± 3.3	35.4 ± 5.1	26.4 ± 7.7	10.9 ± 3.4
	14	11	165.7 ± 9.1	51.3 ± 8.2	33.1 ± 13.6	13.3 ± 4.1
	16	10	178.6 ± 4.9	63.4 ± 6.7	31.4 ± 7.6	13.7 ± 3.9
	18	9	182.0 ± 5.7	67.0 ± 6.0	28.7 ± 8.9	11.7 ± 3.8
Girls	4	6	107.0 ± 4.6	17.9 ± 2.6	29.3 ± 5.7	18.9 ± 2.8
	6	7	119.1 ± 4.1	22.2 ± 3.5	25.9 ± 6.7	17.1 ± 3.1
	8	11	131.5 ± 4.7	28.9 ± 4.0	36.1 ± 15.7	20.9 ± 5.6
	10	5	140.1 ± 4.0	32.7 ± 3.7	31.1 ± 9.5	19.4 ± 4.4
	12	10	153.8 ± 7.2	43.9 ± 8.4	39.1 ± 16.4	20.8 ± 7.2
	14	11	163.4 ± 7.1	53.2 ± 8.5	46.4 ± 14.7	24.3 ± 5.5
	16	9	167.9 ± 5.4	55.9 ± 8.6	48.3 ± 15.0	24.6 ± 6.4
	18	10	166.5 ± 3.9	54.2 ± 6.1	44.8 ± 11.6	24.5 ± 3.7

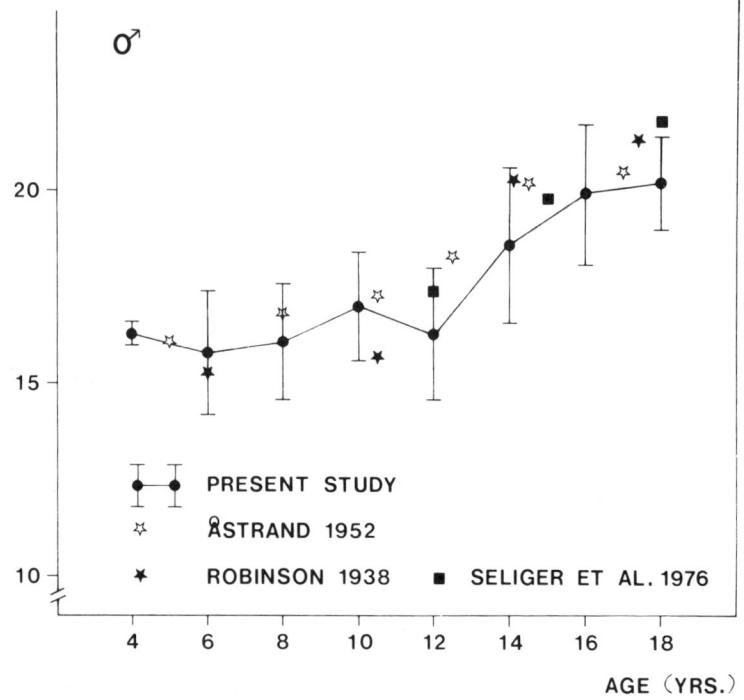

Figure 1A—The mean values (± SD) of the Quetelet-index (kg•m^{-2}) of boys of the different age groups compared with the data from Robinson (1938, U.S.A.), Åstrand (1952, Sweden), and Seliger and Bartinek (1976, Czechoslovakia).

Bartinek (1976), that the data of Åstrand, Robinson, and Seliger and Bartinek, lie within 1 SD of mean values in the current study, indicating that there were no large differences.

There were also no significant differences between the QI indices of the participants as plotted in Figures 1A and 1B and the nonparticipants. All values of this group lie within 1 SD from the mean QI results of the participant group.

The data concerning the aerobic power on the treadmill are shown in Table 3 for both sexes in each age group. The aerobic power, expressed in $\dot{V}O_2$ max/kg, increased for boys up to the age of 8 years and then remained constant with a somewhat higher value for the 16-year-olds. The aerobic power/kg body weight for girls was fairly constant from 6 years on and began to decrease somewhat at about 14 years of age. To compare the aerobic power of this group of children with earlier studies, the mean $\dot{V}O_2$ max per kg (I = SD) of this and other studies are plotted in Figures 2A and 2B.

In studies by Bink and Wafelbakker (1968) and by Seliger and Bartinek (1976) the bicycle ergometer was used. It is generally assumed that the treadmill gives about 7.5 to 10% higher values than the bicycle ergometer (W.H.O., 1968). When these differences were taken into consideration, it became clear that the values of the present study were from 0 to 5% lower than those of Bink and Wafelbakker (1968) and Åstrand (1952) and agree quite well with those of Robinson (1938) and Seliger and Bartinek (1976).

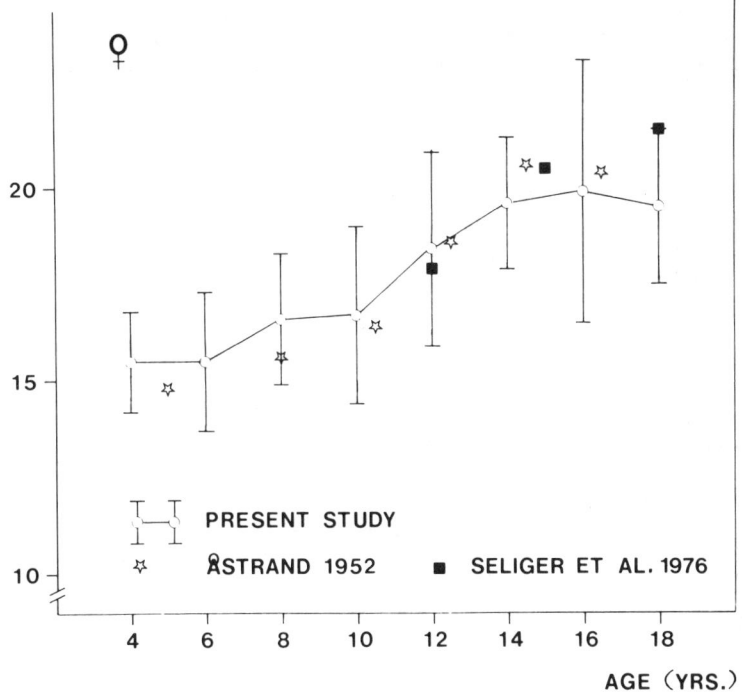

Figure 1B—The mean values (± SD) of the Quetelet-index (kg·m⁻²) of girls of the different age groups compared with the data from Åstrand (1952, Sweden) and Seliger and Bartinek (1976, Czechoslavakia).

Discussion

Selection of Children

Selecting groups of children for the purpose of collecting reference values with respect to physiological exercise parameters is a difficult task. Studying large numbers is prohibitive due to the very time-consuming character of this type of work. Furthermore, cooperation of the subjects is a very important factor. It can be expected that physically fit subjects will have a greater tendency to cooperate than those who are in poor physical condition.

Of special importance was the group that did not respond after two letters. It might be expected that especially this group included children who did not participate because of a low PPC. The literature shows that there is a close relationship between the percentage of fat, physical activity, and the PPC of children. The higher the QI, the lower the PPC (Montoye, 1975; Saris, Binkhorst, Cramwinckel, Van Waesberghe, & Van de Veen, 1980). The QI is therefore used as an indicator for the PPC. The QI values of the children who gave no response were equal to the QI values of the children participating in the study. On the basis of this indicator, it was assumed that no clear selection

Table 3

Aerobic Power (Mean ± SD) and Related Data of Boys and Girls Measured With the Bruce Treadmill Protocol

	Age (years)	n	$\dot{V}O_2$ max (l·min⁻¹)	$\dot{V}O_2$ max (ml·kg⁻¹·min⁻¹)	$\dot{V}_E$ max (l·min⁻¹)	H.R. max (beats·min⁻¹)	R	Lactate (mmol·l⁻¹)
Boys	4	3	0.73 ± 0.14	40.4 ± 5.3	32.7 ± 2.5	206 ± 12.0	1.10 ± 0.08	5.2 ± 0.6
	6	7	1.06 ± 0.16	47.0 ± 6.0	47.7 ± 6.3	203 ± 6.0	1.20 ± 0.07	7.2 ± 2.1
	8	7	1.46 ± 0.17	53.0 ± 3.6	60.0 ± 7.3	207 ± 9.9	1.18 ± 0.07	7.0 ± 1.7
	10	8	1.76 ± 0.23	52.7 ± 5.5	74.8 ± 9.9	205 ± 6.1	1.20 ± 0.04	8.3 ± 0.9
	12	6	1.88 ± 0.33	53.0 ± 4.7	70.7 ± 8.0	206 ± 5.1	1.19 ± 0.11	8.2 ± 1.9
	14	11	2.62 ± 0.49	51.1 ± 5.1	92.6 ± 21.2	203 ± 7.5	1.19 ± 0.07	9.7 ± 1.7
	16	10	3.48 ± 0.44	55.1 ± 6.0	120.3 ± 16.6	202 ± 6.9	1.21 ± 0.05	10.9 ± 1.5
	18	9	3.46 ± 0.37	51.7 ± 3.8	112.0 ± 10.8	198 ± 6.3	1.21 ± 0.04	10.2 ± 2.4
Girls	4	6	0.68 ± 0.18	38.0 ± 7.8	32.0 ± 9.3	209 ± 2.6	1.16 ± 0.06	6.0 ± 1.5
	6	7	1.05 ± 0.16	47.2 ± 3.5	43.0 ± 5.7	205 ± 6.4	1.19 ± 0.09	7.8 ± 2.1
	8	11	1.22 ± 0.17	43.0 ± 4.6	53.3 ± 6.2	203 ± 4.0	1.23 ± 0.06	8.1 ± 2.1
	10	5	1.52 ± 0.09	46.8 ± 4.5	61.0 ± 5.4	205 ± 6.0	1.27 ± 0.05	9.7 ± 2.2
	12	10	2.01 ± 0.25	46.5 ± 5.7	75.4 ± 9.9	208 ± 6.8	1.22 ± 0.04	9.3 ± 1.7
	14	11	2.36 ± 0.42	44.6 ± 4.7	87.6 ± 17.1	200 ± 6.4	1.21 ± 0.07	10.2 ± 1.9
	16	9	2.37 ± 0.31	42.6 ± 4.3	86.3 ± 13.0	196 ± 7.1	1.22 ± 0.07	10.7 ± 3.2
	18	10	2.25 ± 0.31	41.6 ± 5.3	83.8 ± 10.5	200 ± 6.3	1.23 ± 0.05	10.7 ± 2.3

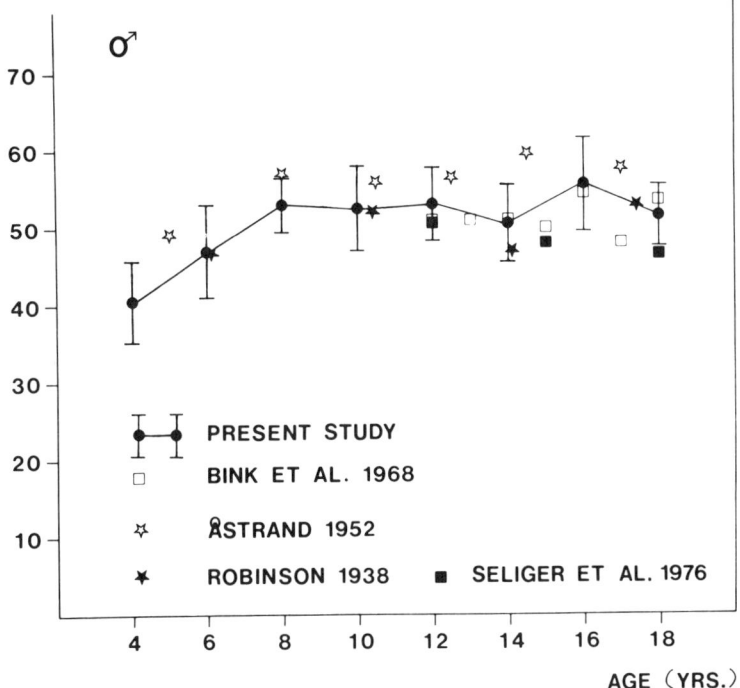

Figure 2A—The mean values (± SD) of maximal oxygen consumption per kg body weight of boys of the different age groups compared with the data from Robinson (1938, U.S.A., treadmill), Åstrand (1952, Sweden, treadmill), Bink and Wafelbakker (1968, bicycle ergometer), and Seliger and Bartinek (1976, Czechoslovakia, bicycle ergometer).

occurred in the sense of a lower participation of children with a lower PPC. The percentage of children participating in this study (65%) seemed satisfactory. At present only Seliger and Bartinek (1976) have published a study of the physical fitness of a randomly selected group. However, they failed to give information about the nonresponse.

Aerobic Power in Children

Through technological developments since the 1930s and 1940s, it is reasonable to assume that the amount and intensity of the physical activity of adults has fallen to a lower level. It is less reasonable to assume this for children because they are more spontaneous by nature and are influenced less by technical advancements. A historical comparison of the degree of physical activity is not possible because such information has become available only in recent years. Åstrand, Engstrom, Eriksson, Karlberg, & Thoren (1963), Ekblom (1971) and others indicate that inactive children have 5 to 15% lower aerobic power than active children. Because data concerning aerobic power were published in the 1930s (Robinson, 1938), a comparison can be made on this basis.

It appears that the only age-limited cross-sectional research performed in the past in The Netherlands is that of Bink and Wafelbakker (1968). The only randomly selected

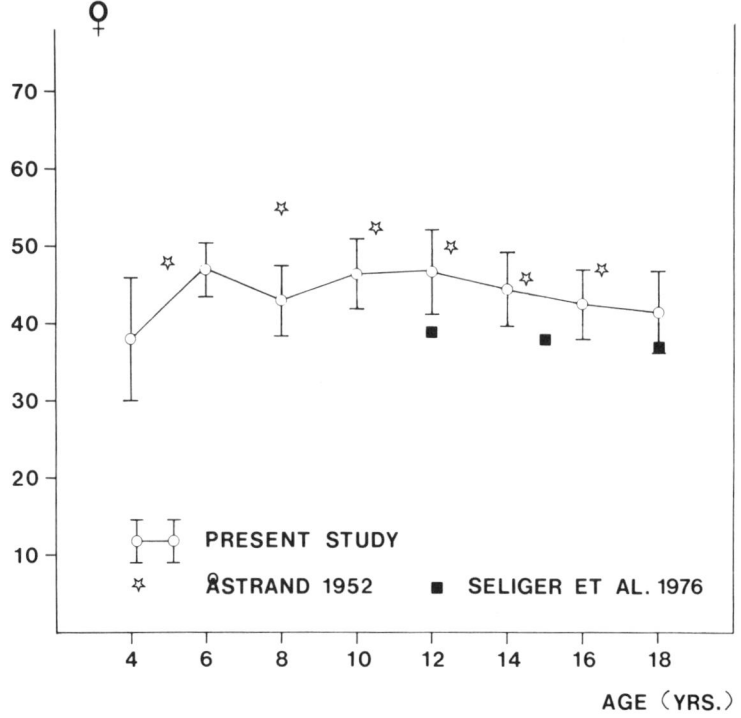

Figure 2B—The mean values (± SD) of maximal oxygen consumption per kg body weight of girls of the different age groups compared with the data from Åstrand (1952, Sweden, treadmill) and Seliger and Bartinek (1976, Czechoslovakia, bicycle ergometer).

study of the PPC in children was performed in Czechoslovakia by Seliger and Bartinek (1976).

Data from that study and the research by Åstrand in Stockholm during the period from 1947 to 1951 and by Robinson in Boston in 1938 are the most suitable earlier data with which to compare the present findings. It has been mentioned primarily that the present data are about 0 to 5% lower than those of Bink and Wafelbakker (1968) and Åstrand (1952).

Which factors could play a role in the differences between the data from this study and that of other studies? Possibly, the most important point of difference between the studies is the selection of the subjects. From the publication of Bink and Wafelbakker (1968), as in the publications of Åstrand (1952), it is suggested that the sample is not representative for the respective age groups because the "poorly" performing subjects were not prepared to participate. This is less clear in the study of Robinson (1938). The 6-year-olds were healthy middle class boys living at home. Unfortunately, no mention was made of the reasons why no maximal values were given for 50% of this young group. The 10-year-olds came from an orphanage, while the 14- and 17-year-olds were students in a private school. The selection procedure in the study of Seliger and Bartinek (1976) was the same as in the current study.

Another possible factor which could explain the differences in aerobic power was the difference in test procedures. Besides the described differences between the treadmill and bicycle ergometer results, there were also differences within the treadmill procedures. In the study by Åstrand (1952) the children walked several times in a period of 3 weeks and therefore had time to get accustomed to the procedure. In the other studies, the measurements were completed in 1 day. Furthermore, the increasing workloads of the Bruce test may have been too high for the younger age groups. Therefore, anaerobic metabolism may be important and consequently force the child to stop before the maximal oxygen consumption is reached due to muscular pain. Comparative research with other test procedures is necessary to evaluate this matter more fully.

Conclusion

Assuming that the aerobic power of the youth in The Netherlands was at the same level as 15 to 40 years ago and comparable with that of the youth in Czechoslovakia around 1968, in Sweden around 1950, and in the U.S.A. around 1935, the current findings indicate that since that time, no clear decline has occurred in the aerobic power of young Dutch people from 4 to 18 years of age. In another way, this conclusion is supported by the observation, described by various investigators (Gilliam & Freedom, 1980; Lange-Andersen, Rutenfranz, Masironi, & Seliger, 1978; Yoshida, Ishiko, & Muraoka, 1981), that extra physical training does not result in an improvement in aerobic power of young children. This could also mean that the general level of physical activity may affect the aerobic power only after a number of years.

Acknowledgment

This study was supported by the Dutch Heart Foundation (Grant 79.015).

References

ÅSTRAND, P.O. (1952). *Experimental studies of physical working capacity in relation to sex and age*. Copenhagen: Munksgaard.

ÅSTRAND, P.O., Engstrom, L., Eriksson, B.O., Karlberg, P., & Thoren, C. (1963). Girl swimmers. *Acta Paediatrica Scandinavica, Supplement, 147*.

BINK, B., & Wafelbakker, F. (1968). Physical working capacity at maximum levels of work of boys 12-18 years of age. *Zschr. Arztl. Fortbild., 62*, 957.

BRUCE, R.A., Blackman, J.R., Jones, J.W., & Strait, G. (1963). Exercise testing in adult normal subjects and cardiac patients. *Pediatrics, 32*, 742.

DURNIN, J.V.G.A., & Womersley, J. (1974). Body fat assessed from total body density and its estimation from skinfolds thickness. *British Journal of Nutrition, 37,* 77.

EKBLOM, B. (1971). Physical training in normal boys in adolescence. *Acta Paediactrica Scandinavica Supplement,* **217,** 60.

GILLIAM, T.B., & Freedom, P.S. (1980). Effects of a 12-week school physical fitness programme on peak $\dot{V}O_2$, body composition and blood lipids in 7- to 9-year-old children. *International Journal of Sports Medicine,* **1,** 73.

KEYS, A., Aravanis, C., & Blackburn, H. (1972). Coronary heart disease, overweight and obesity as risk factors. *Annals of International Medicine,* **77,** 15.

LANGE-ANDERSEN, K., Rutenfranz, J., Masironi, R., & Seliger, V. (1978). *Habitual physical activity and health.* W.H.O. Regional Publications European Series 6.

MONTOYE, H.J. (1975). *Physical activity and health. An epidemiological study of an entire community.* Englewood Cliffs, NJ: Prentice Hall, Inc.

ROBINSON, S. (1938). Experimental studies of physical fitness in relation to age. *Arbeitsphysiologie,* **10,** 251.

SARIS, W.H.M., Binkhorst, R.A., Cramwinckel, A.B., Van Waesberghe, F., & Van de Veen-Hezemans, A.M. (1980). The relationship between working performance, daily physical activity, fatness, blood lipids and nutrition in school children. In K. Berg & B.O. Eriksson (Eds.), *Children and exercise,* **IX,** (pp. 166-174). Baltimore: University Park Press.

SELIGER, V., & Bartinek, Z. (1976). *Mean values of various indices of physical fitness in the investigation of Czechoslovak population ages 12-55 years.* Praha: Czechoslovak Association of Physical Culture.

WORLD Health Organization (1968). Exercise tests in relation to cardio-vascular function. *W.H.O. Technical Report,* Ser. 338, Geneva.

YOSHIDA, T., Ishiko, I., & Muraoka, I. Effect of endurance training on cardio-respiratory functions of 5-year-old children. *International Journal of Sports Medicine,* **1,** 91.

Is a Leveling-Off Criterion in Oxygen Uptake a Prerequisite for a Maximal Performance in Teenagers?

Jan Willem Ritmeester, Han C.G. Kemper, and Robbert Verschuur
University of Amsterdam
Amsterdam, The Netherlands

When measuring oxygen uptake by means of a test (e.g., on a treadmill, as in this study) during which the subject performs maximally until exertion, the following question arises: Did the subjects do their utmost, has the maximal oxygen uptake ($\dot{V}O_2$ max) been reached? Three criteria were considered as an objective control for the attainment of maximal work:

1. A sufficient leveling-off in oxygen uptake during the last minute.
2. A heart beat frequency during the last minute which exceeds 95% of the maximal heart beat frequency as predicted from age.
3. A CO_2/O_2 exchange ratio in the expired air higher than 1.00.

A sufficient leveling-off (criterion 1) can be operationalized in two different ways, namely: (a) a relative criterion: a rise in measured oxygen uptake during the last minute of less than 5%, or (b) an absolute criterion: a rise in measured oxygen uptake during the last minute of less than 150 ml.

In a classical study, Åstrand (Åstrand, 1952) found in boys and girls between 14 and 18 years of age, leveling-off in 50% of his subjects (for both sexes). The two groups reached identical $\dot{V}O_2$ max values (and lactic acid values). Åstrand concluded that leveling-off in oxygen uptake contributes to individual differences and is not a prerequisite for maximal performance. In a more recent study (Cunningham, Macfarlane Van Waterschoot, Paterson, Lefcoe, & Sangal, 1977) leveling-off was reached by only 38% of 66 10-year-old boys. The authors defined leveling-off as less than 2.1 ml/kg•min, which is approximately 3.8% or 71.5 ml, on the average. No differences in maximal oxygen uptake per kilogram body weight between the groups were found and the authors, therefore, reached the same conclusion as Åstrand.

The maximal heart beat frequency was estimated from the pupil's age according to the following formula:

$$f_h \text{ max} = 232 - 2 \cdot A \text{ (A being the calendar age in years).}$$

For the age groups 12 to 17 years this function was the best fit to the curve describing the relationship between maximal heart rate and age as found by Åstrand and Christensen (1964). The standard deviation was approximately 10 beats/min in all age groups.

Procedures

Maximal oxygen uptake ($\dot{V}O_2$ max) of each subject was measured from January to March during regular school hours using a treadmill. Subjects were asked not to eat during the 1½ hr prior to testing. A procedure was followed with a submaximal test preceding a maximal test, slightly modified after the method of Bar-Or and Zwiren (1975). During the submaximal test, the subjects ran three times for 2 min at a time at a constant speed of 8 km/hr, with an increasing slope of 0, 2½, and 5% respectively. In this way subjects got accustomed to running on a treadmill, became acquainted with the mouthpiece plus noseclip, and warmed up.

After a rest-period of 10 to 15 minutes, running was resumed at the same constant speed. In this maximal test the slope was increased every 2 min by 2½ or 5%, depending on the subject's heart rate. The test was continued until complete exhaustion had been reached. Subjects were stimulated by verbal encouragements. Expired air was measured by passing it through a 10 l high speed and low resistance dry gasometer (Parkinson Cowan CDU, Ass., New York, USA) via a two-way low resistance breathing valve with a dead air space of 35 ml. Oxygen uptake was measured each minute throughout the test, using the open circuit method.

Samples of mixed expired air were continuously withdrawn from the gasometer, dried, and analyzed for F_EO_2 by a paramagnetic oxygen analyzer (Servomex) and F_ECO_2 by an infrared carbon dioxide analyzer (Mijnhardt BV). The gasometer, two gas analyzers, and a number of electronic calculators were incorporated into a movable 19-inch unit (ergoanalyzer, Mijnhardt BV, Odijk; The Netherlands). The collected expired air was continuously and automatically analyzed and the calculated oxygen uptake, standardized for temperature, humidity, and barometric pressure (STPD), was printed as output.

Subjects

Subjects were participants in the multiple longitudinal study "Growth and Health of Teenagers" (Kemper et al., 1983). Pupils of one school were measured for 4 successive years, from the 1st or 2nd grade onwards. In a second school, the same grades were followed, but each year a different quarter of the pupils was measured. This design made it possible to estimate confounding effects from time for measurement, birth-cohorts, and repeated testing (Kemper & Van 't Hof, 1978). Of the longitudinal group, 131 girls and 102 boys (82% and 69%, respectively, of the original sample) completed the study. In the control group, 161 girls and 147 boys were measured only once.

Methods

For the two sexes separately, proportions of subjects satisfying each criterion were calculated per age group and per school. Age group was defined as the calendar age at the nearest (last or next) birthday. Effects of testing, sex, and age were investigated. To these data log-linear models were fitted if possible. This had to be done with care, as the mixture of repeated and unique measurements violated the assumptions underlying the test statistics. No statistical text exists applicable to frequency tables containing such a mixture or even only with counts from subjects measured more than twice.

A choice was made between the two operationalizations of the leveling-off criterion. T-tests were performed to test differences between subjects who satisfied the leveling-off criterion and those who did not, in $\dot{V}O_2$ max and $\dot{V}O_2$ max with score variance attributable to body weight partialled out (Katch & Katch, 1974), for each year of measurement separately. The same analysis was applied to the other two criteria and to the combination of all three. An analysis of variance with repeated measurements was not possible as the grouping on the criteria for each subject differed from one year to the next, so interpretations had to be made with care.

Results

Confounding Effects

No evidence was found of testing effects; consequently, changing proportions with age were attributable to age effects alone and there was, in the longitudinal group, no influence of repeated measurement on criterion score (yes or no). No differences between birth cohorts were found.

The Leveling-Off Criterion

In Figures 1 and 2, proportions satisfying the two variants of the leveling-off criterion are shown for the longitudinal sample only. The number of subjects for each age group is given in Table 1.

A significant positive age effect did exist on the 5% criterion for both boys and girls, while on the 150 ml criterion this effect existed for girls only. As can be concluded by comparing Figures 1 and 2, with girls the 5% criterion was in the younger age groups (12 to 15 years) more severe than the 150 ml criterion (40 to 50% vs. 55 to 65%), while at 16 or 17 years of age, there was no difference (75% for both). With boys under 14 eyars of age, the 5% criterion was more severe (40% vs. 55%), but above age 15, the reverse was true (58% vs. 50%). For further analyses the 150 ml criterion was chosen. (See discussion for the reasoning.)

For each time of measurement separately (four) t-tests were performed, with criterion score as grouping variable and as dependent variables $\dot{V}O_2$ max and weight-adjusted $\dot{V}O_2$ max (W-A $\dot{V}O_2$ max). Results are given in Table 2.

One may conclude that a trend existed for boys to attain higher $\dot{V}O_2$ max values when the criterion was *not* satisfied, while for girls there was no difference. When the $\dot{V}O_2$ max was corrected for body weight (W-A $\dot{V}O_2$ max), the difference between the groups was significant (although small: 4%) in both boys and girls: Subjects without leveling-off had higher W-A $\dot{V}O_2$ max values.

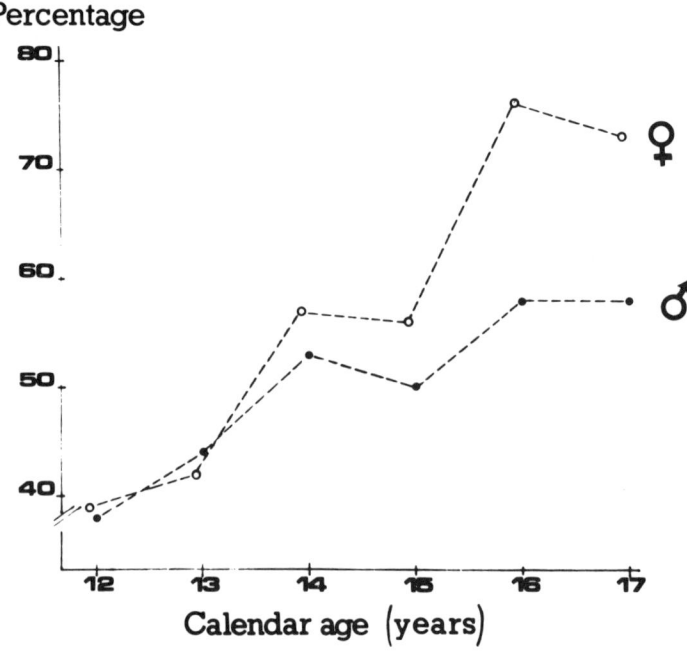

Figure 1—Proportions satisfying the 5% criterion.

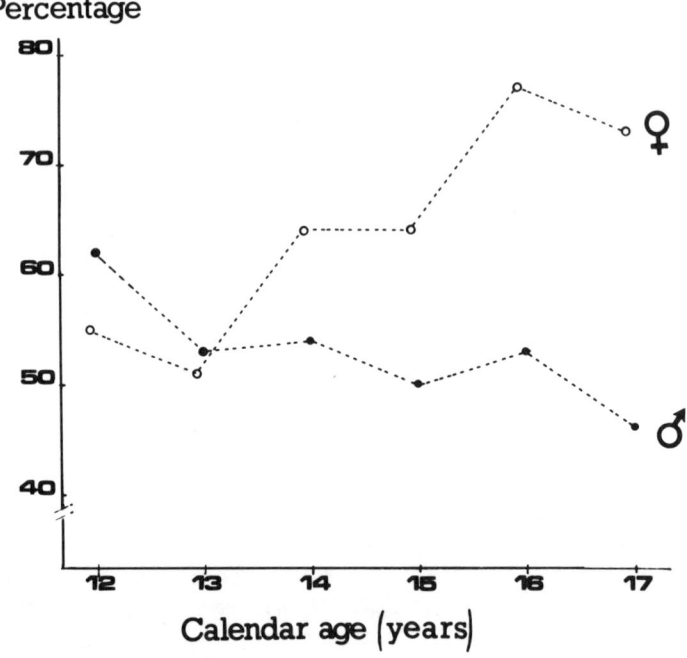

Figure 2—Proportions satisfying the 150 ml criterion.

Table 1

Number of Cases Belonging to Figures 1 to 5
(Proportions of Subjects Satisfying Each Criterion),
for Boys and Girls Separately, per Age Group

Age	12	13	14	15	16	17
Boys	26	72	95	102	76	27
Girls	31	97	129	129	96	30

Table 2

Differences in ml. Between Satisfiers and Not-Satisfiers on $\dot{V}O_2$ max ($\dot{V}O_2$) and W-A $\dot{V}O_2$ max (W-A) With Group Sizes Between Brackets (Identical for the Two Variables With Not-Satisfiers Top and Satisfiers Bottom) for the Two Sexes Separately

Time of Measurement	1	2	3	4
Crit. Sex Variable				
1. M $\dot{V}O_2$	− 82 (47)	− 74 (42)	−254² (54)	−401³ (46)
M W-A	−101¹ (54)	− 53 (56)	−154² (47)	−219² (54)
F $\dot{V}O_2$	− 49 (59)	− 44 (49)	−114 (44)	+ 1 (33)
F W-A	−120² (71)	− 85¹ (80)	− 94¹ (84)	− 85 (93)
2. M $\dot{V}O_2$	+220¹ (18)	+ 89 (17)	+115 (17)	+ 96 (16)
M W-A	+122¹ (83)	+106 (81)	+ 3 (84)	+ 30 (85)
F $\dot{V}O_2$	+ 71 (28)	+ 72 (27)	+ 37 (28)	− 36 (32)
F W-A	+ 44 (102)	+ 99¹ (102)	− 12 (100)	− 37 (94)
3. M $\dot{V}O_2$	−304¹ (11)	+ 21 (4)	(0)	+126 (3)
M W-A	−280³ (90)	+175 (94)	(101)	+ 59 (98)
F $\dot{V}O_2$	− 2 (9)	+ 35 (14)	− 55 (7)	+ 66 (15)
F W-A	− 83¹ (121)	+ 14 (112)	− 64 (121)	− 28 (111)
All 3 Crit.				
M $\dot{V}O_2$	+ 6 (61)	− 38 (48)	−141 (63)	−312² (56)
M W-A	− 72 (40)	− 20 (50)	−122 (38)	−205² (44)
F $\dot{V}O_2$	− 2 (79)	+ 35 (73)	− 55 (64)	+ 66 (66)
F W-A	− 83¹ (51)	+ 14 (53)	− 64 (64)	− 28 (60)

¹ = significant at 5%
² = significant at 1%
³ = significant at 0.1%

Maximum Heart Beat Criterion

In Figure 3, percentages exceeding 95% of the maximal heart beat frequency are shown. The number of cases is given in Table 1. In boys, the percentage rose significantly as they grew older. Table 2 gives the results of the t-tests. The results reveal for boys a trend to achieve higher $\dot{V}O_2$ max values when the heart rate during the last minute exceeded 95% of the predicted maximal heart beat frequency. For girls no reliable differences were found.

The Gas-Exchange Criterion

Proportions satisfying this criterion are given in Figure 4 and the number of cases in Table 1. It can be seen that almost all subjects (90% or more) reached a CO_2/O_2 exchange ratio of 1.0. The apparent rise in boys was not statistically significant.

In Table 2, the results of the t-tests are given. The extreme distribution over the 2 groups on the gas-exchange ratio criterion, with very few cases not attaining a ratio of at least 1.0, and the changing of the sign, made reliable conclusions impossible.

All Three Criteria

The percentage of subjects satisfying all three criteria at the same time is shown in Figure 5. The number of cases is given in Table 1. The positive age effect for girls was significant. Examining the results of the t-tests (see Table 2) no differences were found for girls, while for boys a trend was still visible for not-satisfiers to attain higher $\dot{V}O_2$ max and W-A $\dot{V}O_2$ max values.

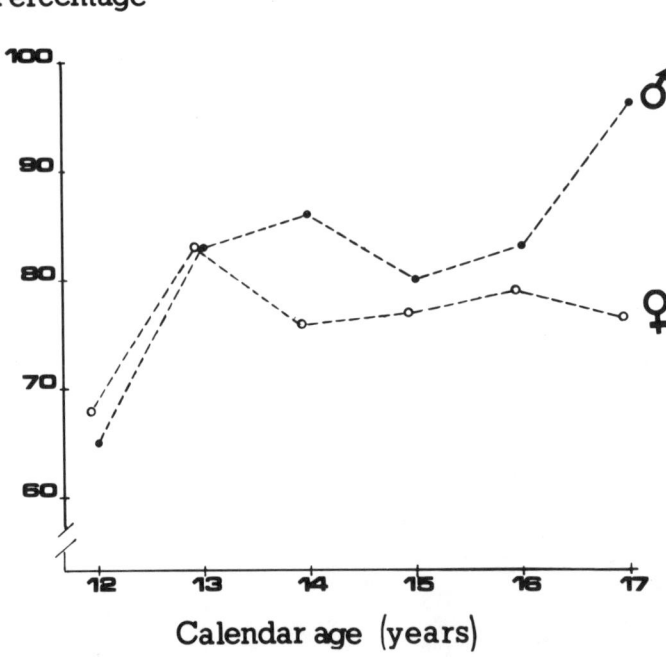

Figure 3—Proportions satisfying the heart beat frequency criterion.

LEVELING OFF IN OXYGEN UPTAKE

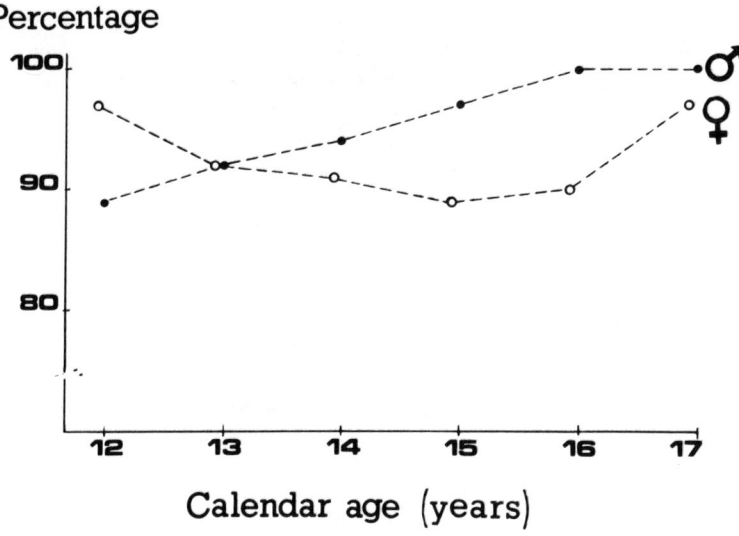

Figure 4—Proportions satisfying the CO_2/O_2 exchange ratio.

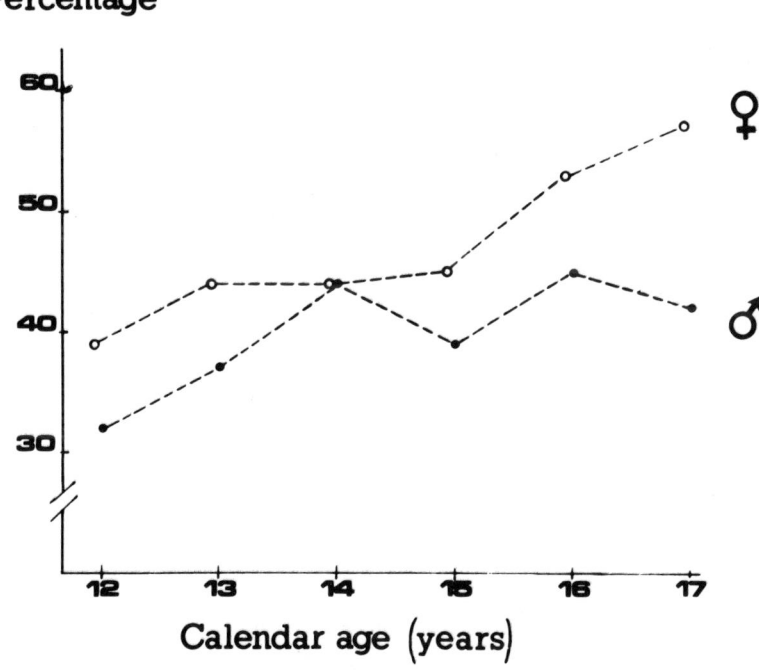

Figure 5—Proportions satisfying all three criteria.

Discussion

In the results, a comparison was made between the age trends on the 5% and 150 ml leveling-off criteria. The conclusions were as expected, because with girls under 17, 5% were on the average less than 150 ml, while with boys the turning point was at 14 years of age ($\dot{V}O_2$ max was a monotonically increasing function of age, mediated by body weight).

Two contrary conclusions can be drawn from the fact that there was an age effect on the 5% criterion:

1. There is a true age effect.
2. The criterion gets easier to satisfy with increasing age.

It is difficult to separate these two. There were clues of an age effect in the other criteria (150 ml in girls and criterion 2 in boys), which could mean the first conclusion is right. On the other hand, the criterion could become easier to satisfy with age because a 5% gain is more of an absolute value. When it comes to choosing between the two variants of the leveling-off criterion, we prefer the absolute, 150 ml gain version because: (a) no artificial age effect will be introduced, and (b) the criterion is identical for everyone irrespective of performance level, age, or sex, which has the intuitive appeal of simplicity.

When examining the results of the tests for the groups satisfying all three criteria vs. those who do not, a few remarks should be made. Compared to the other two criteria, the leveling-off was by far the most severe. Therefore, the results from the t-tests are expected to be similar to those concerning the leveling-off criterion with the heart beat frequency criterion being influenced in the opposite direction.

Conclusions

Contrary to expectations, we found a significant difference in oxygen uptake between children reaching a plateau during the last minute of the test (leveling-off) and those who did not, in favor of the latter. The differences, however, were small, approximately 4% in both boys and girls.

Although in adults leveling-off might be an indication for maximal work, when the subjects are children, the conclusion seems warranted that a leveling-off during the last minute is not a prerequisite for a maximal performance.

References

ÅSTRAND, P-O. (1952). Experimental studies of physical working capacity in relation to sex and age. Copenhagen: Ejnar Munksgaard.

ÅSTRAND, P-O, & Christensen, E.H. (1964). Aerobic work capacity. *Proceedings of the Conference on oxygen in the animal organism* (pp. 298-303). Oxford: Pergamon Press.

BAR-OR, O., & Zwiren, L.D. (1975). Maximal oxygen consumption test during arm exercise-reliability and validity. *Journal of Applied Physiology,* **38**, 425-426.

CUNNINGHAM, D.A., Macfarlane van Waterschoot, B., Paterson, D.H., Lefcoe, M., & Sangal, S.P. (1977). Reliability and reproducibility of maximal oxygen uptake measurement in children. *Medicine and Science in Sports,* **9,** 2, 104-108.

KATCH, V.L., & Katch, F.I. (1974). Use of weight-adjusted oxygen uptake scores that avoid spurious correlations. *Research Quaterly,* **45,** no. 4, 447-451.

KEMPER, H.C.G., Dekker, P.J., Ootjers, M.G., Post, G.B., Snel, J., Splinter, P.G., Storm-van Essen, L., & Verschuur, R. (1983). Growth and health of teenagers in the Netherlands. *International Journal of Sports Medicine,* **4,** 202-214.

KEMPER, H.C.G., & Van 't Hof, M.A. (1978). Design of a multiple longitudinal study of growth and health in teenagers. *European Journal of Pediatrics,* **129,** 147-155.

Max-O$_2$ Reference Values for Children in Relation to Body Mass

Rob A. Binkhorst, Martin A. Van 't Hof, and Annemieke Noordeloos
University of Nijmegen
Nijmegen, The Netherlands

Wim H.M. Saris
University of Limburg
Maastricht, The Netherlands

For comparative purposes, maximal oxygen consumption (Max-O$_2$) is often expressed per unit of body mass (BM) or fat free body mass (FFM). When comparing children of different ages and sexes, it seems, however, more appropriate to take allometric growth (Günther, 1975) into consideration before applying such references.

It was the aim of this study to find the best descriptive formula applicable to both sexes using the allometric equation, Max-O$_2$ = a·M^b in which M is either BM or FFM. The values for a and b and the choice for BM or FFM will be found by minimizing the correlation for the transformed Max-O$_2$ (i.e., Max-O$_2$·M^{-b}) with sex, age, height, BM and FFM.

Methods

Random samples of boys and girls were drawn from 7 different age groups (even ages in the range 6 to 7 years), including a total of 271 children (Saris, Noordeloos, Ringnalda, Van 't Hof, & Binkhorst, 1985). Means and standard deviations with respect to the variables previously mentioned are given in Table 1. The ages did not deviate more than 2 weeks from the target age. Max-O$_2$ was determined on a treadmill according to the Bruce-protocol (Bruce, 1971) using Douglas bags, a paramagnetic O$_2$ analyzer (Taylor Servomex, type OA 272, England), and an infrared CO$_2$ analyzer (Uras, F.R. Germany).

Body fat as fraction of BM was assessed by the four-skinfold method of Durnin and Rahaman (1967) applying a Holtain skinfold caliper. The FFM was calculated as:

$$FFM = (1 - \text{fraction fat}) \cdot BM.$$

Table 1

Anthropometric Data and Aerobic Power of Boys and Girls Between 6 and 18 Years (Mean ± SD)

Age (years)	Sex[1]	n	Height (cm)	Body Mass (kg)	Fat Free Mass (kg)	Max-O_2 ($l \cdot min^{-1}$)
6	b	18	119.9 ± 3.9	22.4 ± 3.4	20.1 ± 2.5	1.04 ± 0.15
	g	13	120.0 ± 4.3	22.2 ± 3.4	18.8 ± 2.2	1.04 ± 0.13
8	b	20	129.9 ± 4.4	27.9 ± 4.4	25.0 ± 3.2	1.41 ± 0.15
	g	20	131.6 ± 4.8	27.5 ± 3.7	22.1 ± 2.3	1.22 ± 0.19
10	b	24	141.9 ± 6.0	33.2 ± 3.9	29.3 ± 2.8	1.73 ± 0.23
	g	17	139.6 ± 6.2	30.8 ± 4.2	24.7 ± 2.5	1.43 ± 0.15
12	b	18	151.3 ± 6.4	39.7 ± 10.1	34.7 ± 6.0	1.96 ± 0.34
	g	22	154.1 ± 7.5	43.3 ± 8.8	33.6 ± 5.3	1.89 ± 0.28
14	b	22	165.0 ± 8.2	51.5 ± 8.7	44.6 ± 5.9	2.61 ± 0.39
	g	22	163.6 ± 6.4	51.0 ± 7.2	38.8 ± 5.0	2.27 ± 0.36
16	b	23	178.6 ± 4.8	62.9 ± 6.6	55.2 ± 5.8	3.39 ± 0.52
	g	17	167.3 ± 5.9	56.7 ± 8.4	42.0 ± 3.5	2.34 ± 0.25
18	b	17	180.4 ± 6.0	66.1 ± 5.2	57.8 ± 4.0	3.38 ± 0.32
	g	18	166.3 ± 6.6	55.1 ± 7.7	41.2 ± 4.5	2.26 ± 0.38

[1]b = boys; g = girls

The trial and error method was used to determine the best value for "b" by varying it from 0.80. to 1.20 in steps of 0.05 for boys and girls together.

Results and Discussion

Table 1 indicates that up to the age of 12 years, there were no large differences between the two sexes. After that age, the differences between boys and girls became larger. This generally reflects the well-known sex differences due to differences in the time and duration of the growth spurt.

Concerning the allometric coefficient with respect to FFM, the smallest correlations were found at a value of b = 1.05 (i.e., $FFM^{1.05}$) for boys and girls together. All correlations including those for the two sexes separately using b = 1.05 were acceptably low (see Table 2). If BM is taken as the standardizing mass parameter, the value of b = 1.00 minimizes the correlations with the considered variables for boys and girls together. The correlation with sex (see Table 2) however, is relatively high (r = − .53). In addition, the correlations with the other variables in the two sexes separately are much larger than for FFM as standardizing parameter. Therefore, the FFM was chosen as the best standardizing mass parameter. The fact that FFM showed it was more generally valid than BM might at least partly be explained by the reasoning that in a random sample, this variable will be influenced minimally by the status of physical training.

Table 2

Correlation Coefficients Between Sex, Age, Height, Body Mass (BM), Fat Free Mass (FFM) and the Best Max-O_2 Transformation (Max-$O_2 \cdot$FFM$^{-1.05}$ or Max-$O_2 \cdot$BM^{-1})

	Max-$O_2 \cdot$FFM$^{-1.05}$			Max-$O_2 \cdot$BM^{-1}		
	Boys + Girls	Boys	Girls	Boys + Girls	Boys	Girls
Sex	−0.08[a]			−0.53[a]		
Age	0.03	0.18	−0.15	0.00	0.23	−0.27
Height	0.04	0.15	−0.14	0.05	0.20	−0.27
BM	0.00	0.11	−0.17	−0.07	0.08	−0.43
FFM	0.03	0.12	−0.19	0.11	0.15	−0.34

[a]The minus sign indicates that girls have lower values than boys.

After fitting, the reference formula resulted in Max-O_2 = 0.048 FFM$^{1.05}$. Table 3 shows the deviations between calculated and measured values for Max-O_2.

For comparative reasons, the results for the value of b = 1.00 with respect to BM and fitted on data for boys and girls separately (i.e., Max-O_2 = 0.051BM for boys and Max-O_2 = 0.044BM for girls) are also presented. Table 4 shows the deviations between the data calculated with these formula and the measured values for boys and girls. Another comparison was made by using a formula developed by McMiken (1976) on data of Klissouras (1971) from boys 7 to 13 years of age: Max-O_2 = 0.077FFM$^{0.92}$. In Table 5 it is shown that the deviations from the actual values were larger than when using our formula with FFM (compare Tables 3 & 5). This might have been due to a number of reasons. The data of Klissouras included: (a) no random sample, (b) a limited number of subjects, (c) a limited age group, and (d) only boys. But, of course, the best fit on the present data was better than the best fit on other data applied to the present data.

Table 3

Relative Deviation of Calculated Max-O_2 (= 0.048 FFM$^{1.05}$) for Boys and Girls From Measured Values: Mean ± SD, in %

Age (years)	Boys (% %)	Girls (% %)
6	7 ± 8	0 ± 7
8	0 ± 9	2 ± 8
10	−3 ± 8	−3 ± 7
12	1 ± 10	1 ± 11
14	−1 ± 10	−1 ± 9
16	−5 ± 13	4 ± 9
18	0 ± 9	5 ± 12

Table 4

Relative Deviation of Calculated Max-O₂ (0.051BM for Boys and 0.044BM for Girls From Measured Values: Mean ± SD, in %

Age (years)	Boys (% %)	Girls (% %)
6	9 ± 10	−3 ± 9
8	1 ± 11	−1 ± 11
10	−2 ± 10	−6 ± 11
12	1 ± 12	−2 ± 14
14	0 ± 11	−1 ± 10
16	−6 ± 13	5 ± 9
18	0 ± 8	6 ± 12

Table 5

Relative Deviation of Calculated Max-O₂ (0.077FFM$^{0.92}$, McMiken 1976) for Boys and Girls From Measured Values: Mean ± SD, in %

Age (years)	Boys (% %)	Girls (% %)
6	15 ± 7	10 ± 6
8	5 ± 8	8 ± 8
10	0 ± 8	3 ± 7
12	2 ± 10	3 ± 10
14	−3 ± 9	−2 ± 9
16	−10 ± 14	2 ± 9
18	−5 ± 9	4 ± 12

Conclusions

No essential differences exist in the level of the reference values from the allometric formula Max-O$_2$ = 0.048FFM$^{1.05}$ for sexes together, and Max-O$_2$ = 0.051BM for boys and Max-O$_2$ = 0.044BM for girls (see Table 3 and 4). FFM, however, was more generally valid, which follows from the correlations in Table 2. If FFM is used, sex differences disappear.

Max-O$_2$ can be predicted from BM or FFM with almost the same standard deviation. Furthermore, this is similar to the prediction from submaximal exercise tests.

Acknowledgment

This study was subsidized in part by The Netherlands Heart Foundation, Grant, No. 79.015.

References

ÅSTRAND, I. (1960). Aerobic work capacity in man and woman with special reference to age. *Acta Physiologica Scandinavica*, Suppl. 169, 1-92.

BRUCE, R.A., Kusumi, F., & Hosmer, D. (1973). Maximal oxygen intake and nomographic assessment of functional aerobic impairment in cardiovascular disease. *American Heart Journal*, **85**, 546-562.

DURNIN, J.V.G.A., & Rahaman, M.M. (1967). The assessment of the amount of fat in the human body from measurements of skinfold thickness. *British Journal of Nutrition*, **21**, 681-689.

GÜNTHER, B. (1975). Dimensional analysis and theory of biological similarity. *Physiological Reviews*, **55**, 659-699.

KLISSOURAS, V. (1971). Heritability of adaptive variation. *Journal of Applied Physiology*, **31**, 338-344.

McMIKEN, D.F. (1976). Maximum aerobic power and physical dimensions of children. *Annals of Human Biology*, **3**, 141-147.

SARIS, W.H.M., Noordeloos, A.M., Ringnalda, B.E.M., Van 't Hof, M.A., & Binkhorst, R.A. (1985). Reference values for aerobic power of healthy 4- to 18-year-old Dutch children. Preliminary results. In R.A. Binkhorst, H.C.G. Kemper, & W.H.M. Saris (Eds.), *Children and Exercise XI* (pp. 151-160). Champaign, IL: Human Kinetics Publishers.

Spontaneous Physical Activity in Preschool Children

Miroslav Kučera
Charles University Prague
Motol, Czechoslovakia

Insufficient physical activity is one of the greatest problems in today's society. In general, the young generation lacks adequate physical activity. This is evidenced by the fact that 36% engage in adequate physical activity while 64% have inadequate physical activity. Only 2% engage in maximal activity (sport training of high intensity), 50% engage in limited activity (only 2 hr daily), and 12% has insufficient physical activity (less than 1 hr).

What is an adequate workload—that is, what constitutes inadequate physical activity for children? It may be assumed that the child's spontaneous activity without any guidance or prodding from parents corresponds to the child's needs or to the phylogenic needs for activity. However, the determination of the required activity is very complicated and, in many cases, it is deduced rather than objectively observed. Within the framework of a lengthy research program, an attempt was made to determine the quantitative needs for physical activity of younger children.

Methodology

Time and motion studies of the physical activity of subjects were performed with the help of a hidden camera. The child was observed without such knowledge and without any limitations on activity or disturbances by the observer. All activities characterized by dynamic motion were recorded, and the static types of physical activity were ignored. In addition, the heart rate was telemetered (Seliger, Trefny, Bartunkova, & Pauer, 1974). Periods of standing, sitting, lying, and playing some children's games, when the heart rate failed to increase by 50% above its resting level, were considered to be times of inactivity (e.g., playing with dolls, building castles in the sand, children's card games, etc.). Telemetry of the heart rate was conducted using standard procedures (Anderson, 1971; Kučera, Zika, Revenda, & Tikal, 1973; McArdle, Foglia, & Patti, 1967). The transmitting device was the WAS 400 (CS) or NCA (USA). The pulse rates were recorded for 1 min at 10-min intervals with a polygraphic device.

The study of these healthy children was carried out in a summer camp in the woods near a pond, which was used as a training center for young sportsmen. The basic equip-

Table 1

Physical Characteristics of Subjects

	Boys (n = 23)		Girls (n = 17)	
	M	SD	M	SD
Age (years)	4.29	0.76	4.08	0.64
Height (cm)	107.05	2.78	104.89	3.89
Weight (kg)	18.58	1.92	17.57	2.88

ment of the summer camp at their disposal included: the pond for bathing, a boat for rowing, a playground for basketball, handball, volleyball, football, and tennis, a pit for jumping, sand, a brook, table tennis tables, rings, a rope, and the forest. The observed children were present with their parents on holidays; however, they were left alone during the observations. The physical activities of 40 preschool children were observed. The characteristics of these subjects are presented in Table 1.

All subjects were physically healthy with no period of hospitalization longer than 21 days in their medical histories. There was no preselection of subjects; therefore, all children present in the camp were studied.

The physical activities were monitored between 8 a.m. and 6 p.m. with a break of 1 hr at noon (between 12 and 1 p.m., which is the time for the main meal in Czechoslovakia).

Results

The activities listed in Table 2 constituted a mean period of 6 hr and 5 min (365.1 min) of activity for the boys and 5 hr and 27.9 min (327.9 min) for the girls. These time periods comprised 67.5 and 60.5% for the boys and girls, respectively, of the total 9 hr of observation. Boys were active in a mean of 11.8 different types of activities and girls in 9.4 activities. The principal kinds of activities engaged in are shown in Table 2 with the percentage of subjects engaged in each activity.

The data for individual subjects are presented in Table 3 and 4 for the boys and girls, respectively. The heart rates are shown in Figure 1. The mean values at rest were 95.8 beats/min for boys and 98.0 beats/min for girls. During activities, the maximal heart rates were 172.0 and 165.3 beats/min for the boys and girls, respectively, while the minimal values were 150.7/min for boys and 152.0/min for girls. The mean heart rates during the entire day (9 hr of observations) wee 161.2/min for boys and 158.8/min for girls (without considering the noon hour recess). In Figure 2, the heart rate data are shown as relative values, with the resting heart rate as 100%.

The differences between boys and girls were not statistically significant ($p>.05$). Figure 3 further illustrates heart rate values for a child while alone: She was active for the entire first day of observation; the next morning she was with her mother (Figure 4).

Table 2

Principal Types of Activity Engaged in and the Percentage of Time Spent in Each

Activity Engaged In	Boys (n = 23) % of subjects	Girls (n = 17) % of subjects
Kicking a ball	15.0	0.0
Playing with a ball (other than kicking it)	22.1	15.4
Playing in the woods	6.0	12.0
Running	25.0	33.0
Skipping	12.6	17.2
Jumping in the sand	12.0	8.0
Climbing on furniture, apparatus, or trees	21.0	6.0

Table 3

Observed Physical Activity for the Boys Aged 3 to 5 Years Between 8:00 a.m. and 6:00 p.m. (n = 23)

Total Time of Activity (min)	Different Types of Activities	Heart Rates (beats/min)				
		Rest	Maximal	Minimal	Mean	SD
480.41	15	90	158	125	140.5	10.4
388.55	16	95	172	148	159.2	4.7
304.28	8	91	160	132	147.3	8.9
311.20	9	98	180	156	170.7	8.1
446.15	16	102	182	164	176.2	7.2
426.20	14	91	165	148	153.5	5.8
412.10	16	99	180	160	173.1	7.8
355.10	10	96	172	154	166.6	8.0
335.30	11	102	181	162	173.2	6.9
315.50	9	95	172	148	162.5	7.5
366.10	14	92	160	150	155.7	4.1
385.10	14	94	170	150	161.5	6.5
370.20	12	101	184	163	156.2	7.2
312.10	10					
312.25	8					
335.42	8					
444.13	12					

Table 3 Cont.

Table 3 (Cont.)

Observed Physical Activity for the Boys Aged 3 to 5 Years Between 8:00 a.m. and 6:00 p.m. (n ⁵ 23)

Total Time of Activity (min)	Different Types of Activities	Heart Rates (beats/min)				
		Rest	Maximal	Minimal	Mean	SD
398.36	12					
320.25	11					
382.20	12					
274.16	12					
352.50	12					
370.50	12					
n 23	23	13	13	13	13	13
Mean 365.1	11.8	95.8	172.0	150.7	161.2	7.1
SD 52.8	2.5	4.2	9.0	11.5	10.7	1.6

Table 4

Observed Physical Activity for the Girls Aged 3 to 5 Years Between 8:00 a.m. and 6:00 p.m. (n = 23)

Total Time of Activity (min)	Different Types of Activities	Heart Rates (beats/min)				
		Rest	Maximal	Minimal	Mean	SD
448.53	10	85	152	122	134.6	12.4
297.25	9	102	158	148	154.8	3.2
396.15	12	100	166	158	161.6	3.0
380.10	10	95	154	144	149.5	4.2
350.10	10	95	155	146	150.7	3.6
360.10	8	97	160	154	156.6	2.5
320.12	8	98	162	155	158.4	2.4
415.11	11	99	164	156	159.6	2.7
301.20	8	100	166	158	163.7	2.7
250.15	8	100	168	161	166.5	4.9
265.42	12	102	182	162	170.8	7.9
295.35	8	101	182	150	168.1	8.7
302.10	12	101	180	163	170.5	6.7
352.10	10					
260.20	8					
315.16	8					
265.42	9					
n 17	13	13	13	13	13	13
Mean 327.9	9.4	98.0	165.3	152.0	158.8	4.9
SD 57.9	1.5	4.5	10.3	10.8	10.0	3.0

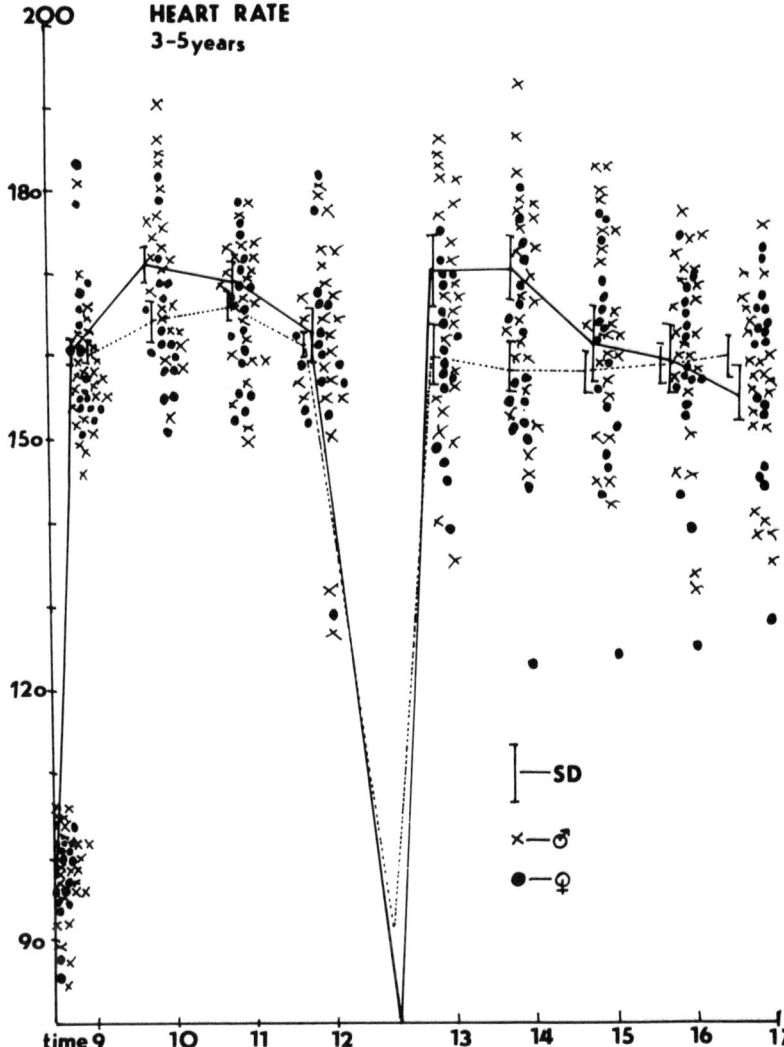

Figure 1—Heart rates (beats/min) during spontaneous physical activity in 3- to 5-year-old-boys (boys = x and girls = .).

Discussion

It is very difficult to answer the question directly concerning the amount of activity required in early childhood. On the basis of the analysis of the spontaneous open air activity, an attempt was made to express the amount of active movement by healthy children. This type of activity corresponds best to the natural style of a child's life. The movements of preschool children are rich, intensive, and gay. There are many kinds of activities engaged in (11.8 in boys and 9.4 in girls) resulting in high heart

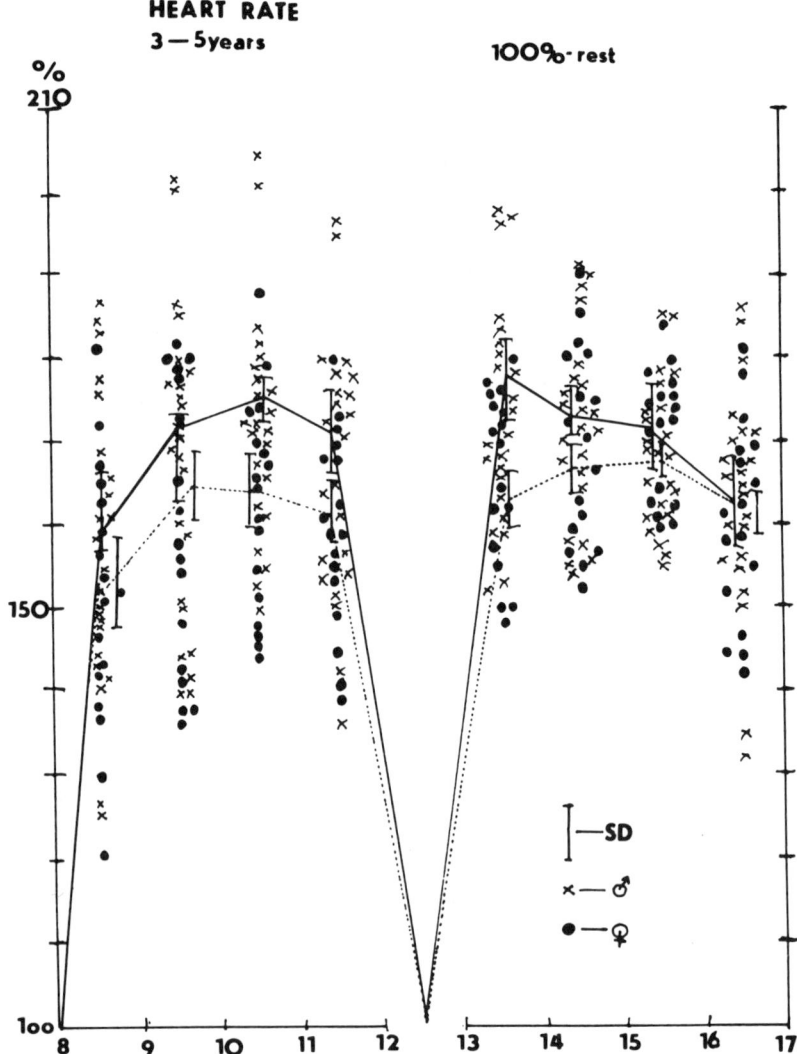

Figure 2—Relative heart rate during spontaneous physical activity in 3- to 5-year-old boys (boys = x and girls = .). The resting heart rate of values are 100%.

rates (between 150.7 and 172.0 beats/min for boys and between 152.0 and 165.3 beats/min for girls). The daily activities accompanied by high-level heart rates (over 150% of the resting heart rate) occupied 67.5% of the time for boys and 60.5% for girls. These heart rate responses averaged 161.2 beats/min and 158.8 beats/min for the boys and girls, respectively. Expressed as values relative to the resting heart rates, these were 150 to 160% higher. This type of calculation may be used for comparison with other age groups.

SPONTANEOUS PHYSICAL ACTIVITY IN PRESCHOOL CHILDREN 181

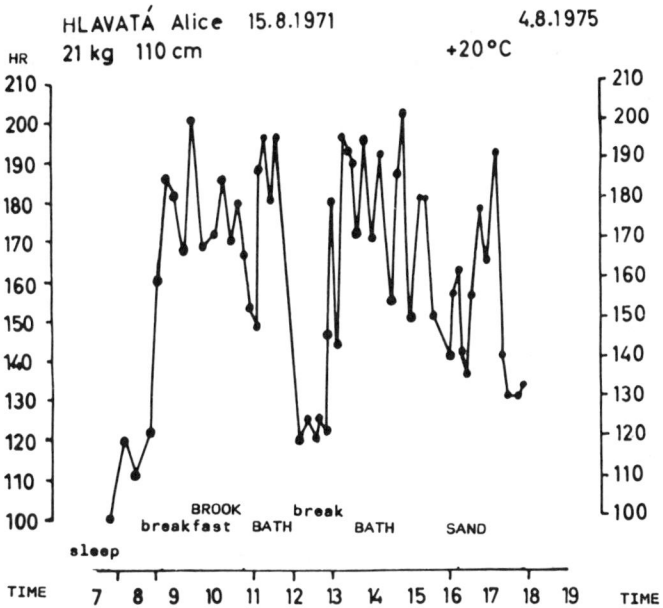

Figure 3—Heart rate during spontaneous activity in a 4-year-old girl.

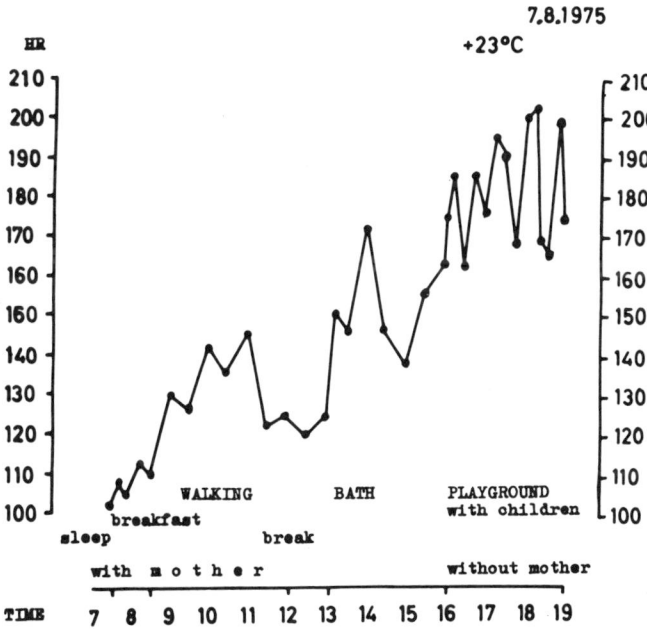

Figure 4—Heart rate during the day of the same girl (see Figure 3) while accompanied by her mother during part of the observation day.

The activities selected by the children confirm the popularity of ball games: 37% of the boys and 15% of the girls engaged in activities using a ball. The nature of children is such that monotonous activities are not acceptable, but rather that children prefer frequent changes in activities. The changes are dependent on the possible choices and the knowledge of the available activities. The physical condition and the possibilities for creative activities on the part of the child are very important in this process.

Conclusion

The children of this young age group, in a stage of maximal growth and development, should be sufficiently stimulated to be physically active. Also the quality and quantity of activity may be calculated from the spontaneous activity of observed children.

References

ANDERSON, G.J. (1971). Continuous prehospitalization monitoring of cardiac rhythm. *American Heart Journal,* **82**, 642-646.

KUČERA, M., Zika, K., Revenda, M., & Tikal, V. (1973). Follow up of the physical education at school by telemetry. *Telesna vychova mladeze,* **39**, 161-167.

McARDLE, W.D., Foglia, G.F., & Patti. A.V. (1963). Telemetered cardiac response to selected running events. *Journal of Applied Physiology,* **23**, 566-570.

SELIGER, V., Trefny, Z., Bartunkova, S., & Pauer M. (1974). The habitual activity and physical fitness of 12-year-old boys. *Acta Pediatrica Belgica,* **28** (suppl.), 54-59.

The Relation Between Physical Activity and Energy Intake of 8- and 13-Year-Old Children in Sweden

Jan Sunnegardh, Lars-Eric Bratteby, Stig Sjölin, Ulla Hagman, and Anna Hoffstedt
University of Uppsala
Uppsala, Sweden

In healthy individuals, throughout life, the energy intake is well adjusted to the energy requirements. In adults, differences in energy intake are mainly explained by differences in physical activity. The energy intake per kg body weight is higher in growing individuals than in adults; also, most studies on energy intake in children have shown a sex difference, with boys eating more than girls. These differences in energy intake between children and adults and between groups of healthy children are to a large extent due to differences in energy requirements for growth and development. However, the habitual physical activity also exerts a major influence on the energy requirements in children, but its importance relative to that of other factors in different age groups is essentially unknown. The aim of the present study was to investigate the relation between physical activity and energy intake of 8- and 13-year-old Swedish boys and girls.

Methods

As part of a nationwide food consumption study undertaken during 1980-81, an investigation was performed on 131 children born in 1967 and 1972. They were living in Uppsala in the central part of Sweden, a university and industrial town, and in Tierp, a small municipality in a rural area of this region. The municipalities of Uppsala and Tierp have a population of about 175,000. Initially, 155 children were randomly selected for this study, and the total drop-out was thus 16%. One child, a 13-year-old boy was inaccessible, and all of the other 23 nonparticipants refused to continue participation in the study. The study was approved by the Ethical Committee of the Medical Faculty of Uppsala University and informed consent was given by the children and their parents. The mean ages of the children and age ranges, and their mean weight and height with standard deviation (SD) are given in Table 1. The younger children are referred to in the following as the 8-year-old boys and girls, and the older ones as the 13-year-olds.

Table 1

Mean Ages, With Ranges in Parentheses, and Means and Standard Deviations (SD) of Height and Weight of Four Subgroups of Children Based on Age and Sex

Sex	Age (years) mean (range)	Height (cm) mean ± SD	Weight (kg) mean ± SD
Boys (n = 29)	8.7 (8.3 – 9.8)	132.1 ± 6.0	27.6 ± 3.6
Girls (n = 34)	8.7 (8.3 – 9.3)	133.8 ± 5.9	30.4 ± 6.9
Boys (n = 33)	13.8 (12.8 – 14.2)	164.2 ± 7.6	50.7 ± 11.9
Girls (n = 35)	13.7 (13.4 – 14.1)	163.9 ± 4.7	52.0 ± 9.1

Physical Activity

Questionnaire Method

On the same occasion that a dietary interview was conducted, the children answered a questionnaire concerning their habitual physical activity. Questions were asked about the duration and type of their most usual leisure-time activities, their activities during school breaks, mode of transportation to school, and sleeping habits. They were also questioned about their attitudes towards sports and physical education, their impression of their habitual physical activity and skill in physical performance, and about the frequency and duration of any regular physical training. The amount of physical activity on school days was estimated from the reported duration of specified daily activities, and by using different scores for measured (Durnin & Passmore, 1967) and estimated oxygen consumption at these activities. In two children, one boy and a girl, both 13 years of age, no activity score could be calculated because of insufficient answers.

Actometry

Eight different actometers were used. They were based on automatically winding calendar wrist watches (Certina), adjusted as described by Schulman and Reisman (1959). The instruments were tested repeatedly on a rotating plate which moved the instrument in two opposite directions intermittently. The interinstrumental variation, which was less than 0.5%, was not corrected for in the calculations. Recordings were obtained over a period of 24 hours and only during school days, with the instrument fastened on the wrist of the dominant arm and on the ankle of the contralateral leg. The sum of the arm and leg actometry measurements is referred to as the actometry value. During the day of actometry, an activity protocol was kept by the children, their

Table 2

Correlation Coefficients (r) and Significance Levels (p) of the Linear Regressions Between Actometry and Classified Physical Activity During Actometry in 17 Children

Sex	Age (years)	Subject No.	r	p
Boy	8	1	0.89	<.001
		2	0.60	n.s.
		3	0.69	<.05
		4	0.77	<.01
Girl	8	5	0.84	<.001
		6	0.81	<.001
		7	0.91	<.01
		8	0.94	<.0001
Boy	13	9	0.89	<.001
		10	0.76	<.01
		11	0.64	<.05
		12	0.76	<.05
Girl	13	13	0.83	<.001
		14	0.89	<.001
		15	0.75	<.05
		16	0.89	<.01
		17	0.69	<.05

parents and their school teachers, who also entered the actometry readings into the protocol. In 17 of these protocols, the activities were specified at least hour by hour and could be used for a detailed comparison with the actometric results (see Table 2). A close correlation was found between actometry values and classified physical activity in 16 of these 17 children. For technical reasons, actometry was not performed in 2 of the boys and 4 of the girls in the 8-year group, and in 3 of the boys and 4 of the girls in the 13-year group.

Energy Intake

Interviews for 24-hr dietary recalls were conducted with all children. In addition, in the younger age group, the 7-day food recording method was used, and in the 13-year-old children a dietary history interview was conducted. The same dietician (U.H.) performed all interviews. In the calculation of energy intake, food composition tables (Swedish National Food Administration, 1981) were used. In the 7-day food recording study, six records were incomplete and were thus omitted.

Statistical Methods. Student's t-tests, and the Pearson product moment correlation coefficient analysis were used to test mean differences and quantify relationships. A probability value of $p<.05$ was considered as statistically significant.

Results

Physical Activity

Questionnaire Method. The 8-year-old boys and girls had a mean daily activity score of 2210 ± 383 (SD) and 1905 ± 201, respectively, while the corresponding figures for the older boys and girls were 1997 ± 386 and 1783 ± 288, respectively (see Figure 1). In both the younger and older age groups, boys had a significantly higher mean daily activity score than girls of the same age. The mean activity of the 8-year-old boys was 14% higher than that of the 8-year-old girls, and the older boys had a mean activity score 11% higher than that of the girls of the same age group. The younger children had a significantly higher mean activity score than the older ones of the same sex ($p<.05$ in both sexes).

Actometry. The mean actometry values of the boys and girls 8 years of age were 156 ± 29 and 134 ± 28, and of the older boys and girls 144 ± 41 and 116 ± 26, respectively (see Figure 2). The mean actometry value of the younger boys was 14% higher than that of the girls of the same age and among the older children, this difference was 19%. Within the same sex, the younger children had a higher mean actometry value than the older ones, but this difference was statistically significant only for the girls ($p<.05$). Based on the actometry values expressed per hour awake, the younger boys were significantly ($p<.05$) more active than the older ones.

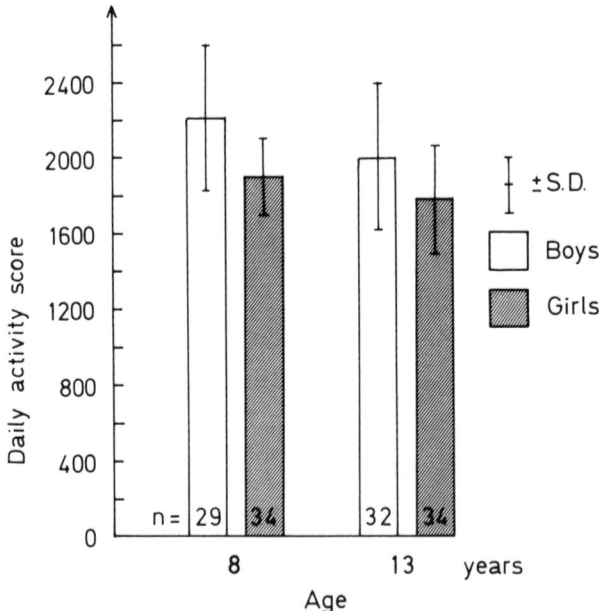

Figure 1—Means and SDs of daily activity score based on the questionnaire method. Student's t-test for independent means on sex differences in younger children $p<.0005$, in older children $p<.05$, and on age differences in both sexes $p<.05$.

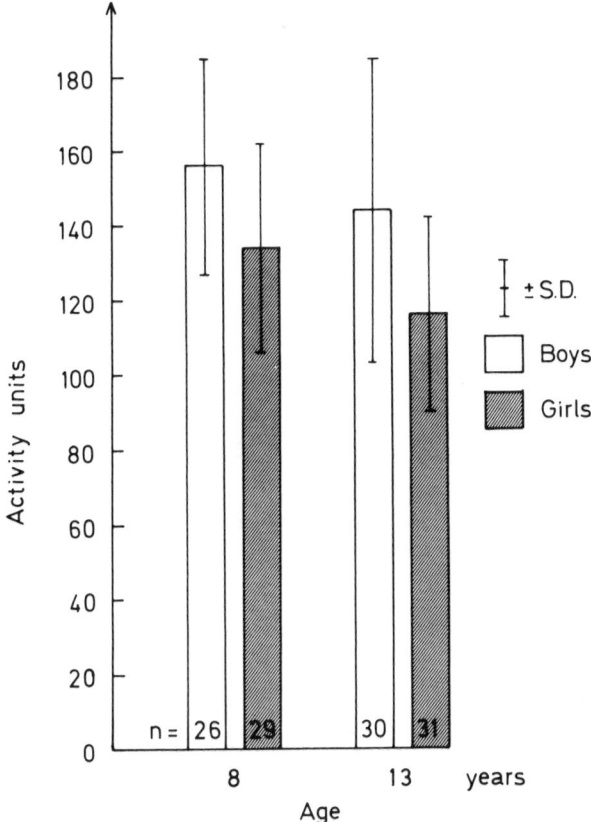

Figure 2—Means and SDs of actometry values. Student's t-test for independent means on sex differences in younger children $p<.01$, in older children $p<.005$, and on age differences in boys n.s. and in girls $p<.05$.

Energy Intake. The energy intake in absolute values (MJ) and related to body weight (MJ/kg) is shown in Tables 3, 4, and 5. In the 24-hr recall study, the 8-year-old boys had the highest mean energy intake per kg body weight and per day. The difference was significantly greater when the energy intake of the younger boys was compared with that of the older boys ($p<.05$), but was not quite so in comparison with the girls of the same age. The younger girls had a significantly higher mean energy intake per kg body weight per day than the older ones ($p<.0001$). Using the 24-hr recall method, the mean energy intake of the 8-year-old boys was found to be 12% higher than that of the 8-year-old girls; the difference between boys and girls in the older age group was 30% (see Table 3). In comparison with these results from the 24-hr recall method, a significantly higher mean energy intake was found in both younger boys ($p<.005$) and younger girls ($p<.05$) with use of the 7-day recording method. With this latter method, the mean energy intake per kg body weight and per day was 16% higher in the 8-year-old boys than in the girls of this age ($p<.01$) (see Table 4). The

Table 3

Mean Energy Intake/Day From 24-Hr Recall Interviews

Sex	Age (years)	MJ/day mean ± SD	MJ/kg mean ± SD
Boys	8	7.7 ± 2.06 (n = 29)	0.28 ± 0.075 (n = 28)
Girls	8	7.3 ± 1.65 (n = 34)	0.25 ± 0.076 (n = 33)
Boys	13	11.2 ± 3.64 (n = 33)	0.23 ± 0.088 (n = 33)
Girls	13	7.9 ± 2.28 (n = 35)	0.16 ± 0.030 (n = 34)

Student's t-test for independent means, mean energy intake/kg/day, for sex the difference in younger children was n.s., in older children $p<.0001$, based on age the difference in boys $p<.05$ and in girls $p<.0001$.

Table 4

Mean Energy Intake per Day, From 7-Day Food Recordings in 8-Year-Old Children

Sex	MJ/day mean ± SD	MJ/kg mean ± SD
Boys	9.1 ± 1.35 (n = 25)	0.33 ± 0.045 (n = 24)
Girls	8.2 ± 1.45 (n = 32)	0.28 ± 0.079 (n = 31)

Student's t-test for independent means, MJ/kg/day, $p<.01$.

mean energy intake estimated by the dietary history method was very similar to that resulting from the 24-hr recall method. Using the dietary history method, the mean energy intake per kg body weight and per day of the older boys was 26% higher than that of the older girls ($p<.0005$) (see Table 5).

Discussion

Actometry has been shown to give reliable and valid information on physical activity in children (Saris & Binkhorst, 1977). The high correlation between the intensity grading of physical activity and the actometry recordings in this study confirms this finding. The measurements cannot, however, be converted directly into traditional energy

Table 5

Mean Energy Intake per Day, From Dietary Histories in 13-Year-Old Children

Sex	MJ/day mean ± SD	MJ/kg mean ± SD
Boys	11.2 ± 2.85 (n = 33)	0.23 ± 0.070 (n = 33)
Girls	8.5 ± 2.51 (n = 35)	0.17 ± 0.063 (n = 34)

Student's t-test for independent means, MJ/kg/day, $p<.0005$.

values such as Joules or Calories, and care should be taken when comparing actometry values between children with very different body dimensions. The actometry method can be used for comparisons of habitual physical activity between groups of individuals. A reliable estimate of the habitual physical activity of an individual, however, requires much more prolonged recording than was used in this study.

The questionnaire method permits a general description of the habitual activity of an individual and requires only a short time to perform. However, it has the disadvantage of not being objective and of not measuring the vigor of a given physical activity.

Measurements of the intake of energy with use of different methods of studying dietary intake also present considerable methodological problems, and the results obtained by different methods are not always comparable (Räsänen, 1979; Sjölin, 1971).

In this study, differences were found both in physical activity and in energy intake between boys and girls of both age groups, the greatest physical activity and energy intake being noted in boys. Within the same sex, the younger children were more active and had a greater energy intake per kg body weight and per day than the older ones. These age and sex differences are well documented in earlier reports concerning physical activity (Gilliam, Freedson, Greenen, & Shahraray, 1981; Huenemann, Shapiro, Hampton, & Mitchell, 1967; Ku, Shapiro, Crawford, & Huenemann, 1981; Rutenfranz, Berndt, & Knauth, 1974; Shephard, Jequier, Lavallee, & La Barre, 1980; Spady, 1980) and energy intake (Berge, 1978; Berge, 1980; Burke, Reed, van den Berg, & Stuart, 1959; Räsänen & Ahlström, 1975; Räsänän, Ahola, Viikari, & Åkerblom, 1981; Samuelsson, 1971). To our knowledge, however, no comparison of these differences has been previously published.

In the younger children of this study, the relative differences between boys and girls in physical activity and energy intake were almost identical, no matter which method was used for measuring physical activity or energy intake (see Figure 3). This finding supports the assumption that the sex difference in energy intake in younger children is largely because of a difference in physical activity. The question whether this difference in physical activity is due mainly to biological or to sociocultural factors still remains unanswered.

The same pattern of sex differences in physical activity and energy intake was found in the older children of this study, but the agreement between the different methods was not as close as in the younger children (see Figure 3). Thus, the results of the

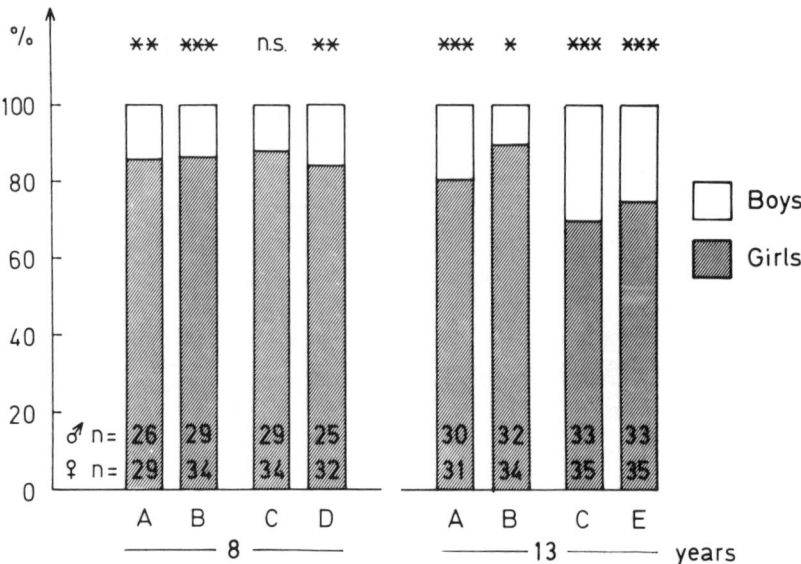

Figure 3—Sex differences (%) in actometry values (A), daily activity score (B), and energy intake/kg/day—24-hour recall (C), 7-day food recording (D), and dietary history (E). The mean values for boys are normalized to 100%. Student's t-test for independent means, $p<.05$ = *, $p<.01$ = **, $p<.005$ = ***.

questionnaire method showed a smaller sex difference than was found by actometry. This is probably explained by the insufficiency of the questionnaire method in recording intensity of physical activity. In this study, the mean actometry value of 13-year-old boys having physical education was significantly higher than that of the boys not having such lessons, while there was no significant difference in 13-year-old girls having and not having physical education (see Figure 4). This indicates that 13-year-old boys participate in physical education with more intense motor activity than girls of the same age. Such a difference is not possible to reveal by our questionnaire method.

It is obvious, however, that the difference in habitual physical activity between 13-year-old boys and girls is smaller than the corresponding difference in energy intake. In this age group, boys have a higher energy intake than girls, as a result of greater energy requirements, not only due to a higher physical activity. The 13-year-old boys of this study should have been at their peak height velocity, while the girls should have passed this stage (Karlberg, & Taranger, 1976). Therefore, these boys should have had a greater energy requirement for growth than the girls. Moreover, the girls ought to have had a lower basal energy requirement than the boys of the same age, attributed to a higher fat content of their tissues, and a lower energy requirement due to heat loss because of more efficient insulation by their larger subcutaneous fat layer.

The intention of this study was not to evaluate the contribution of factors other than habitual physical activity to differences in energy requirements between 8- and 13-year-old boys and girls. The findings indicate, however, that energy balance during puberty is more complex than it is a few years earlier in childhood. In order to make separate quantitative estimations of energy requirements during the pubertal years due to basal

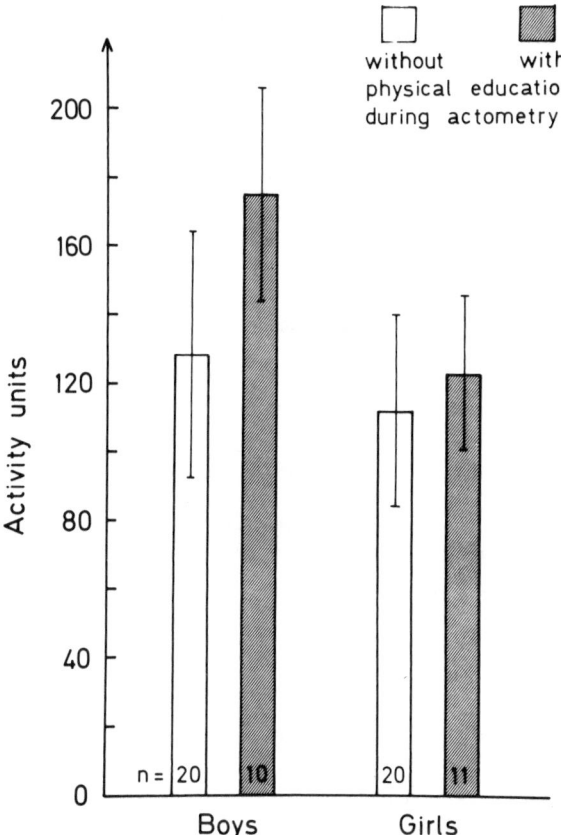

Figure 4—Mean actometry values of 13-year-old boys and girls with and without physical education during the day of actometry recording. Student's t-test for independent means on sex difference in boys $p<.001$, in girls n.s.

(maintenance) metabolic demands, growth and development, and habitual physical activity, it is clearly necessary to perform longitudinal studies of energy intake, body dimensions, and habitual physical activity during this stage of development, using methods of estimating physical activity expressed in traditional energy units (Joules, Calories). Such a study would also have clinical implications, forming a basis for better understanding of the energy (im)balance in such conditions as anorexia nervosa, obesity, and diabetes mellitus—which so often start or are aggravated during puberty.

Conclusions

Among the 8-year-old children in the present study, the physical activity of the boys was 14% higher than that of the girls, and the difference was almost identical to the sex difference in energy intake. This finding supports the assumption that the sex difference in energy intake in this age group is mainly due to a difference in physical activity.

A higher physical activity and higher energy intake were also found in the 13-year-old boys compared with the girls of the same age, but the difference in physical activity was smaller (approximately 20%) than that in energy intake (approximately 30%). These results may imply that the higher energy intake of boys of this age group, compared with girls of the same age, is also due to a significant extent to factors other than the difference in physical activity.

Acknowledgment

This study was conducted in collaboration with the Swedish National Food Administration and supported by grants from the Folksman Insurance Company.

References

BERGE, S. (1978) Dietary surveys among school children in Lom and Skjak. *Forskningsresultater*, **21**, Landsforeningen for kosthold och helse, Oslo.

BERGE, S. (1980). Dietary survey among school children in Gjövik. *Forskningsresultater*, **23**, Landsforeningen for kosthold og helse, Oslo.

BURKE, B.S., Reed, R.B., Van den Berg, A.S., & Stuart, H.C. (1959). Caloric and protein intakes of children between 1 and 18 years of age. *Pediatrics*, Vol. 4, Part II, Nov., 922-940.

DURNIN, J.V.G.A., & Passmore, R. (1967). *Energy, work and leisure*. London: Heineman.

GILLIAM, Th.B., Freedson, P.S., Greenen, D.I., & Shahraray, B. (1981). Physical activity patterns determined by heart rate monitoring in 6-7 year-old children. *Medicine and Science in Sports and Exercise*, **13**, 65-67.

HUENEMANN, R.L., Shapiro, L.R., Hampton, M.C., & Mitchell, B.W. (1967). Teenagers' activities and attitudes toward activity. *Journal of American Dietetic Association*, **51**, 433-440.

KARLBERG, P., & Taranger, J. (1976). The somatic development of children in a Swedish urban community. *Acta Paediatrica Scandinavica*, Suppl. 258.

KU, L.C., Shapiro, L.R., Crawford, P.B., & Huenemann, R.L. (1981). Body composition and physical activity in 8-year old children. *The American Journal of Clinical Nutrition*, **34**, 2770-2775.

RÄSÄNEN, L., & Ahlström, A. (1975). Nutrition survey of Finnish rural children II. Food consumption. *Annales Academiae Scientarum Fennicae*, **169**, 1-40.

RUTENFRANZ, J., Berndt, I., & Knauth, P. (1974). Daily physical activity by time budget studies and physical performance capacity of school boys. *Acta Pediatrica Belgica*, **28**, 79-86.

RÄSÄNÄN, L., Ahola, M., Viikari, J., & Åkerlund, H.K. (1981). A multicenter study of the level of coronary risk factors in Finnish children. *Naringsforskning*, **25**, 113-148.

RÄSÄNEN, L. (1979). Nutrition survey of Finnish rural children VI. Methodological study comparing the 24-hour recall and the dietary history interview. *The American Journal of Clinical Nutrition*, **32**, 2560-2567.

SAMUELSSON, G. (1971). An epidemiological study of child health and nutrition in a Northern Swedish country. I. Food consumption survey. *Acta Paediatrica Scandinavica*, suppl. 214.

SARIS, W.H.M., Binkhorst, R.A. (1977). The use of pedometer and actometer in studying physical activity in man. Part I: Reliability of pedometer and actometer. *European Journal of Applied Physiology,* **37,** 219-228.

SARIS, W.H.M., & Binkhorst, R.A. (1977). The use of pedometer and actometer in studying physical activity in man. Part II: Validity of pedometer and actometer for measuring the daily physical activity. *European Journal of Applied Physiology,* **37,** 229-235.

SCHULMAN, J.L., & Reisman, J.M. (1959). An objective measure of hyperactivity. *American Journal of Mental Deficiency,* **64,** 455-456.

SHEPHARD, R.J., Jequier, J-C., Lavallée, H., La Barre, R., & Rajic, M. (1980). Habitual physical activity: Effects of sex, milieu, season and required activity. *Journal of Sports Medicine,* **20,** 55-66.

SJÖLIN, S. (1969). Food consumption surveys in children and adolescents. *Symposia of the Swedish Nutrition Foundation,* **7,** 68-77.

SPADY, D.W. (1980). Total daily expenditure of healthy, free ranging school children. *American Journal of Clinical Nutrition,* **33,** 755-766.

SWEDISH National Food Administration (1981). *Food composition tables.* Helsingborg.

Habitual Physical Activity in Dutch Teenagers Measured by Heart Rate

Robbert Verschuur and Han C.G. Kemper
University of Amsterdam, The Netherlands

Physical activity is generally held to be an important factor in the growth and development of children and adolescents (Rarick, 1973). However, in our western industrialized society, there is a strong tendency toward hypokinesia due to automatization and mechanization. Research in The Netherlands has revealed a relatively good fitness and activity level in 12- and 13-year-old boys (Kemper et al., 1975). In an older group of 15- to 19-year-old youngsters, however, almost 50% had physical problems (Nijenhuis, 1975).

The multiple longitudinal study "Growth and Health of Teenagers" was initiated in order to study the course of the physical and mental development of teenagers in relation to their life style, and to see whether there is a period of deterioration in their health status. The present study was part of this larger project and was designed to describe the longitudinal development of habitual physical activity between ages 12 and 18 years. Recording of the heart rate has shown to be feasible as an indirect measure of energy expenditure in persons who are not largely sedentary (Bradfield, 1971).

Methods

This study was carried out at two secondary schools in the Amsterdam area. At the start all pupils of the first and second forms of both schools participated. In one school, all pupils were studied longitudinally and measured once per year. In the other school, every year a different 25% of the selected population was measured as a control in order to determine the effects of repeated measurements. Of the longitudinal group, 131 girls and 102 boys completed the 4 years of study. If effects of repeated measurements were absent, data were grouped according to age combining different years of measurement.

One of the instruments applied to measure habitual physical activity was an 8-level heart rate integrator (HRI, Depex, De Bilt, The Netherlands) which has proven to be a reliable and simple method of recording heart rate (Saris, Snel, & Binkhorst, 1977). The HRI was applied once per year, for a continuous period of 48 hr during 2 randomly selected school days, in the period from January through March. Scores were collected after each school day and each leisure time period. The HRI was the size of a package of cigarettes and weighed 220 grams. Each R-R interval was measured, analyzed, and stored in one of the eight registers of the integrator, corresponding to 40 to 69, 70 to 99, 100 to 124, 125 to 149, 150 to 176, 177 to 199, 200 to 225, and 225 to 300 beats/min. The 8th register range (225 to 300 beats/min) was used as a quality control of the ECG transmission and stored erroneous signals. The HR recordings had to meet the following three "quality" criteria in order to be considered reliable.

1. Score register 8/score register $(1+\ldots+7) < 10\%$

2. $-10\% < \dfrac{\text{estimated - real time}}{\text{real time}} \times 100 < +10\%$

   The estimated time was calculated by dividing the number of counts per register by a set value of 55, 82.5, 112.5, 137.5, 163, 188, 212.5, and 262.5, respectively.

3. The mean HR should fall within the range of 60 to 180 beats/min during the school period and 55 to 130 beats/min during the leisure time period (including sleep).

The 24-hr HR-scores were calculated only if at least one school and one leisure time measurement were reliable. In case of two reliable school or leisure time measurements, the scores of each register were averaged.

Energy expenditure was calculated from HR recordings using the individual HR-$\dot{V}O_2$ relationship, determined during a three-level submaximal treadmill test (Kemper & Verschuur, 1980). HR and $\dot{V}O_2$ in the 1st (0% inclination, 8 km/hr) and 3rd stage (5% inclination, 8 km/hr) were used. The relationship was considered reliable when the $\dot{V}O_2$ at a HR of 137.5 beats/min (midvalue of register 4) was between 5.7 and 40 ml/kg•min and at a HR of 188 beats/min (midvalue of register 6) between 20 and 80 ml/kg•min. This relationship was used only to calculate energy expenditure above a HR of 125 beats/min (register 4 to 7). The oxygen uptake at midvalue of the registers 4 to 7 was converted into energy expenditure using a factor of 4.92 kilocalories (Weir, 1949).

The energy expenditure in registers 1 to 3 was calculated by multiplying the recorded time of the HR in these registers by a fixed value for the energy expenditure of 25 cal/kg•min. This was based on calculations of the basal metabolic rate according to the equation of Harris and Benedict (Carpenter, 1939) and the net energy expenditure during standing (unloaded) (Bink, Bonjer, & Van der Sluijs, 1966).

Energy expenditure was expressed per kilogram body weight (EE/BW) as a measure of daily activity and per kilogram fat free mass (EE/FFM) to indicate the load on the active tissue. Indices of intensive activities were the time spent (T) and the EE/BW above 50% and above 75% of the individual's maximal oxygen uptake measured directly on the treadmill (Kemper & Verschuur, 1980).

Results

Comparison of the daily energy expenditure in the longitudinal and control groups did not show an interfering effect of repeated measurements with the HRI. In girls as well as in boys, almost 40% of the average 24-hr HR scores could not be calculated

Table 1

Number of Girls and Boys with Reliable HR-Recordings and HR-$\dot{V}O_2$ Relationships

Age	Girls n	Boys n
12	14	5
13	45	37
14	59	54
15	70	67
16	54	48
17	19	13
Total number	261	224

due to unreliable recordings. For the calculation of daily energy expenditure, an additional 5 to 10% of the measurements were excluded because of an unreliable HR-$\dot{V}O_2$ relationship. The number of reliable measurements is shown in Table 1.

The development of height and weight was compared with the results of a cross-sectional survey of a representative group of adolescents in The Netherlands carried out in 1965 (Van Wieringen, Wafelbakker, Verbrugge, & Haas, 1968) and in 1980 (Roede & Van Wieringen, 1982). The height of the present longitudinal sample was quite comparable to the 1980 sample and 2 to 5 cm taller than in 1965. The weight was not different from the 1965 sample and the same or lower than in 1980.

The percentage body fat of total body weight increased in girls from 23% at age 12 to 28% at age 17. In boys it remained almost constant during the age range at 15 to 16%.

Daily Energy Expenditure

Mean and standard error of total daily energy expenditure (TEE) from ages 12/13 to 17/18 years is shown in Figure 1. TEE of the girls remained fairly constant, 9.6 to 10.4 MJ/day (2300 to 2500 kcal/day). TEE of the boys increased from 8.1 MJ/day (1940 kcal/day) at age 12/13 to 11.9 MJ/day (2850 kcal/day) at 17/18 years of age. Because the number of subjects at age 12/13 (n=5) and 17/18 (n=13) was quite small, these data should be interpreted with caution. The girls had a higher TEE than the boys until they were 14/15 years old. However, this difference was not significant. From age 15/16 on the TEE of the boys was significantly higher than that of the girls.

The EE/BW of the girls (see Figure 2) gradually decreased from 200 KJ/kg•day (48 kcal/kg•day) at age 12/13 to 175 KJ/kg•day (42 kcal./kg•day) at 17/18 years of age. The EE/BW of the boys (see Figure 2) was almost constant from age 12/13 to 14/15, ca. 205 KJ/kg•day (49 kcal/kg•day) and decreased to 182 KJ/kg•day (43 kcal/kg•day)

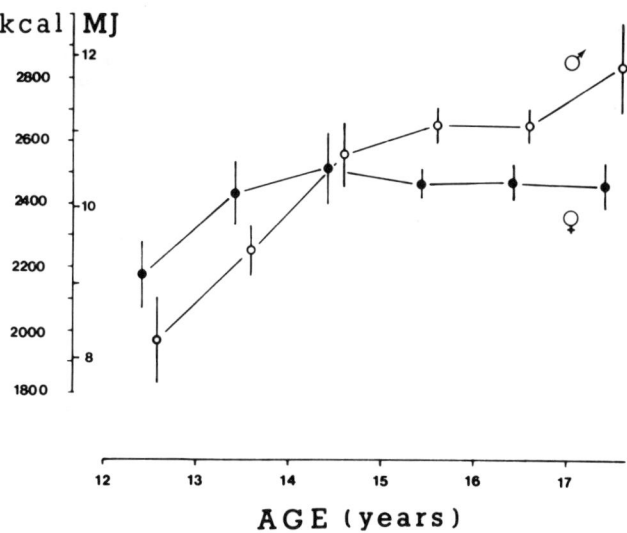

Figure 1—Mean and standard error of total daily energy expenditure (TEE) in girls and boys, estimated from 48-hr HR recordings, vs. chronological age.

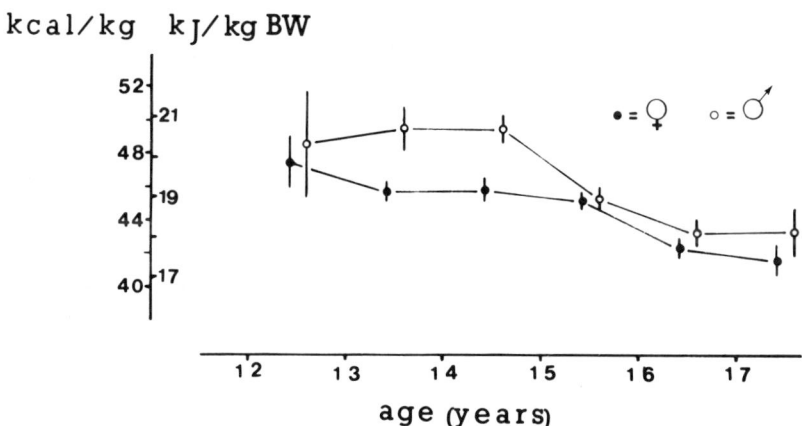

Figure 2—Mean and standard error of daily energy expenditure per kilogram body weight (EE/BW) in girls and boys, estimated from 48-hr HR recordings, vs. chronological age.

at age 17/18. Only at age 13/14 and 14/15 did the boys have significantly higher values than the girls.

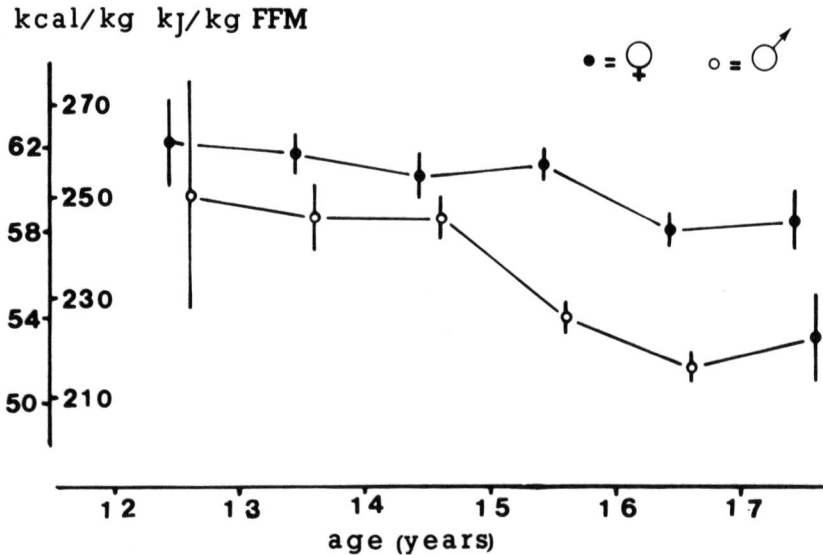

Figure 3—Mean and standard error of daily energy expenditure per kilogram fat-free mass (EE/FFM) in girls and boys, estimated from 48-hr HR recordings, vs. chronological age.

The EE/FFM of the girls (see Figure 3) remained almost constant from age 12/13 to 15/16, approximately 255 KJ/kg·day (61 kcal/kg·day) and decreased to 243 KJ/kg·day) (58 kcal/kg·day) at age 16 to 18. The EE/FFM of the boys (see Figure 3) was relatively constant until age 14/15, 248 KJ/kg·day (59 kcal/kg·day) and dropped to 218 KJ/kg·day (52 kcal/kg·day) at 16 to 18 years of age. The girls spent significantly more energy than the boys from age 15/16 to 17/18. The difference was approximately 12 to 13%.

Peak Energy Expenditure

T > 50% for the girls (see Figure 4) decreased gradually from about 70 min/day at 12/13 to 40 min/day at 17/18. In boys (see Figure 4) the decrease was larger, from about 80 min/day at age 12/13 to 14/15 to about 30 min/day at 17/18 years of age. However, the difference between girls and boys was never significant. The development of T > 75% was very similar—a decrease from about 12 min/day to 6 min/day in both sexes.

EE/BW > 50% for the girls (see Figure 5) decreased gradually from 11 kcal/kg·day at 12/13 to 5 kcal/kg·day at 17/18. In boys the EE/BW > 50% (see Figure 5) remained constant until age 14/15 (13 kcal./kg·day) and dropped to the same level as the girls at age 16 to 18. The boys have a significantly higher value at 13/14 and 14/15 years of age. EE/BW > 75 developed similarly in girls and boys—a decrease from approximately 2.5 kcal/kg·day at 13/14 to about 1.0 kcal/kg·day at 16/17 years of age.

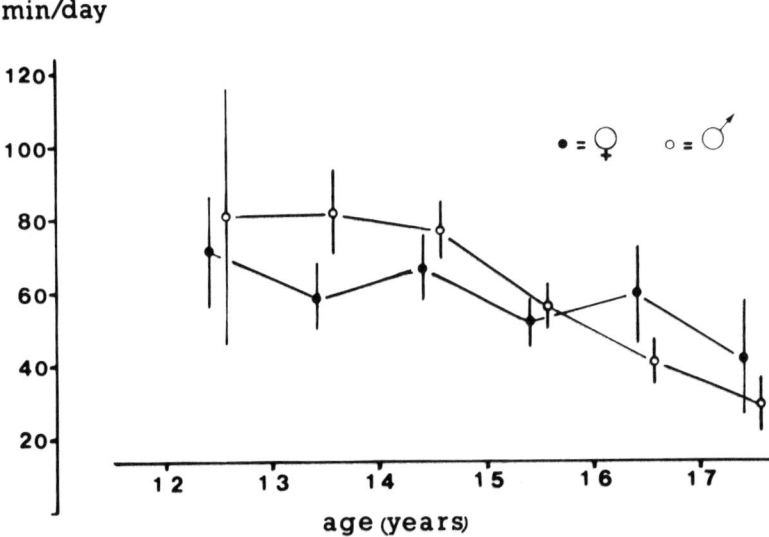

Figure 4—Mean and standard error of the time the heart rate is above 50% of the maximal oxygen uptake (T > 50) in girls and boys, estimated from 48-hr HR recordings, vs. chronological age.

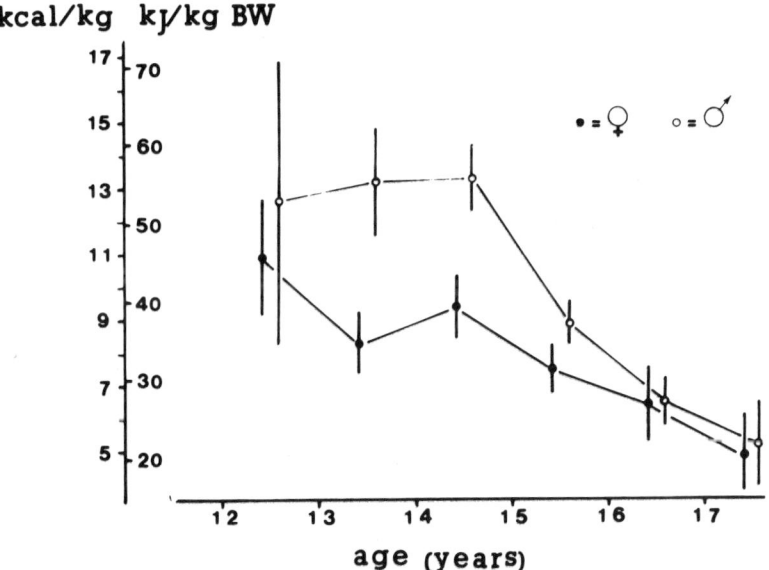

Figure 5—Mean and standard error of daily energy expenditure per kilogram body weight above 50% of the maximal oxygen uptake (EE/BW > 50) in girls and boys, estimated from 48-hr HR recordings, vs. chronological age.

Discussion and Conclusions

Reliability

The number of unreliable HR recordings was relatively high in comparison to the data of Saris (personal communication) even though the quality criteria were broader in this study. However, this high percentage of drop-outs was expected. A choice had to be made between either spending less time on electrode attachment and checking, or measuring only about 25% of the subjects. Because the latter option would have introduced a difference in treatment, the former procedure was selected.

Daily Energy Expenditure

The values of the TEE were comparable to those found in other studies (Durnin, 1971; Durnin & Passmore, 1967) except for the 12/13-year-old boys which seemed low. This could have been due to the small number ($n=5$) of 12-year-old subjects. Saris et al. (1982) found an average daily expenditure estimated from HR recordings in 10-year-old boys of 9.4 MJ/day (2251 kcal/day).

Total daily energy expenditure provided very little information about the level of activity because it was largely dependent on body weight. In children and adolescents, body weight changes considerably due to growth. The development of EE/BW, which is more indicative of the level of activity, showed that the increase in TEE in boys was due mainly to increases in weight, rather than activity. The difference between girls and boys in TEE development was caused by differences in their growth patterns. Girls had their growth spurt at an earlier age (median age: 12.6 years) than the boys (median age: 14.0 years); therefore, the girls were taller and heavier than boys up to 14/15 years of age. At that age, the growth of the girls was almost complete, whereas boys continued to grow until 17/18 years of age.

The EE/BW of the 12-year-olds in this study was lower than the values of 6-, 8-, and 10-year-old girls and boys recalculated from Saris and associates (1982). However, in their study a steady decline was observed. If their values are extrapolated to 12 years, the present values are very similar. According to EE/BW, boys were more active than girls until about 15 years of age. From 15/16 to 17/18 years, there were no differences between the sexes. The EE/FFM even indicated that from 15/16 to 17/18 years the load on the active tissue was higher in girls than in boys. The energy expenditure was calculated with a fixed value of 25 kcal/kg•min for the time the HR spent in the registers 1 to 3, which was determined to be approximately 90% of the total time. According to McArdle, Katch, and Katch (1981) basal metabolic rate is related to body surface area or fat-free mass rather than total body mass because fat is metabolically less active. Because girls and boys start to differ considerably in body composition during this age period could have been an influence.

If the energy expenditure had been calculated with a fixed value related to fat-free mass, boys would have had approximately 13% higher energy expenditure in comparison with the girls. That would mean that boys were significantly more active than girls at all ages but 12/13, according to their EE/BW, and that the load on their active tissue (EE/FFM) was, in general, the same as in the girls.

Peak Energy Expenditure

The time spent on intensive forms of physical activity decreased with age in girls and boys. However, the decrease was larger in boys (64 to 83%) than in girls (40 to 45%). According to the recommendations for adults (ACSM, 1978), in order to keep a reasonable level of fitness, one should be physically active for at least 60 min at an energy expenditure of 50% of the $\dot{V}O_2$max, 3 to 5 times per week. This would mean that the girls and boys in this study spent enough time at least until 15/16 years of age. However, both girls and boys had a relatively high aerobic power of 52 and 59 ml/kg•min, respectively, at age 12/13 years. It is likely that in order to keep this high level of fitness, more training than indicated by ACSM would be necessary. From these time figures, one would expect an identical development in aerobic fitness for girls and boys. However, the boys maintained their high $\dot{V}O_2$max/BW, whereas that of the girls gradually declined with age from 52 to 44 ml/kg•min. Even if the aerobic power is expressed in relation to fat-free mass, girls' aerobic power declined with age although less (7% instead of 15%). One explanation is that even though the amount of time spent with a HR above 50% $\dot{V}O_2$max was not different in girls and boys, the energy expended per kg body weight was higher in boys. Durnin and Passmore (1967) also concluded that 13/14-year-old Scottish boys did the same activities with higher intensity than girls.

Conclusion

During the teens, the level of activity decreased in both girls and boys. At least until age 14/15 years, boys are more active than girls, this difference decreasing with increasing age. However, the load on the active tissue is only slightly different. Although the time spent on high intensity activities is similar in girls and boys, the boys do the same activities with a higher intensity.

References

ACSM (American College of Sports Medicine). (1978). Position statement on the recommended quantity and quality of exercises for developing and maintaining fitness in healthy adults. *Medicine and Science in Sports,* **10**(3), vii-x.

BINK, B., Bonjer, F.H., & Van der Sluys, H. (1966). Assessment of the energy expenditure by indirect time and motion study. In K. Evang & K. Lange Anderson (Eds.), *Physical activity in health and disease* (pp. 207-215). Oslo: Scandinavian University Book.

BRADFIELD, R.B. (1971). A technique for determination of usual daily energy expenditure in the field. *American Journal of Clinical Nutrition,* **24**, 1148-1154.

CARPENTER, T.M. (1939). *Tables, factors and formulas for computing respiratory exchange and biological transformations of energy.* Washington: Carnegie Institute.

DURNIN, J.V.G.A. (1971). Physical activity by adolescents. In C. Thorén (Ed.), *Acta Paediatrica Scandinavica,* Supplement **217**, 133-135.

DURNIN, J.V.G.A., & Passmore, R. (1967). *Energy, work and leisure.* London: Heinemann Education Books LTD.

KEMPER, H.C.G., & Verschuur, R. (1980). Measurement of aerobic power in teenagers. In K. Berg & B.O. Eriksson (Eds.), *Children and exercise IX* (pp. 55-63). Baltimore: University Park Press.

KEMPER, H.C.G., Verschuur, R., Ras, J.G.A., Snel, J., Splinter, P.G., & Tavecchio, L.W.C. (1975). Biological age and habitual physical activity in relation to physical fitness in 12- and 13-year-old schoolboys. *Journal of Pediatrics,* **119**, 169-179.

McARDLE, W.D., Katch, F.I., & Katch, V.L. (1981). *Exercise physiology.* Philadelphia: Lea & Febiger.

NIJENHUIS, H.W.A. (1975). *Youth employment and health.* Organization for health research, T.N.O., Den Haag, Uitg. V.R.B., Groningen.

RARICK, G.L. (1973). Preface. In G.L. Rarick (Ed.), *Physical activity. Human growth and development.* New York: Academic Press.

ROEDE, M. & Wieringen, J.C. van. (in press). Design and results from the Dutch third nation wide survey on growth. *Tijdschrift voor Sociale Geneeskunde.*

SARIS, W.H.M., Noordeloos, A.M., Cramwinckel, A.B., Boeyen, I., Elvers, J.W.H., Van Veen, M., Köning, K.G., & Binkhorst, R.A. (1982). Aerobic power, daily physical activity and some cardiovascular disease risk indicators in children ages 6-10 years. In W.H.M. Saris (Ed.), *Aerobic power and daily physical activity in children* (pp. 153-176). Unpublished doctoral dissertation, Catholic University of Nijmegen, The Netherlands.

SARIS, W.H.M., Snel, P., & Binkhorst, R.A. (1977). A portable heart rate distribution recorder for studying daily physical activity. *European Journal of Applied Physiology,* **37**, 19-25.

WEIR, J.B. (1949). New methods for calculating metabolic rate with special reference to protein metabolism. *Journal of Applied Physiology,* **109**, 1.

WIERINGEN, J.C. van, Wafelbakker, F., Verbrugge, H.P. & Hass, J.H. de. (1968). *Groeidiagrammen Nederland (Growth diagrams The Netherlands).* Groningen: Wolters-Noordhoff.

Physical and Psychological Effects of Physical Training on Handicapped Children

Monique H.W. Dresen
University of Amsterdam and The Free University
Amsterdam, The Netherlands

Disorders in both physical performance and learning behavior have often been commented upon in the literature (Getman & Hendrickson, 1961; Kagan, Rasman, Day, Arbert, & Phillips, 1964; Lievens, 1974).

The results from preceding studies (Dresen, De Groot, Brandt Corstius, Krediet, & Meijer, 1982; Dresen, Vermeulen, Netelenbos, & Krot, 1982) showed that handicapped children spent less time in daily life on heavy physical activity and had a significantly lower physical work capacity, a lower physical efficiency as well as lower classroom-attention scores than a comparative group of nonhandicapped children. Both low physical work capacity and low physical efficiency can be considered detrimental to the execution of the activities of daily life (ADL). A low classroom-attention level may have negative effects on learning and/or performance (Samuels & Turnure, 1974).

Regular physical exercise can induce an improvement in physical work capacity and physical efficiency as well as body composition (Hollmann & Hettinger, 1980) and can increase the capacity to perform ordinary daily activities (Katz, 1967).

Therefore, the question which presents itself is, Can physical training for handicapped children induce an improvement in physical variables like physical work capacity, physical efficiency, body composition, and (indirectly) classroom attention? In this article, effects of two kinds of physical training programs are reported, namely, an intensification of physical activity incorporated into the scheduled school physical education lessons and an increase in the number of physical education lessons per week.

Methods

Subjects

In these studies, 2 groups of physically handicapped children were involved. Group A consisted of 11 handicapped children (7 boys and 4 girls) and Group B of 18 handicapped children (13 boys and 5 girls). The mean ages of the children in Groups A and B at the start of the study were 139 (range: 104 to 174) and 135 (range: 76 to 168) months, respectively.

Procedures

The overall experimental procedure involved a pretest, a training program and a posttest. The subjects in both Groups A and B were subdivided into a control and an experimental group. The experimental group of Group A consisted of 6 children and that of Group B, 9 children.

Measurements of Physical Parameters

Physical Work Capacity and Physical Efficiency. In order to obtain the physical work capacity (PWC) and physical efficiency of the handicapped children, oxygen uptake and heart rate were measured at different increasing work loads on an electrically braked bicycle ergometer. A work load schedule based on the International Biological Program (Weiner & Lourie, 1969) was applied.

Linear regression functions of oxygen uptake (STPD) (ml·$^{-1}$·kg^{-1}) on heart rate (beats·min^{-1}) (i.e., physical work capacity) and of oxygen uptake (STPD) (ml·min^{-1}) on work load (W) (i.e., physical efficiency) were calculated. In addition, the oxygen uptake (ml·min^{-1}·kg^{-1}) at a heart rate of 170 beats·ml^{-1} (PWC$_{170}$) (using the regression lines) was estimated.

Anthropometric Variables. Body height, body weight, and the sum of four skinfold thicknesses (biceps, triceps, supra iliaca, and subscapula) were measured.

Measurements of Classroom Attention

Assessment of the level of the pupils' classroom attention was based on previously designed observation instrument (for a detailed description see Dresen, Vermeulen, Netelenbos, & Krot, 1982). Classroom-attention measurements were repeated at least 5 times on several days at the same time each day. The classroom-attention score for 1 observation period was obtained by expressing the total number of times "attentive behavior" was recorded as a percentage of the total observations per session. The mean percentage score (of at least 5 repeated observations) was used as the classroom-attention score.

Training Program

The physical training program for Group A was conaucted within the framework of the regular school physical education lessons (3 lessons/week). During all the lessons, for the children of the experimental group only, the intensity of the activity during the physical education lessons was increased. The intensity was evaluated for both subgroups by means of (continuous) heart rate recordings, an attempt being made to reach and to maintain a heart rate of 160 beats·min^{-1} or higher as long as possible during each lesson. The physical training program in Group B consisted of one additional physical education lesson per week for the children of the experimental group. The experimental group had three lessons of physical education per week, the control group only two. The actual intensity of activity during the physical education lessons was measured in both experimental and control groups by means of (continuous) heart rate recordings.

Results

No significant differences were found between control and experimental groups in either Group A or Group B before the start of the training program (pretest) on any of the measured parameters.

Training Program

As was intended in Group A, the intensity of the training program (the time spent at a heart rate of 160 beats·min^{-1} or higher per lesson) with respect to games, swimming, and judo lessons was higher for the experimental group than the control group (see Table 1). In Group B, the experimental group had one additional physical education lesson per week. The mean intensity of physical activity per lesson between experimental and control groups did not differ significantly (see Table 2).

Table 1

Intensity and Duration of the Training Program in Group A

Training Program	Experimental (n = 6)	Control (n = 5)
Games (about 30 min a week)		
presence	78%	88%
time, $f_H \geqslant 160$ beats·min^{-1} per lesson (min)	19.1 + 6.0*	10.3 ± 8.0
Swimming (about 40 min a week)		
presence	60%	60%
time, $f_H \geqslant 160$ beats·min^{-1} per lesson (min)	15.0 ± 7.6*	6.8 ± 3.2
Judo (about 50 min a week)		
presence	91%	97%
percentage of observations with $f_H \geqslant 160$ beats·min^{-1}	27 ± 18 *	4 ± 6

Mean values and standard deviations of the times for which subjects have heart rates at or above 160 beats·min^{-1} per lesson during games and swimming lessons. During judo lessons the relative number of observations at which heart rates were found at or above 160 beats·min^{-1} is given. The mean percentage of the scheduled lessons which were attended by the children, is indicated by "presence." Significant differences between experimental and control group are indicated by * (t-test, one-tailed, p<.05).

Table 2

Duration, Number and Intensity of Physical Education Lessons in Group B

Characteristics of Lessons	Experimental Group (n = 9)	Control Group (n = 9)
Mean duration per lesson (min)	27 ± 4	26 ± 3
Number of lessons per week	3	2
Mean heart rate per lesson (beats·min^{-1})	146 ± 34	130 ± 33
Presence	92%	88%

The mean percentage of the scheduled lessons which were attended by the children is indicated by "presence."

Physical Parameters

Physical Efficiency (Oxygen Uptake Relative to Work Load). A significant difference in level between experimental and control groups was found (see Table 3). In Group B, no significant changes in the mean values of the individual differences between post- and pretests with respect to slope and level values between groups were found.

Table 3

Mean Values and Standard Deviations of the Differences Between Post- and Pretest With Respect to Slope and Level of the Relationship Between Oxygen Uptake (STPD) and Work Load for Control (n = 5) and Experimental (n = 6) Group in Group A

Variable	Post-/Pretest	
	Experimental	Control
Relation oxygen uptake—work load		
Slope [ml·min^{-1}·W^{-1}]	0.1 ± 2.9	0.6 ± 1.8
Level [ml·min^{-1}]	-82 ± 57*	9 ± 98

Significant differences between control and experimental groups are indicated by * (t-test, one-tailed, $p < .05$).

Table 4

Mean Values and Standard Deviations of the Individual Differences Between Post- and Pretest Concerning Body Height, Body Weight, and Sum of Four Skinfold Thicknesses in Control and Experimental Group in Both Group A and B

	Group A Post-/Pretest		Group B Post-/Pretest	
Body Height (mm)	9 ± 7	19 ± 13	10 ± 6	14 ± 9
Body weight (kg)	0.8 ± 0.5*	2.0 ± 0.9	0.7 ± 0.8*	2.5 ± 2.3
Sum of four skinfold	-2.2 ± 6.7*	4.6 ± 2.7	-0.8 ± 3.6*	2.7 ± 2.7

Significant differences between experimental and control group are indicated by * (t-test, one-tailed, $p < .05$).

Physical Work Capacity (Oxygen Uptake Relative to Heart Rate). No significant changes in the mean values of the individual differences between post- and pretest with respect to slope values and PWC_{170} were found between subgroups in both Groups A and B.

Anthropometric Variables. The mean values of the individual differences between post- and pretest with respect to body weight and sum of skinfold thicknesses did differ significantly between experimental and control group in both Groups A and B (see Table 4).

Classroom Attention

In Group A the mean values of the individual differences between post- and pretest for the experimental group was 6.2% (SD: 4.7) and for the control group -3.1% (SD: 10.1). The difference between experimental and control group with respect to these mean difference values differed significantly (t-test, one-tailed, $p < .05$). In Group B the mean values of the individual differences between experimental and control groups did not differ significantly.

Discussion

An intensification of physical activity was shown to induce a significant improvement in physical efficiency, body composition, and classroom-attention of handicapped children. No effect of these increases was found for physical work capacity.

One additional physical education lesson per week is insufficient to improve physical work capacity, physical efficiency, or classroom-attention scores of handicapped children. An improvement in body composition of handicapped children can be induced both by an intensification of physical activity as well as by an increase in the amount of physical education per week.

In the literature, the results of studies dealing with training effects on physical efficiency and physical work capacity are not uniform. An improvement in efficiency after an increase in (training) intensity was reported for handicapped children by Rieckert, Bruhn, Schwalm, and Schnizer (1977) and for nonhandicapped children by Daniels and Oldridge (1971). However, in studies of Lundberg and Pernow (1970) and Bar-Or, Inbar, and Spira (1976) no effect was found in the efficiency after an increase in, respectively, intensity and amount of physical activity for handicapped adolescents. An increase in physical work capacity after an increase in intensity for handicapped subjects was found by Berg (1970), Bar-Or, Inbar, and Spira (1976), and Lundberg, Ovenfors, and Saltin (1967). In studies by Kemper, et al. (1978), Bar-Or and Zwiren (1973), and Johnson (1969) no physiological effects as a result of mere increase in the number of physical education lessons per week were found for nonhandicapped boys or girls. According to studies reported in the literature and the studies described here, a high level of training intensity is necessary to produce an effect on physical work capacity of children.

An increase in the amount of work per week and in intensity of physical activity does seem to be sufficient to induce positive effects on body weight and sum of skinfold thicknesses of handicapped children. According to Åstrand and Rodahl (1970), the *amount* of work is more important than the *intensity* of work for caloric expenditure.

An explanation for the increase in classroom-attention level could be that the children, as a result of the increase in physical efficiency, get less tired during execution of the activities of daily life. A decrease in fatigue could also have positive effects on classroom attention.

References

ÅSTRAND, P.O., & Rodahl, K. (1970). *Textbook of work physiology.* New York: McGraw-Hill Book Company.

BAR-OR, O., & Zwiren, L.D. (1973). Physiological effects of increased frequency of physical education classes and of endurance conditioning on 9- to 10-year old girls and boys. In O. Bar-Or (Ed.), *Pediatric work physiology.* Proceedings of the Fourth International Symposium. Tel-Aviv: Wingate Institute.

BAR-OR, O., Inbar, O., & Spira, R. (1976). Physiological effects of a sports rehabilitation program on cerebral palsied and post-poliomyelitic adolescents. *Medicine and Science in Sports,* **8**, 157-161.

BERG, K., (1970). Adaptations in cerebral palsy of body composition, nutrition and physical working capacity at school age. *Acta Paediatrica Scandinavica*, (Supplement) **204**, 1-93.

DANIELS, J., & Oldridge, N. (1971). Changes in oxygen consumption of young boys during growth and running training. *Medicine and Science in Sports,* **3**, 161-165.

DRESEN, M.H.W., Groot, G. de, Brandt Corstius, J.J., Krediet, G.H.B., & Meijer, M.G.H. (1982). Physical work capacity and daily physical activities of handicapped and non-handicapped children. *European Journal of Applied Physiology,* **48**, 241-251.

DRESEN, M.H.W., Vermeulen, H., Netelenbos, B.J., & Krot, H. (1982). Physical work capacity and classroom-attention of handicapped and non-handicapped children. *International Journal of Rehabilitation Research,* **5**, 5-12.

GETMAN, G.N., & Hendrickson, H.H. (1961). The needs of teachers for specialized information on the development of visuo-motor skills in relation to academic performance. In W.M. Cruickshank (Ed.), *A teaching method for brain injured and hyperactive children.* Syracuse: University Press.

HOLLMANN, W., & Hettinger, Th. (1980). *Sportmedizin-, Arbeits- und Trainingsgrundlagen.* Stuttgart: Schattauer Verlag.

JOHNSON, E.L. (1969). Effects of 5-day a week vs. 2- and 3-day a week physical education class on fitness skill, adipose tissue and growth. *Research Quarterly,* **40,** 93-98.

KAGAN, J., Rasman, B.L., Day, D., Arbert, J., & Phillips, W. (1964). Information processing in the child; Significance of analytic and reflective attitudes. *Psychological Monographs: General and Applied,* **78,** 32-37.

KATZ, L.N. (1967). Physical fitness and coronary heart disease. *Circulation,* **35,** 405-414.

KEMPER, H.C.G., Verschuur, R., Ras, K.G.A., Snel, J., Splinter, P.G., & Tavecchio, L.W.C. (1978). Investigation into the effects of two extra physical education lessons per week during one school year upon the physical development of 12- and 13-year old boys. In J. Borms, & M. Hebbelinck, *Pediatric work physiology. Medicine and Sport,* **11,** Basel: Karger.

LIEVENS, P. (1974). The organic psychosyndrome of early childhood and its effects on learning. *Journal of Learning Disabilities,* **7/10,** 626-631.

LUNDBERG, A., Ovenfors, C.O., & Saltin, B. 1967. Effect of a physical training on schoolchildren with cerebral palsy. *Acta Paediatrica Scandinavica,* **56,** 182-188.

LUNDBERG, A., & Pernow, B. (1970). The effect of physical training on oxygen utilization and lactate formation in the exercising muscle of adolescents with motor handicaps. *Scandinavian Journal of Clinical and Laboratory Investigation,* **26,** 89-96.

RIECKER, H., Bruhn, L., Schwalm, U., & Schnizer, W. (1977). Ein Ausdauertraining im Rahmen des Schulsports bei vorwiegend spastisch gelähmten Kindern (Endurance training in physical education lessons for spastic handicapped children). *Medizinische Welt,* **28,** 1694-1701.

SAMUELS, S.J., & Turnure, J.E. (1974). Attention and reading achievement in first grade boys and girls. *Journal of Educational Psychology,* **66,** 29-32.

WEINER, J.S., & Lourie, J.A. (Eds.) (1969). *Human biology; A Guide to Field Methods.* I.B.P. Handbook No. 9. Oxford: Blackwell.

Work Efficiency of Children During Submaximal Bicycle Exercise

Klaus Klausen, Birger Rasmussen, Lone K. Glensgaard and Ole V. Jensen
University of Copenhagen, Denmark

When maximal aerobic power (e.g., ml $O_2$2·min^{-1}) is determined in adults by extrapolation from measurements of heart rate during steady state at submaximal work intensity on a bicycle ergometer, the calculation is usually based on a standard net efficiency of the exercise of about 23%. Values of about 21% are used if the work intensity during the test is as low as 50-70 W (I. Åstrand, 1960). In recent studies (unpublished), it was found that the aerobic power of children 9 to 14 years of age was often very low when calculated either according to the age-corrected I. Åstrand's nomogram (1960) or according to the extrapolation principle described by Asmussen and Molbech (1959). Hence, the purpose of the present investigation was to measure the mechanical efficiency during submaximal bicycle exercise in children.

Methods

The subjects were 53 children from a Copenhagen primary school. They were divided into 4 groups according to sex and age. Average values of age, height, and weight of the 4 groups are given in Table 1.

Exercise was performed on the Monark bicycle ergometer. The ergometer was specially designed to allow for a proper adjustment of the saddle height to each child. Further, the weight of the pendulum bob was reduced so that the scale reading was doubled at any given work load in order to improve the adjustment of the ergometer. Each child exercised with a pedaling frequency (RPM) of 50 revolutions/min at zero load and at 2 submaximal work loads ($\dot{W}1$ and $\dot{W}2$), giving a heart rate (HR) of about 120 and 160 beats/min, respectively. After a resting period, the 2 submaximal work loads were repeated at an RPM of the child's own choice. Finally, the maximal HR (HRmax) was determined by having the children exercise to exhaustion with increasing work load over a period of 2 to 4 min. The sequence of events is shown in Figure 1. Oxygen uptake ($\dot{V}O_2$ and CO_2 output ($\dot{V}CO_2$) were measured by the Douglas bag method. HR was registered continuously from electrodes placed on the chest. The RPM was measured continuously by means of a microswitch placed on the crank of the bicycle

Table 1

Mean Age, Height, Weight, Basal Metabolic Rate (BMR), and Maximal Heart Rate (HRmax)Xx

n	Sex	Age (years)	Height (cm)	Weight (kg)	BMR (KJ·min⁻¹)	HRmax (beats·min⁻¹)
13	M	9.6 ± 0.13	137.1 ± 1.66	30.9 ± 1.40	3.54 ± 0.020	197.2 ± 3.16
13	M	13.4 ± 0.09	157.5 ± 2.33	43.4 ± 1.61	4.24 ± 0.022	206.3 ± 2.25
13	F	9.9 ± 0.14	137.5 ± 2.02	30.9 ± 1.33	3.33 ± 0.019	201.1 ± 1.60
13	F	13.6 ± 0.10	160.9 ± 2.00	50.7 ± 1.88	4.31 ± 0.021	199.4 ± 1.86

All means are given ± 1 se.

ergometer. Basal metabolic rate (BMR) was predicted for each child from the surface area according to Carpenter's tables (1924).

The efficiency of exercise was calculated in three different ways:

1. The *net efficiency* (EF_N) was calculated from the equation:

$$EF_N = \frac{\dot{W}}{\dot{M} - m}, \quad (1)$$

where, $\dot{W}$ is the work intensity calculated from the work load on the ergometer and the registered RPM, M is the metabolic rate during exercise calculated from $\dot{V}O_2$ and a caloric equivalent of O_2 estimated from the actual respiratory exchange ratio (R), and m is the BMR.

2. The *zero load efficiency* (EF_O) was calculated from the equation:

$$EF_O = \frac{\dot{W}}{\dot{M} - \dot{M}_O}, \quad (2)$$

where M_O is the metabolic rate during zero load exercise calculated from $\dot{V}O_2$ at zero load and the caloric equivalent of O_2.

3. The *apparent efficiency* (EF_A) was calculated from the equation:

$$EFA = \frac{\dot{W}_2 - \dot{W}_1}{\dot{M}_2 - \dot{M}_1}, \quad (3)$$

where $\dot{W}_2$ and $\dot{W}_1$ are the work intensities giving a HR of about 160 and 120 beats/min, respectively, and $\dot{M}_2$ and $\dot{M}_1$ are the corresponding metabolic rates.

Results

Average group values of BMR and HRmax are included in Table 1. The HRmax was defined as the highest 5 = s QRS-count during the max-test, usually obtained a few seconds before the subjects stopped the exercise.

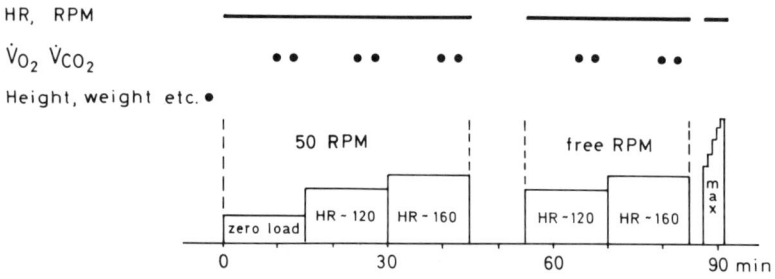

Figure 1—Sequence of events during a complete test of a subject.

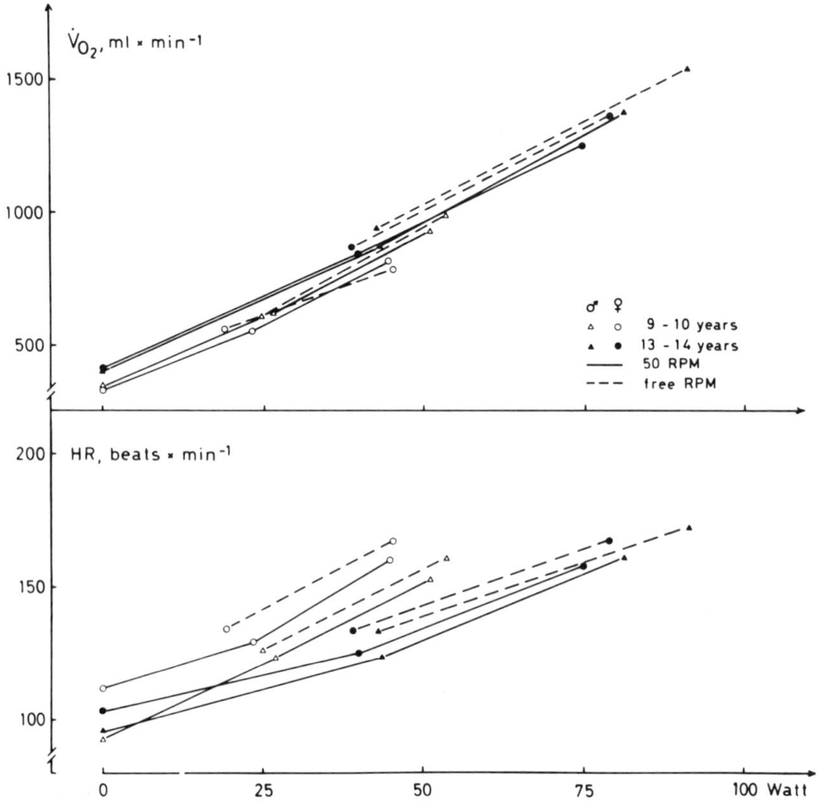

Figure 2—Mean values of $\dot{V}O_2$ and HR in relation to work intensity. The standard error (se) of the work intensity for all means given in the figure ranges from ± 2 to ± 4 W. The se of the $\dot{V}O_2$ values range from ± 13 to ± 59 ml·min^{-1}. The se's of the HR values range from ± 3.1 to ± 7.3 at zero load, whereas at all other work loads the se's ranged only from ± 1.6 to ± 3.9.

The RPM-registration revealed that all 4 groups of subjects on the average exercised at a higher RPM than the requested 50 RPM. Thus, at zero load the actual RPM (± 1

se) was 54.1 ± 0.59 and at W_1 and W_2, it was 52.4 ± 0.49 and 54.3 ± 0.58, respectively. When the children were asked to exercise at an RPM of their own choice, the average RPMs at the 2 work loads, W_1 and W_2, were 66.8 ± 1.39 and 67.3 ± 1.33, respectively.

The average $\dot{V}O_2$ during exercise at zero load in the 4 groups ranged from 331 to 396 ml $O_2 \cdot min^{-1}$, and as can be seen in Figure 2, the two oldest groups (filled symbols) clearly had the highest values. There was an almost linear relation between work intensity and $\dot{V}O_2$, although in all groups the increase in $\dot{V}O_2$ from zero load to W_1 was slightly less steep than that from W_1 to W_2. $\dot{V}O_2$ at free RPM tended to be slightly higher than at 50 RPM at the same work intensity, and the young groups (open symbols) tended to have a lower $\dot{V}O_2$ at a given work load than the older groups. All the group average HR's are also plotted against work intensity in Figure 2. Note that for all groups, there was a steeper increase in HR from W_1 to W_2 than from zero load to W_1. The two young groups (open symbols) had a higher HR at a given work intensity than the older groups, and in all groups free-choice RPM's yielded a slightly higher HR than 50 RPM.

Average values (±1 se) of the mechanical efficiency of bicycle exercise calculated according to the three equations are presented in Table 2. In all 4 groups of subjects, the EF_N values calculated from the work load giving a HR of about 120 beats/min (W_1) were lower than those obtained by calculation from the work load giving a HR of about 160 beats/min (W_2). Furthermore, the EF_N from the 9- to 10-year-old children tended to be lower than the EF_N from the 13- to 14-year-old children, and finally, comparable values showed that the EF_N tended to be lower at free-choice RPM than at 50 RPM. The EF_O was always highest when calculated from W_1, and girls in both age groups tended to have higher values than the boys. The EF_A values did not show

Table 2

Mean Values of Net-Efficiency (EF_N), Zero-Load Efficiency (EF_O), and Apparent Efficiency (EF_A)

	Age	9-10 Years		13-14 Years	
	Sex	M	F	M	F
EF_N %	50 $\dot{W}_1$	17.5 ± 1.00	17.6 ± 0.80	19.9 ± 0.79	19.4 ± 0.85
	RPM $\dot{W}_2$	19.9 ± 0.42	20.1 ± 0.48	20.6 ± 0.45	21.5 ± 0.55
	Free $\dot{W}_1$	17.6 ± 1.64	15.5 ± 1.29	17.5 ± 0.45	17.5 ± 0.92
	RPM $\dot{W}_2$	19.3 ± 0.60	19.0 ± 0.51	20.1 ± 0.38	20.1 ± 0.54
EF_O %	50 $\dot{W}_1$	27.7 ± 0.67	30.9 ± 1.32	27.2 ± 1.14	29.2 ± 1.17
	RPM $\dot{W}_2$	25.2 ± 0.54	27.5 ± 0.87	24.4 ± 0.50	27.6 ± 1.17
EF_A %	50 RPM	23.4 ± 0.87	23.4 ± 1.14	21.9 ± 0.91	25.6 ± 1.20
	Free RPM	22.3 ± 0.83	24.3 ± 1.02	23.8 ± 0.82	23.9 ± 0.75

All mean values are given ± 1 se. For further information, see text.

any systematic difference either between age groups or between groups of girls and boys of the same age.

Discussion

The net efficiency (EF_N) is the value normally used for evaluation of the mechanical efficiency of bicycle exercise. In normal adult subjects the EF_N will usually be about 23% (Åstrand, 1958, 1960; Åstrand, Åstrand, & Rodahl, 1959; Åstrand, 1952; Ryming, 1953) although somewhat lower values (19 to 22%) were obtained in older subjects, and in subjects who were tested at work intensities as low as about 50 W. The EFN values obtained at 50 RPM in the present experiments (see Table 2) are slightly lower than those reported by I. Åstrand (1960) at comparable work intensities. The reason for this could be that the BMR of children is lower than the BMR of adults (cf. Equation 1). However, the EF_A (cf. Equation 3 and Table 2) in the present experiments ranges from 21.9 to 25.6, while values calculated from I. Åstrand's data on adults (1960) range from 23.9 to 26.6 These calculated values are in accordance with values previously reported by Asmssen (1952), for example.

It has previously been reported that the EF_N in adults is very low at work intensities below 60 W (I. Åstrand, 1960). If all the individual EF_N determinations in the present study were pooled and averaged in groups with 16.4 W intervals, the EF_N would increase gradually from about 13% in the 16.4 W group to a level of 21% at about 60 W (see bottom of Figure 3). This gradual increase of EF_N was similar to that found by I. Åstrand (1960). It should, however be emphasized that as can be seen from Figure 2, all the EF_N values in the present experiments were obtained at HR values ranging from about 125 to 170, whereas the low EF_N in I. Åstrand's experiments were obtained at a much lower HR. Thus, if a normally recommended test for HR of about 130 beats/min is applied to small children, the EF_N may be as low as 13%, which means that the aerobic capacity of a child may be underestimated by about 40 to 45%. Even if the test load is above 60 W, the average EF_N of the children as mentioned above seems to be almost 10% lower than the EF_N found in adults (i.e., 21%). Part of the explanation for this difference in EF_N is probably that the children are tested on the same bicycle ergometers as those which are used for testing of adults. This implies that most children are slightly handicapped by the mechanical characteristics of the ergometer. Some of the important factors are (a) the forward tilt of the trunk (Klimt & Voigt, 1971), (b) the horizontal distance between the saddle and the crank axle (Müller, 1939), and (c) the length of the crank (Klimt & Voigt, 1974).

The reason for the extremely low EF_N values obtained at the lowest work intensities was probably due to the energy cost of moving the legs, fixation of the trunk, and the internal friction in the ergometer, which, all in all, amounts to a considerable amount of the total energy cost at low-work intensities. Thus, from the upper half of Figure 2 and Table 1, it can be calculated that the $\dot{V}O_2$ during bicycling at zero load on the average is about 90% higher than the BMR. The relatively high $\dot{V}O_2$ at zero load also explains the high EF_O values in Table 2, and as can be seen from the upper third of Figure 3, the EF_O is highest (above 30%) when calculated from $\dot{V}O_2$ at zero load and the $\dot{V}O_2$ at low-work intensities.

The EF_A is almost a constant (about 23%) when plotted against work intensity, as appears in the middle third of Figure 3. This means that there is a linear relation be-

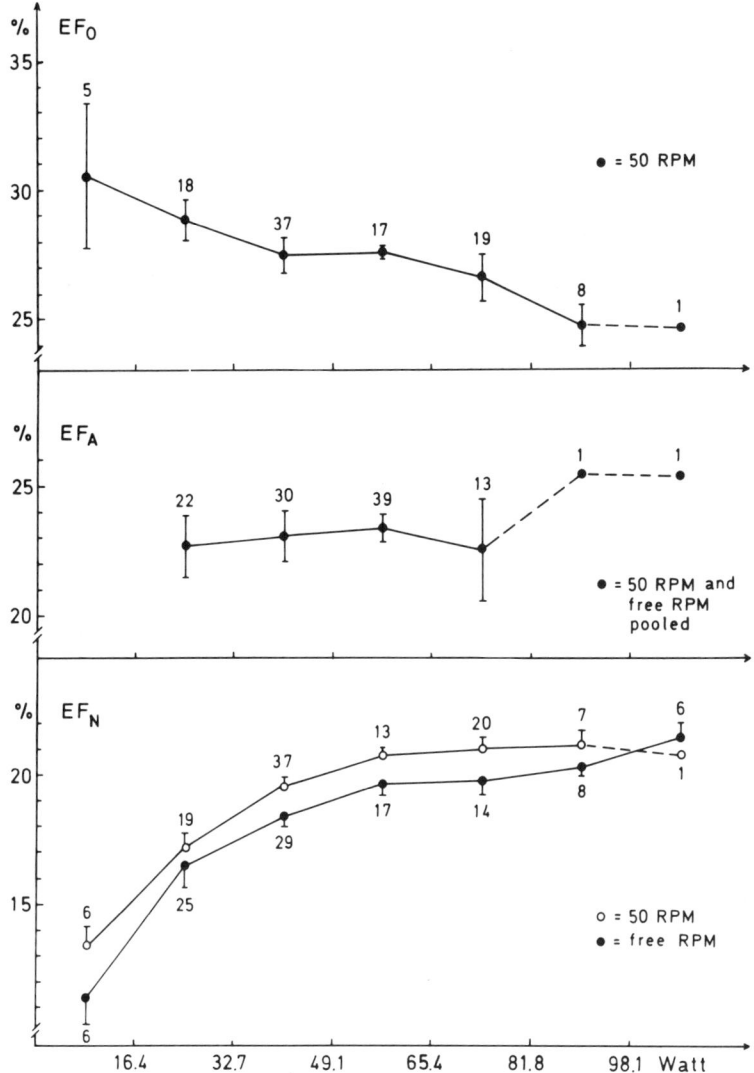

Figure 3—Mean values of zero load efficiency (EF_O), apparent efficiency (EF_A), and net efficiency (EF_N) in relation to work intensity. Vertical lines indicate 1 se. The number at each symbol indicates the number of individual determinations included in the symbol in question. For further explanation, see text.

tween $\dot{V}O_2$ and work intensity. However, as already mentioned, the EF_A in the present study tended to be lower than in previous experiments on adults (Asmussen, 1952; I. Åstrand, 1960; Nielsen, 1969). The constant EF_A implies that maximal aerobic power in children may be calculated from 2 submaximal exercise tests, provided that HRmax and the $\dot{V}O_2$ at rest are known. The HRmax in children has been measured by several researchers (P.-O. Åstrand, 1952; Hermansen & Oseid, 1971; Lindemann,

Rutenfranz, Mocellini, & Sbresny, 1973; Seliger et al., 1971; Robinson, 1983; Wilmore & Sigerseth, 1967; Wirth et al., 1978). The HRmax in the present experiments agreed with previous findings and implied that the aerobic power may be over- or underestimated by 10 to 15%, if a standard HRmax of about 200 is used. As far as the $\dot{V}O_2$ at rest is concerned, it can be seen from Figure 2 that a linear extrapolation from $\dot{V}O_2$ at W_2 and W_1 to zero on the average gives a $\dot{V}O_2$ of about 310 ml•min^{-1}, that is, a value about 60% higher than the BMR in Table 1. Thus, a BMR value about 60% higher than can be predicted from the children's surface area should be used in the calculation of $\dot{V}O_2$max.

Finally, it should be pointed out that the present experiments have shown that children were not able to maintain a constant RPM. They tended to pedal at an RPM about 8% higher than requested, which will give an underestimation in the calculation of $\dot{V}O_2$max of 8%. It is further interesting to note that when they had a free choice of RPM, they pedaled even faster (at an average of 67 RPM) in spite of the fact that this caused a decrease in EF_N, as can be seen from Table 2 and the black circles at the bottom of Figure 3.

Acknowledgment

This investigation was supported by a grant from The Danish Sports Research Council.

References

ASMUSSEN, E. (1952). Positive and negative muscular work. *Acta Physiologica Scandinavica*, **28**, 364-382.

ASMUSSEN, E., & Molbech, S. (1959). Methods and standards for evaluation of the physiological working capacity of patients. Communication from the testing and observation institute. Danish National Association for Infantile Paralysis, No. 4.

ÅSTRAND, I. (1958). The physical working capacity of workers 50-64 years old. *Acta Scandinavica*, **42**, 73-84.

ÅSTRAND, I. (1960). Aerobic work capacity in men and women with special reference to age. *Acta Physiologica Scandinavica*, Suppl., **49**, 169, 1-92.

ÅSTRAND, I., Åstrand, P.-O., & Rodahl, K. (1959). Maximal heart rate during work in older men. *Journal of Applied Physiology*, **14**, 562-566.

ÅSTRAND, P.-O. (1952). *Experimental studies of physical working capacity in relation to sex and age*. Copenhagen: Munksgaard.

CARPENTER, T.M. (1924). *Tables, factors, and formulas for computing respiratory exchange and biological transformations of energy.* (2nd ed.). Washington: Carnegie Hall.

HERMANSEN, L., & Oseid, S. (1971). Direct and indirect estimation of maximal oxygen uptake in pre-pubertal boys. *Acta Paediatrica Scandinavica*, Suppl., **217**, 18-23.

KLIMT, F., & Voigt, G.B. (1971). Untersuchungen zur Standardisierung der Sattelhöhe bei ergometrischer Fusskurbelarbeit bei 6-, 8- und 10-jährigen Knaben (An investigation with the aim to standardize the saddle height during leg exercise on a bicycle ergometer in 6-, 8- and 10-year-old boys). *Pädiatrische Grenzebieten*, **10**, 167-175.

KLIMT, F., & Voigt, G.B. (1974). Untersuchungen zur Standardisierung der Drehzahl und der Kurbellänge bei Arbeit am Fahrradergometer von Kindern im Alter von 6 bis 10 Jahren (An investigation with the aim to standardize the pedaling frequency and the length of the crank during bicycle ergometer exercise in children 6 to 10 years of age). *European Journal of Applied Physiology,* **33,** 315-326.

LINDEMANN, H., Rutenfranz, J., Mocellin, R., & Sbresny, W. (1973), Metodische Untersuchung zur indirekte bestimmung der maximalen O_2-aufnahme (Methodical investigation of indirect estimation of maximal oxygen uptake). *European Journal of Applied Physiology,* **32,** 25-53.

MÜLLER, E.A. (1939). Der Einfluss der Sattelstellung auf das Arbeitsmaximum und den Wirkungsgrad beim Radfahren (Influence of saddle position on maximal work capacity and on the efficiency of bicycling). *Arbeitsphysiologie,* **10,** 1-7.

NIELSEN, B. (1969). Thermoregulation in rest and exercise. Doctoral thesis, Copenhagen.

ROBINSON, S. (1938). Experimental studies of physical fitness in relation to age. *Arbeitsphysiologie,* **10,** 251-323.

RYMING, I. (1953). A modified Harvard step test for the evaluation of physical fitness. *Arbeitsphysiologie,* **15,** 235-250.

SELIGER, V., Cermak, V., Handzo, P., Horak, J., Jirak, Z., Macek, M., Pribil, M., Rous, J., Skranc, O., Ulbrich, J., Urbanek, J. (1971). Physical fitness of the Czechoslovak 12- and 15-year-old population. *Acta Paediatrica Scandinavica,* Suppl., **217,** 37-41.

WILMORE, J.H., & Sigerseth, P.O. (1967). Physical work capacity of young girls, 7-13 years of age. *Journal of Applied Physiology,* **22,** 923-928.

WIRTH, A., Träger, E., Scheel, K., Mayer, D., Diehm, K., Reischle, K., & Weicker, H. (1978). Cardiopulmonary adjustment and metabolic response to maximal and submaximal physical exercise of boys and girls at different stages of maturity. *European Journal of Applied Physiology,* **39,** 229-240.

Energy Intake and Energy Expenditure in Top Female Gymnasts

Marie-Agnes van Erp-Baart, Lilly W.H.M. Fredrix, and Rob A. Binkhorst
University of Nijmegen, The Netherlands

Tresi C.L. Lavaleye, Peter C.J. Vergouwen
Dutch Sports Federation, Arnhem

Wim H.M. Saris
University of Maastricht, The Netherlands

It is well known that gymnasts need a low body weight to perform well and that their food intake generally is low. Because they train daily for hours, a larger energy intake (EI) might be expected. Therefore, it was decided to study EI as well as energy expenditure (EE) of a group of female gymnasts in The Netherlands to obtain information about their energy balance.

Methods

A group of 11 top female gymnasts belonging to the national selection group participated in this study. They trained 3 hr/day, 5 days/week in a national sports center. During the week they lived with foster parents and during weekends they returned home. Anthropometric data for the subjects are given in Table 1. The percentage of body fat was assessed from skinfold measurements according to the method used by Durnin and Ramahan (1967). This body fat value in comparison with their peers was low (25%, Kemper et al., 1983).

Data on EI were collected using a 7-day record which was analyzed by means of a computerized program (Elvers, 1980). Daily EE minus EE during the training hours was obtained by measuring each individual's hours resting metabolic rate (RMR). To this measured RMR the net EE of daily activities obtained from a questionnaire (Q) was added. RMR was determined with a closed spirometer system using an energy equivalent for O_2 of 20.3 kJ (4.825 kcal).

The Q was divided into two parts: that is, weekend and weekday. Mean values for net EE of activities are given in Table 2.

Table 1

Anthropometric Data of 11 Subjects. Mean ± SD

Age (years)	Height (cm)	Weight (kg)	Body Fat (%)	Lean Body Mass (kg)
15.4 ± 1.4	158 ± 8	48 ± 8	16.4 ± 2.7	40.0 ± 5.4

Table 2

Net Energy Expenditure for Daily Activities From Literature
(See text for further explanation.)

Activity	kJ·min^{-1}	Activity	kJ·min^{-1}
Running	36	Walking	10
Swimming	25	Shopping	10
Football	25	General moderate	8
Sport at school	25	Domestic	7
Tennis	21	Playing organ	2
Chopping wood	19	General light	2
Dancing	17	Sleeping	= RMR
Bicycling	11		

Mean data of Durnin & Passmore (1967), van der Sluys & Dirken (1970), Reiff (1967), and Kemper (1983).

EE during the training hours was estimated using two methods. First, a time-and-motion study was performed. During each training session 1 subject was observed and the activities and the time spent in each were recorded. The activities were divided into three categories: heavy, moderate, and light. For heavy activities, net EE was obtained from data in the literature (see Table 3). Because EE were lacking data on acrobatics, floor and ballet, a net EE of 192, 96, and 50 kJ·min^{-1}, respectively, was estimated based on the observations in the present study and data in Table 3. For moderate (e.g., warming-up, preparing the apparatus) and light (e.g., sitting, standing, walking slowly) net EE was fixed, respectively, at 17 and 6 kJ·min^{-1} (see Table 2).

Second, EE during training was estimated using the heart rate (HR) method, in which EE was calculated from the recorded HR and the individual's relationship of HR and EE as obtained at different working levels on a treadmill (Saris, 1982).

HR was recorded on a heart rate memory (HRM) system (Saris, Snel, Baecke, Waesberghe, & Binkhorst, 1977). To predict EE from HR below 100 beats·min^{-1} the individual's RMR plus 0.029 kJ·kg BW^{-1} (Van der Sluys & Dirken, 1970) was taken, as was suggested by Saris (1982). From the mean HR above 100 beats·min^{-1} and the HR-EE relationship on the treadmill, the remainder of the EE during training was

Table 3

Net Energy Expenditure for Gymnastics From Literature
(See text for further explanation.)

Activity	kJ•min^{-1}	Literature
Vaulting-horse	380	H&H
Parallel bars	68	H&H
Trampoline	54	H&H
Press up	38	D&P
Balancing beam	15	H&H

H&H = Hollmann & Hettinger (1976)
D&P = Durnin & Passmore (1967)

calculated. In summary, the 24-hr EE was the sum of the individual's 24-hr RMR plus net EE of daily activities (from the questionnaire) plus net EE during training (from the time-and-motion study or from the HR method).

For statistical analysis, Student's t-test for paired data was used.

Results

Energy Intake

Table 4, first column, shows the EI of the group per 24 hr in total, per kg BW, and per kg FFM. No significant differences were found in EI between the weekdays and the weekends: 7,211 ± 1,576 kJ and 7,440 ± 2,136 kJ, respectively. From the

Table 4

Mean ± SD of Energy Intake (EI and DF&NB) and Energy Expenditure (EE) of Top Female Gymnasts

Units	EI	DF&NB*	EE (T&M)	EE (HR)
kJ•24 hr^{-1}	7277 ± 1530	9614	8502 ± 861	9125 ± 865
kJ•BW^{-1}	158 ± 43	185	180 ± 28	193 ± 28
kJ•FFM^{-1}	184 ± 47	247	215 ± 30	230 ± 30

*Recommended by the Dutch Food and Nutrition Board for girls of this age with normal physical activity.

EE (T&M) : EE determination including time-and-motion study. EE (HR) : EE determination incuding heart rate method. (See method for further explanation.)

standard deviation (S.D.) it can be seen that large interindividual differences existed. One girl indicated she was on a weight-reducing diet. Table 4, second column shows the recommended daily allowances of the Dutch Food and Nutrition Board (1981).

Energy Expenditure

Mean resting metabolic rate for this group was 5,317 kJ•24 hr^{-1}. This was not significantly different from standard data applicable for this age group; e.g. 5,697 kJ (Talbot, 1938) and 5,447 kJ De Wijn, 1974).

Time-and-motion study during training showed that the mean time spent on a training session was 3 hr and 15 min. The intensity of the training was on the average 15% heavy, 8% moderate, and 77% light. The mean total EE/min of all girls was calculated to be 15 kJ•min^{-1} for the training.

The mean total EE/min during the training predicted from HR measurements was 19 kJ•min^{-1}. The 24-hr EE's are presented in Table 4. The third column shows the values utilizing the time-and-motion study. The last column shows the results using the HR-method. The values are the weighted means of week and weekend days. There were significant differences between these periods (p<.001): for the values obtained with the time-and-moton study, it was 8,937 ± 869 kJ•24 hr^{-1} for weekdays and 7,394 ± 890 kJ•24 hr^{-1} for weekend days, while the values from the HR-method were 9,769 ± 7,394 ± 890 kJ•24 hr^{-1}, respectively.

Discussion

The data in Table 4 show that EE was estimated to be higher than EI. Values differed significantly (EI vs. EE (T&M) : p<.01 and EI vs. EE (HR) : p<.001). It was assumed that the differences were due mainly to the difficulty in assessing EE during training correctly, because there were no significant differences between EI and EE during the weekends (EI = 7,440 kJ•24 hr^{-1} and EE 7,394 kJ•24 hr^{-1}) during which practically no training was performed. A systematic difference of about 623 kJ between EE employing the time-and-motion method and EE utilizing the HR method was found. The difference between EI and EE might be attributed to the fact that the HR method usually overestimates EE (Saris, 1982). Another possibility is that some girls reduced their EI in order to meet the social acceptability within this group that needed to be lean for their best performances. Finally, it is generally assumed that EE yields about 418 to 1,672 kJ higher values than EI (Workshop, Amsterdam, 1983).

Compared with the scarce data in the literature, the results show that EI of the present group (see Table 4) was not greatly different from other groups. In Japan, Matsuko and Kitagawa (1983) found an intake of 165 kJ•kg BW^{-1} or 198 kJ•kg FFM^{-1}. This group trained 6 days/week, 4 hr/day. Caldarone et al. (1982) in Italy found that a group of young female artistic gymnasts had a mean intake of 8,999 kJ•day^{-1}. They trained 3 times/week, 1 to 3 hr/day. However, in Russia Zabourkin, Volkov, & Psjendin (1977) advised that the intake should be 251 kJ•kg BW^{-1} per day. However, no information was given about intensity and frequency of training.

Related to the recommended daily allowances of the Dutch Food and Nutrition Board (see Table 4), EE values in kJ per kg BW were comparable to these standards. EI, however, was about 25 to 30 kJ•kg BW^{-1} lower than that recommended.

It is tentatively concluded that a part of the differences between EI and EE can be accounted for by methodological problems. However, the actual difference between the mean EI and EE indicates that a number of these gymnasts has a real energy imbalance. In our opinion, this aspect is an important nutritional problem in these types of sport.

Acknowledgments

Thanks is given to Peter Hollander and Gert Kok of the Interfaculty of Human Movement Science and Education, The Free University, Amsterdam, for assisting with the treatment of the H.R.M. data.

References

CALDARONE, G., Amicis, A.D., Berlutti, G., Alicicco, E., & Catasta, G. (1982). Nutrition of athletes: The role of confectionary in the diet of young girls in training. *Journal of Sports Medicine*, **22**, 120-124.

DURNIN, J.V.G.A., & Passmore, R. (1967). *Energy, work and leisure.* London: Heinemann Books.

DURNIN, J.V.G.A., & Ramahan, J. (1967). The assessment of the amount of fat in the human body from measurements of skinfold thickness. *British Journal of Nutrition*, **21**, 681.

DUTCH Food and Nutrition Board. (1981). *Nederlandse Voedingsmiddelentabel (Food tables).* Voorlichtingsbureau voor de Voeding (The Netherlands Bureau for Food and Nutrition Information) (Ed.). 's-Gravenhage.

ELVERS, J.W.H. (1980). *Geautomatiseerd voedingsonderzoek (Computerized dietary research).* Stichting G.V.P.-project (Health Education Project) (Ed) Nijmegen.

HOLLMANN, W., & Hettinger, Th. (1976). *Sportmedizin, arbeitsund training grundlagen (Sportmedicine, work and training principles).* Stuttgart: Schattauer Verlag (Schattauer Editor).

KEMPER, H.C.G., Dekker, H., Ootjers, G., Post, B., Ritmeester, J.W., Snel, J., Splinter, P., Storm-van Essen, L., & Verschuur, R. (1983). Growth and health of teenagers. Amsterdam: University of Amsterdam.

MATSUOKA, H., & Kitagawa, K. (1983). Investigation of a certain diet program and its effects on the various body functions of female college gymnasts (English title). *Research Journal of Physical Education of Chukyo University*, **24**, 27-37.

REIFF, G.G., Montoye, H.J., Remington, R.D., Napier, J.A., Metzener, H.L., & Epstein, F.H. (1967). Assessment of physical activity by questionnaire and interview. In M.J. Karvonen & A.S. Barry (Eds.), *Physical activity and the heart* (Chapter 31). Springfield: Thomas.

SARIS, W.H.M., Snel, P., Baecke, J., Waesberghe, F. van, Binkhorst, R.A., (1977). A portable miniature solid-state heart rate recorder for monitoring daily physical activity. *Biotelemetry*, **4**, 131-140.

SARIS, W.H.M. (1982). Aerobic power and daily physical activity in children. Unpublished doctoral thesis, University of Nijmegen.

SLUYS, H. van der, & Dirken, J.M. (1970). *Dagelijks energieverbruik van de Nederlandse industrie-arbeider (Daily energy expenditure of the Dutch industrial worker)*. Groningen: Wolters-Noordhoff.

TALBOT, F.B. (1938). Basal metabolism standards for children. *American Journal of Diseases of Children,* **55**, 455-9.

WIJN, J.F. de. (1974). Energy expenditure at rest and for work. In *International Course in Food Science and Nutrition*. Gent. (unpublished)

WORKSHOP. (1983). *Reappraisal of methods of estimating energy expenditure and body composition*. The 4th European Nutrition Conference in Amsterdam. May.

ZABOURKIN, E.M., Volkov, A.G., & Psjendin, A.I. (1972). Pitánieje gimnástov (Nutrition of gymnasts). *Gimnastika,* **II**, 40-43.

The Organization of Developmental Studies

Martin A. van 't Hof
University of Nijmegen, The Netherlands

Development may either be studied by using cross-sectional or longitudinal designs. Advantages and disadvantages of both approaches are discussed in the literature. As is often the case in such a dilemma, the solution is found in a combination of the competing approaches. In this situation, the so-called multiple longitudinal design (Kemper, Dekker, Ootjens et al., 1983) or mixed longitudinal design (Prahl-Andersen, Kowalski, & Heydendael, 1979) presents an acceptable alternative.

Before discussing the characteristics of the mixed longitudinal approach, the problems associated with pure cross-sectional and pure longitudinal designs will be discussed.

Longitudinal and Cross-Sectional Studies

A pure longitudinal design, including the individual follow-up of a sample of children born during a relatively small time span gives the opportunity to analyze individual growth curves and also mean growth curves. The shape of individual and mean growth curves may be different, especially when growth spurts have an effect on these curves (see Figure 1). Due to many individual differences concerning the moment of spurt, the situation at the start of the spurt, the duration of the spurt, and the magnitude of the spurt, the mean growth curve is much flatter than the underlying individual growth curve. Thus, in general, mean growth curves will not present complete information about the developmental process. Therefore, the term "growth curve" will be reserved for individual follow-up, while the term "age curve" will be used for mean curves.

A pure cross-sectional study may only result in such an age curve because there is no individual follow-up. This is a limitation of the cross-sectional design.

The question arises whether age curves as obtained by a cross-sectional or by a longitudinal study are comparable. Figure 2 shows that this is not always the case. There may be (considerable) differences between both types of age curves, due to differences in the developmental history of the involved birth cohorts. The cross-sectional age curve in Figure 2 does not reflect any aspects of individual or group development. This does not imply, however, that this cross-sectional age curve is useless. Especially in preparing policy decisions, these kinds of curves may be relevant. For example,

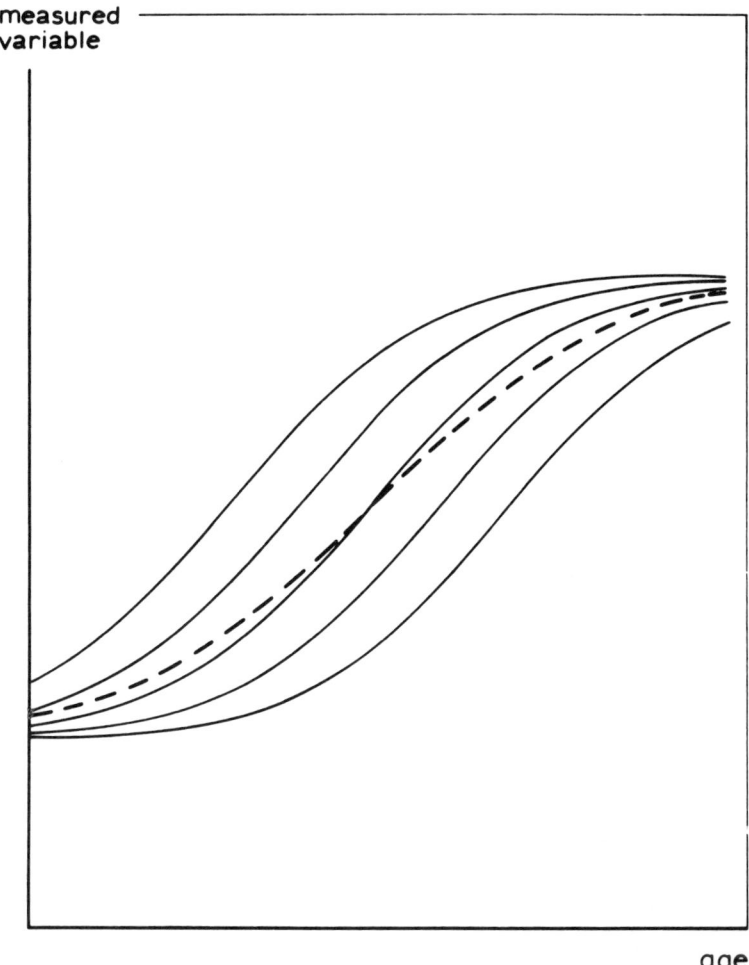

Figure 1—Example showing how an average age curve (dotted line) may deviate from each of the individual subject curves (solid lines).

if the measured variable (see Figure 2) indicates the utilization of municipal sports facilities, it may be assumed from Figure 2 that central sports facilities must be included for the types of sports which are of interest to persons of 20 to 30 years of age. None of the longitudinal age curves present a basis for such a conclusion. Such comparisons may lead to the conclusion that longitudinal designs are relevant for the study of developmental processes and that cross-sectional studies are helpful in social decision making. Because the study of developmental processes is the topic of this article, the longitudinal design and its methodological problems will be discussed in more detail in the next sections.

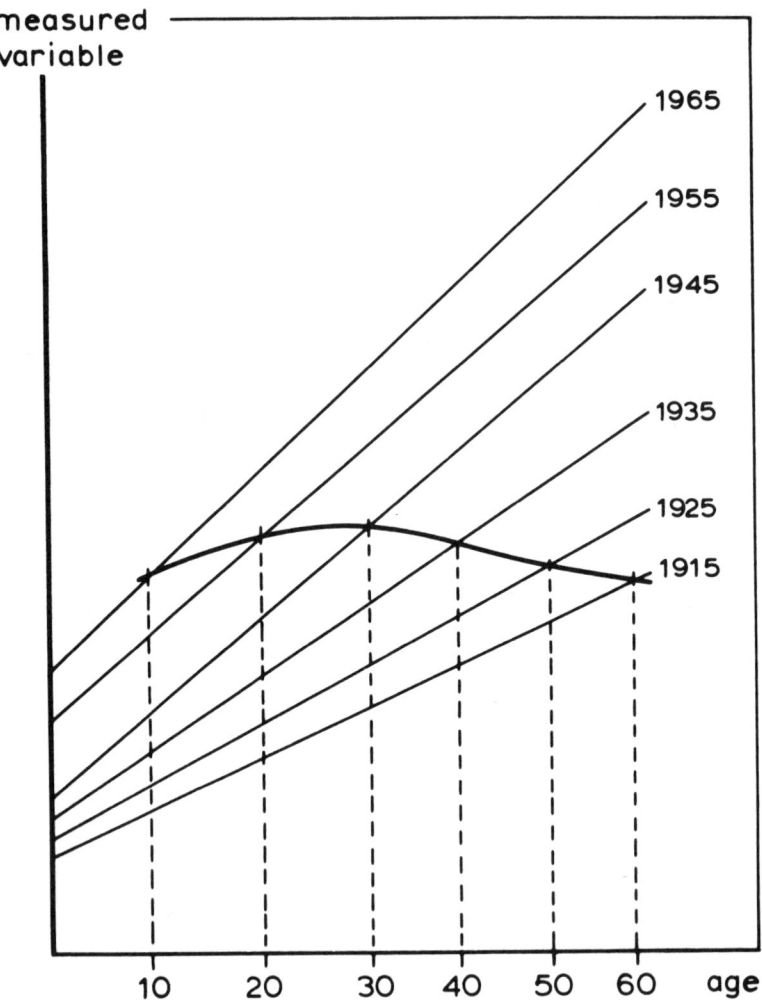

Figure 2—Example of an average age curve based on cross-sectional data collected in 1975 (the bent curve) that deviates from each of the involved average cohort age curves (straight lines).

Methodological Problems in Longitudinal Studies

A longitudinal study of developmental processes requires high quality data, with several specific characteristics.

The Accuracy of the Measurements

Measurement techniques including a large random error (relative to the differences in real change over time) are unsuitable for the study of development. Growth velocity curves will not be interpretable and do not reflect development but mainly error. The term "accuracy" in this context has to be considered very widely. For instance, a biochemical determination may have a high reproducibility on one blood sample, but if the biochemical content of the blood shows large daily fluctuations, the total measurement procedure may not be considered as accurate. Motor tests and biochemical parameters are often less accurate in this respect.

The Stability of the Measurements in Time

Due to calibration problems and subjectivity in rating systems, measurement techniques may show *symstematic differences* over time. Especially if during the course of a study it is necessary to change observers, stability may become a problem. The so-called time-of-measurement effects (Schaie, 1965) are related to this kind of instability. If time of measurement effects are present, growth velocities may be either underestimated or overestimated and the obtained individual growth curve is not correct. Special attention with respect to stability is necessary for measurements such as skinfolds and biochemical parameters.

Test and Learning Effects

Test effects arise where an achievement on the part of the participants is required. Measurement results may be distorted due to positive or negative changes in motivation during the study (test effects) or due to increasing aptitude for the performance of the test (learning effects). In both cases, the obtained growth curves do not depict pure development. In particular, motor tests and inquiries are sensitive to these kinds of influence.

Drop-Outs From the Study

Not only may the number of observations become insufficient, but a bias may also arise when there are a number of drop-outs from the study. The number of drop-outs (study mortality) will be smaller when the duration of participation and the number of measurement occasions per participant are reduced. The bias, due to selectivity in drop-out, does not affect the validity of the individual growth curves but does influence the population characteristics, calculated on the basis of the remaining sample. For example, children showing an increase in test results may stay in the study, while those showing disappointing results may withdraw. The remaining individual growth curves are correct but an overestimation of growth velocity will result. Mainly measurements associated with socially desirable qualities are subjected to selectivity, such as performance in motor tests or fatness.

Prevention of Methodological Problems in Longitudinal Studies

There is no certain way to avoid the methodological or measurement problems already mentioned. Measures of prevention with respect to this are partly available. Accuracy of the measurements may be improved by (a) standardization of the measurement protocol, (b) ongoing training of the observers, (c) duplicate or triplicate independent observations, (d) an adequate data processing system, and (e) a quick feedback of errors (Veling & Wennmacker, 1983). Stability of the measurements in time may be obtained by a frequent check-up on the calibration of the instruments and simultaneous measurement sessions in the case of succeeding observers. Test effects may be prevented by motivation promoting actions of the observer and learning sessions before the actual tests. Selectivity in drop-out can be prevented by personal attention and arrangements for individual participants. Not all these preventive measures are applicable in all situations, and, of course, not all actions are sufficiently effective. In addition, there is also the danger that preventing selectivity in drop-out leads to test effects. This does not mean that longitudinal studies are destined to fail, for many of the assumed problems may only be of marginal importance. The only way to deal with these aspects is to check the quality of the data after they have been collected. This will be discussed in the next section.

Data Quality Control in Longitudinal Studies

The accuracy of the measurements may be checked afterwards using the so-called interperiod correlation matrix analysis. An example of an interperiod correlation matrix is given in Table 1. The analysis includes the estimation of the reproducibility in terms of the test-retest correlation (see Figure 3). For the calculation of individual growth velocities in a (narrow) birth cohort, a reproducibility of at least 0.95 is required. Interperiod correlation matrix analysis is only reliable for at least four measurement occasions per participant (Prahl-Andersen, Kowalski, & Heydendael, 1979).

The stability of measurements in time may only be estimated properly in a mixed longitudinal design. Mixed longitudinal includes the longitudinal study of several cohorts during a certain time period (Van 't Hof, Roede, & Kowalski, 1977).

An example of a mixed longitudinal design is presented in Figure 4. The cohorts are studied longitudinally, and at each measurement occasion a certain cross-section is also present. The mixed longitudinal design may be regarded as a mixture of several (pure) longitudinal studies and several cross-sectional designs. The power of the mixed

Table 1

Example of an Interperiod Correlation Matrix

	Year 1	Year 2	Year 3	Year 4	Year 5	Year 6
Year 1	—	0.96	0.90	0.83	0.80	0.77
Year 2	0.96	—	0.94	0.87	0.81	0.79
Year 3	0.90	0.94	—	0.92	0.81	0.80
Year 4	0.83	0.87	0.92	—	0.86	0.88
Year 5	0.80	0.81	0.86	0.93	—	0.95
Year 6	0.77	0.79	0.80	0.88	0.95	—

Note. From "Symmetric Matrix for Stature in the Leuven Boys Study" (Ostijn, Simons, Beunen et al., 1980). Reprinted with permission.

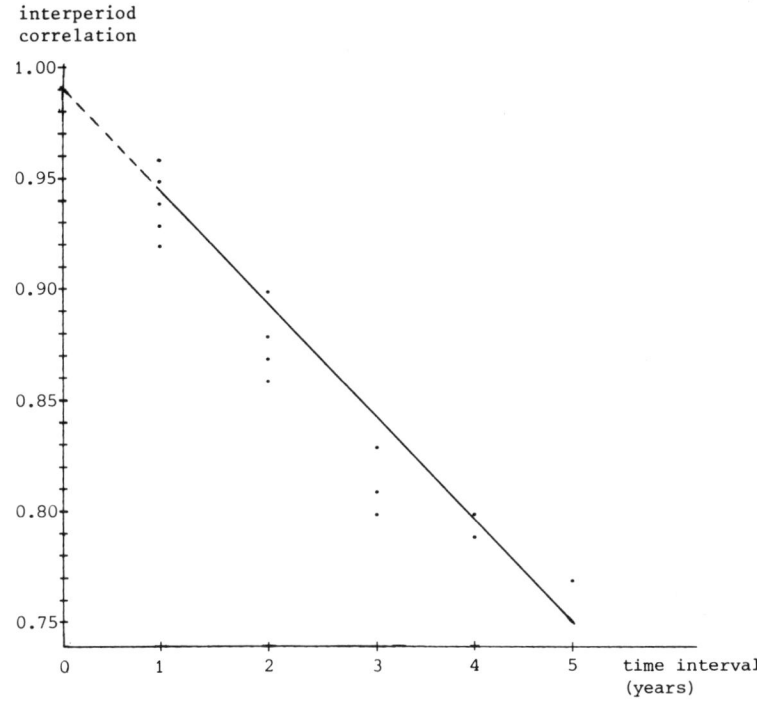

Figure 3—Interperiod correlation matrix analysis. Extrapolation of the regression line through the correlation coefficients plotted against their time interval (see Table 1) gives a direct measurement-remeasurement correlation of .99.

longitudinal approach is illustrated in Figure 5. The terminology in this respect is not quite standardized. The term mixed longitudinal is sometimes used for a design in which drop-outs are replaced by new participants. In such a design mixed longitudinal indicates a mixture of repeated and independent measurements. The term multiple longitudinal (for the first mentioned design) is introduced to avoid this confusion.

Test effects may be estimated using control groups, that is, new samples of the same population of the same age and measured at the same time (see Table 2). The difference between the longitudinal groups and the control groups exists in the measurement history of the study. Control groups may be inserted at each measurement occasion but also a lower frequency may be helpful for the assessment of test effects and their relation to the number of tests per individual (e.g., see Table 3).

Drop-out selectivity may partly be evaluated in a longitudinal study by comparing remaining participants with those who have withdrawn. Such a comparison is often made on the information collected at the first measurement occasion, hoping that this information contains some indication of the cause of withdrawal. A more realistic approach would be to use the last obtained information or even the last increments as a criterion for drop-out selectivity. An efficient matching procedure between remaining and withdrawn children or a layered analysis must be used for this check. For this problem, no general recommendations are available at this moment.

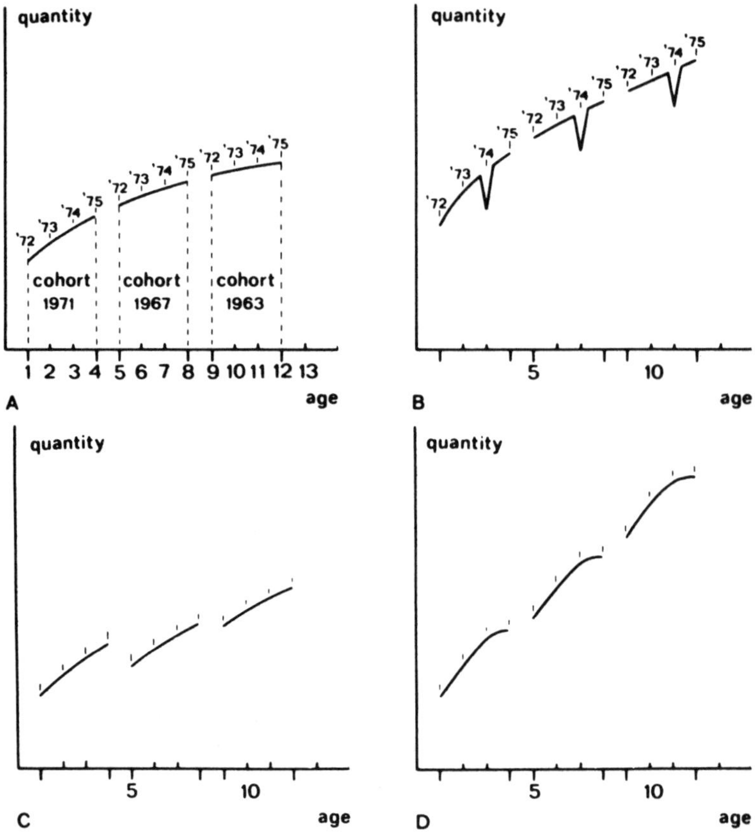

Figure 4—Several mixed longitudinal age curves shown in (A) neither cohort nor time-of-measurement effects, (B) a time-of-measurement effect in 1974, (C) cohort effects, and (D) both cohort and time-of-measurement effects.

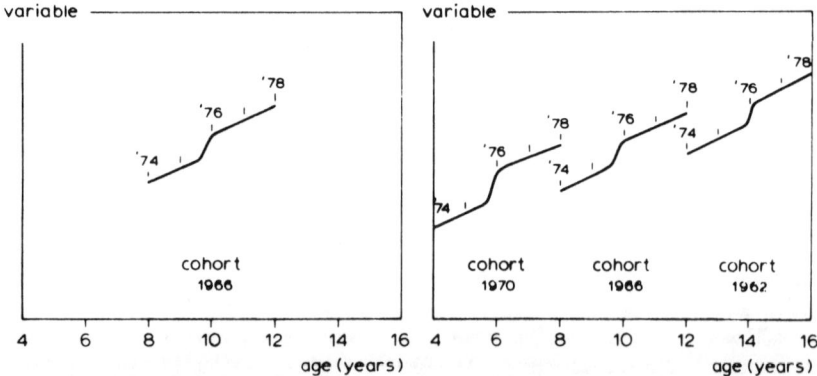

Figure 5—Time-of-measurement effect. The average age curve (left) suggests a growth spurt occurring at an age of 10. When average age curves of other cohorts are also available (right), the combined evidence indicates that a time of measurement effect is more likely.

Table 2

Observed Test Effects in the Motor Tests

	Second Measurement	After Several Measurements
Plate tapping	3%	6%
Arm pull	2%	9%
Leg lifts	5%	10%
Shuttle run	2%	4%

Note. The test effects are given as a percentage of first measurements. All test effects are in the direction of a better performance. From Ostijn, Simons, Beunen et al., 1980. Reprinted with permission.

Table 3

Example of a Mixed Longitudinal Design

Age (Years)	Cohort 1978	Cohort 1979	Cohort 1980
6			x '86 x
7		x '86 x	x '87 o
8	x '86 x	x '87 o	x '88 x
9	x '87 o	x '88 x	o '89
10	x '88 x	o '89	
11	o '89		

The design covers an age range of 6 to 11 years, including several control groups. Each x represents a measurement occasion. A control group is indicated by o.

Conclusions

As a result of the preceding principles relative to the organization of longitudinal studies, one may decide with respect to the design to (a) use a multiple longitudinal design (mixed longitudinal), (b) insert control groups, or (c) keep the number of measurements as low as possible (but use at least four measurements).

With respect to the data quality control each variable has to be checked according to (a) absence of time of measurement effects (using the mixed longitudinal character of the data), (b) absence of test effects (using the control groups), (c) absence of dropout selectivity (using the last collected information), and (d) sufficient reproducibility of the measurement (interperiod correlation matrix analysis).

Variables which do not pass these tests are not valid for pure developmental analysis. Unfortunately, the validity of a variable which fulfills all these conditions is still uncertain. Some studies are especially designed to measure test effects (e.g., screening programs), time of measurement effects (e.g., community health education programs), or to predict participation (e.g., attendance studies). In all such situations, the validity checks, of course, should be adapted to the nature of the study.

References

KEMPER, H.C.G., Dekker, H., Ootjens, G., et al. (1983). *Growth and health of teenagers.* University of Amsterdam.

OSTIJN, M., Simons, J., Beunen, G., et al. (1980). *Somatic and motor development of Belgian secondary schoolboys.* Leuven University Press, Leuven.

PRAHL-ANDERSEN, B., Kowalski, C.J., & Heydendael, P. (Eds.) (1979). *A mixed longitudinal interdisciplinary study of growth and development.* New York: Academic Press.

SCHAIE, K.W. A general model for the study of developmental problems. *Psych. Bulletin,* **64**, 92-107.

VAN 'T HOF, M.A., Roede, M.J., & Kowalski, C.J. (1977). A mixed longitudinal data analysis model. *Human Biology,* **49**, 165-179.

VELING, S.H.J., & Wennmacker, J.L.M. (1983). *NYLDAS user manual.* Nijmegen: Social Medicine Department.

The Problems of Analyzing Longitudinal Data From the Study "Growth and Health of Teenagers"

Han C.G. Kemper, Hans Dekker, Gré Ootjers,
Bertheke Post, Jan Willem Ritmeester, Jan Snel,
Paul Splinter, Lucienne Storm-van Essen,
and Robbert Verschuur
University of Amsterdam, The Netherlands

Since 1968 a series of research experiments has been carried out at the University of Amsterdam to measure the influence of physical education (p.e.) at school upon the physical and psychological developmental characteristics of boys in secondary schools (Kemper, 1973; Kemper, Poulus, & van der Helm, 1971; Kemper et al., 1975). The current longitudinal study was based on these previous investigations of 12- and 13-year-old schoolboys.

In general, no clear effects of intensified or additional p.e. could be shown. The results, however, were restricted to a specific sample: only boys in the age range 12 to 13 years and pupils of one secondary school in Amsterdam. There were also indications that differences in biological development and in habitual physical activity of the students could have masked any effect (Kemper et al., 1975). Moreover, it appeared that because the majority of the boys at that age showed relatively good health, they might have been less sensitive to training effects than boys in poor physical condition.

This present investigation was designed to describe the course of the physical and mental development of teenagers and to find out whether there is a period of deterioration in the health status of growing youngsters in The Netherlands. In order to explain changes in physical and mental development, measurements were taken of normal daily diet and habitual physical activity. More specifically, the study was designed to answer the following questions:

1. How do boys and girls grow and develop during the period of 12 to 18 years of age?
2. Does the style of living change, particularly in those aspects that seem important for health, such as habitual physical activity and daily food intake?
3. What relationships exist between growth and development and the physical and mental characteristics of the style of living?

The ultimate purpose of this study was to contribute to the improvement in health education of teenagers in The Netherlands.

Methods and Procedures

Design

In studies of growth and development, the following three classical designs have been used to a great extent, namely, the cross-sectional, the time-lag, and the longitudinal design. Concerning such studies, each measurement taken on a subject at a particular moment is influenced by three factors:

1. *Age of the subject* which is defined as the lapse of time between birth and time of measurement. Age effects produced the mean growth curve.
2. *Birth cohort to which the subject belongs* refers to the group of individuals born in the same year. Cohort effects can be used in studying secular trends.
3. *Time of measurement* is the moment at which the measurement is taken. Time-of-measurement effects have to do with changes in environmental conditions that may occur over a period of time (such as changes in methods of measurement).

None of these designs allows the three effects (age, time of measurement, and cohort) to be isolated (Schaie, 1965).

Multiple Longitudinal Design. In the literature, descriptions can be found of several designs which try to face the problem of confounding effects (Kowalski & Prahl-Andersen, 1979; Rao & Rao, 1966; Tanner, 1962).

The design of the current study is "multiple longitudinal" which implies the idea of repeated measurements on more than one cohort (Kemper & Van 't Hof, 1978), and has the advantage that it can isolate the main effect, for example, the age effect from interfering effects such as time-of-measurement and cohort effects.

Cluster Effects. In this case, the measurements were taken during 4 successive years from 1976 to 1979. Original measurements were obtained on children from the 1st and 2nd forms of a secondary school in Amsterdam. These 2 groups are referred to as clusters. The clusters were composed of children with an average age of 13 (C1) and 14 (C2) years in 1976 (see Figure 1). During the course of the study, the composition of these clusters remained the same. Pupils who stayed in a class for a 2nd year remained a member of their original cluster.

There were 4 times of measurement, but, because there were 2 longitudinal studies which ran parallel to each other with a lag of 1 year in age, the study consisted of 5 age groups. Because there was an overlap in age, the 2 clusters can be compared with each other at 3 ages. A systematic difference between the 2 clusters at these 3 ages was called a "cluster effect."

Time-of-Measurement Effects. At the same time, it was possible to distinguish one of the interfering factors in a longitudinal study, namely the factor time-of-measurement (Veling & Van 't Hof, 1980). For example: 14-year-old children were measured in 1976 (C2) as well as in 1977 (C1). If it was found that there was no cluster effect, the time of measurement was blamed for a possible difference between the two groups of children. If it appeared that there was no time-of-measurement effect and no cluster effect either, then the data were arranged in age groups and an estimated 5-year development pattern in a period of 4 years (Bell, 1954) was developed.

Testing or Learning Effects. Another problem that occurs with repeated measurements is a testing or learning effect. Many variables, physical as well as

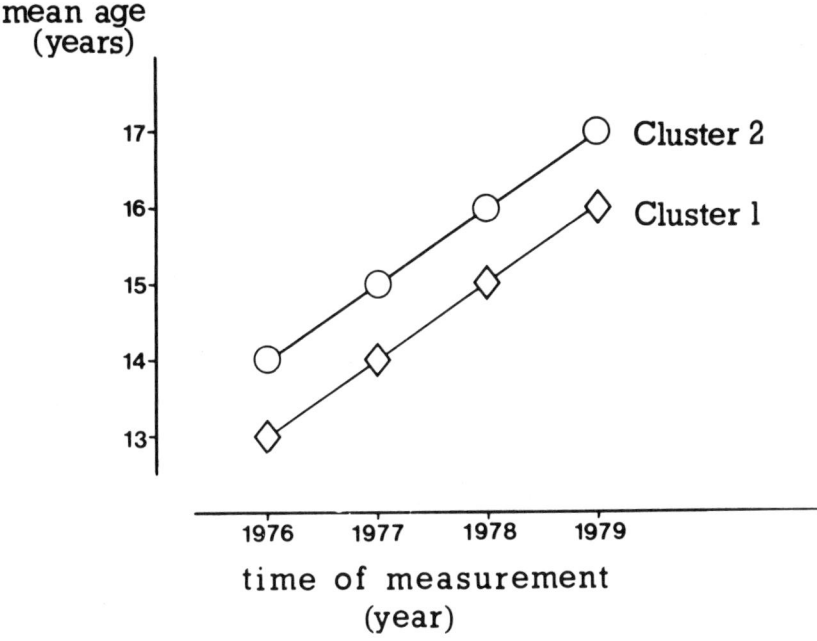

Figure 1—Design of the multiple longitudinal study with 2 clusters.

psychological, require a certain motivation or habituation of the subject when measuring. This introduces differences between periods of measuring that are solely due to changes in attitude towards the measurement procedure itself. Such testing effects may be positive (i.e., when habituation or learning is important) or negative (i.e., when motivation decreases). Repeated measurements may therefore have a disturbing influence on the quantity measured and diminish the external validity of the results. Systematic testing effects can be estimated if the design also includes a control group in which repeated measurements are not made. The design of this study provided the following: At a second school comparable with the first, an identical arrangement in clusters was made, but during the 4 years of the study, every time another quarter of the pupils was measured (see Figure 2). These measurements are comparable with those of the first school, except that they were not repeated measurements but came from independent samples. In this design, when comparing data from both schools, systematic divergence of mean values in the course of the study is an indication of a testing effect. At the first measurement, when the measurements were taken in both schools for the first time, a possible school effect can be noticed. For example: If we found that in 1976 the children from one school did not differ from peers from the other school (i.e., there was no school effect), then differences found later on may be attributed to a testing effect.

Both time-of-measurement effect and testing effect, if they are established for a certain characteristic, will seriously hinder the interpretation of individual and mean growth curves. When neither cluster nor time-of-measurement nor testing effects were found, the data were arranged in age groups to study the development of the children. The

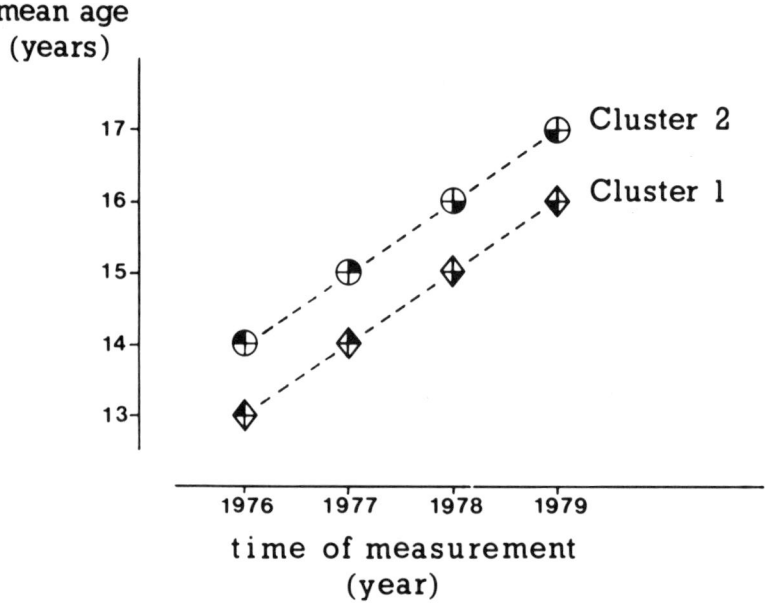

Figure 2—Design of the control groups: 2 clusters, 8 groups of independent observations.

age groups were composed of 2 clusters, only the 2 clusters contained 3 birth cohorts. Tests were conducted for cluster effects, but not for cohort effects because differences between cohorts in 1 cluster were not expected. Afterwards it was noticed that birth cohort seemed to be more important than the cluster. So it would have been better to divide the sample into 3 birth cohorts (i.e., 12-, 13-, and 14-year-olds at the start of the study) instead of in 2 clusters with a mean age of 13 and 14 years.

Tails of the Mean Age Curve. The average age curve of, for example, the sum of four skinfolds (see Figure 3) was more accurate in the middle part (ages 14 and 15) because observations of all three cohorts were available. The tails of the curve (ages 12 and 17), however, were estimates based on only a small group of children from one cohort. If, for example, the youngest or oldest groups deviated from the norm, it influenced the average age curve. To avoid this kind of misinterpretation, graphical plots were made of the mean values of each cohort and the cohorts were inspected for any typical deviations at the tails that could influence the developmental curves substantially.

Drop-Outs. During the study, a number of pupils withdrew from the sample. The main reason for this secession was that they left the school. Because of the chance of selective drop-out, this group was compared with that group of pupils which stayed in the sample for 4 years. This comparison was made on the basis of measurements from the 1st year (1976) and used univariate or multivariate t-tests.

Individual Growth. The purpose of longitudinal studies is to investigate individual changes in time. This becomes difficult when the stochastic measurement error exceeds the change in time. The degree to which this occurs in a variable may be studied on the basis of interperiod correlation matrices (Veling & Van 't Hof, 1980). An in-

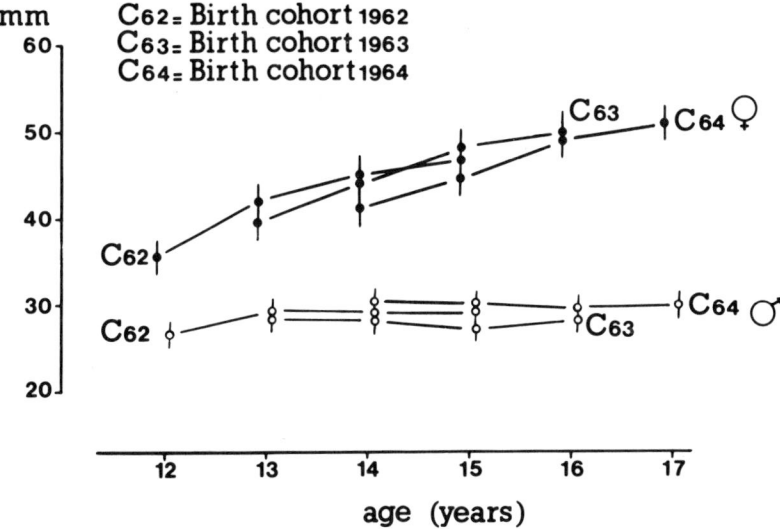

Figure 3—Sum of 4 skinfolds. The tails of the average age curve are based on the data of only 1 cohort.

terperiod correlation (IPC) is a coefficient of correlation between 2 periods of measurement for the variable. Van 't Hof and Kowalski (1979) have shown that under fairly realistic conditions, the IPCs can be approximated by a linear function of the time interval (see Figure 4). The intercept of the straight line is the correlation coefficient between 2 (independent) measurements (having an intermediate time interval equal to zero) and may be interpreted as the instantaneous measurement-remeasurement reproducibility. Therefore, it is a measure of the reliability of the measurement in question. The slope of the line or the decay in correlation per yearly time interval gives an impression of the interindividual change over time of the measurement in question. The "ideal" IPC matrix shows a line with an intercept of about 1 and a steep descent.

Schools

The current study was carried out at two secondary schools in The Netherlands, in Amsterdam and in Purmerend, a suburb of Amsterdam. Care was taken to ensure that the same measurements were done in the same period of each school year. To increase the reliability of the measurements, each measurement was carried out by the same tester during the 4 years.

Subjects

Subjects were all the pupils enrolled in the 1st and 2nd form of the two schools in the school year, 1976/1977. At the start of the study in August 1976, the longitudinal

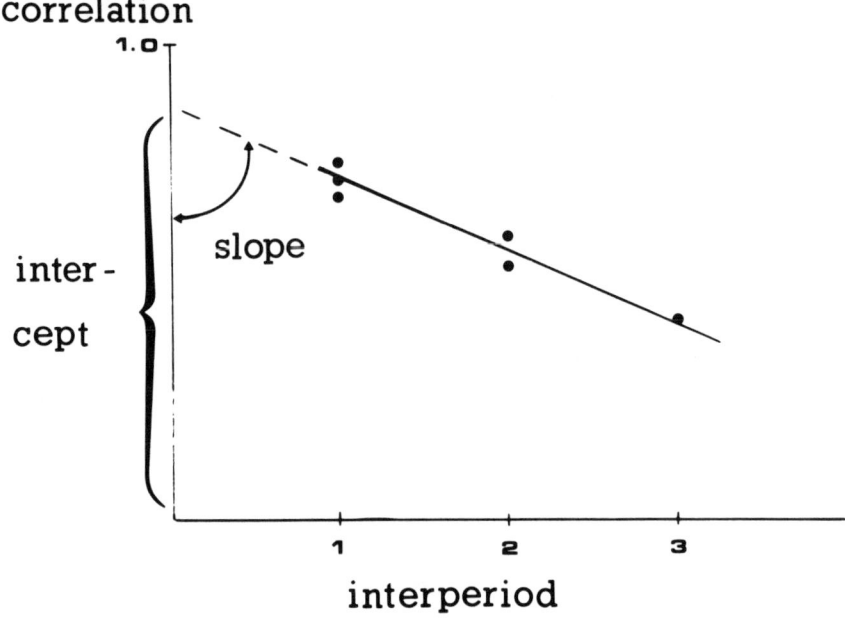

Figure 4—Principles of a plot of the interperiod correlation coefficients of a variable.

group from the Pius X Lyceum consisted of 307 pupils: 159 girls and 148 boys. Of 233 pupils, 131 girls and 102 boys completed the 4-year study. The total drop-out percentage was 24%, girls 18%, and boys 31%. Of these, only 2% refused to continue to participate. The remaining 22% dropped out because of transfer to other places and/or other types of school. The Ignatius College acted as the control school. Every year a random sample was taken of 25% of the population of pupils who were enrolled in the 1st and 2nd forms in the school year 1976/1977. At the end of the study, a total of 133 boys and 150 girls was measured only once.

Because the subjects were not selected by age but comprised all the pupils in the 1st and 2nd forms of each school, they differed in age. Most of them were born in 1963 and 1964. The 15th of September was selected as the reference date for classifying pupils into age groups.

Measurements

The methods of measurements can be divided in 5 groups:

1. 18 physical measurements: height, weight, bone diameters, skinfold thicknesses, circumferences (Weiner & Lourie, 1969), and posture (Seroo, Storm-van Essen, & Kemper, 1982).
2. 20 physiological measurements: strength, speed, flexibility (Kemper, Verschuur, & Bovend'eerdt, 1979), aerobic power (Bar-Or & Zwiren, 1975), ventilation, and cardiovascular risk indicators.
3. 10 psychosocial measurements: personality traits (Bücking, Van Egmond, Elsenga, & Haanstra, 1975; Hermans, 1979), sociometric status (Defares, 1970; Gardner,

Thomson, 1958), and attitudes toward school (De Groot, 1968) and toward physical education (Adams, 1963; Splinter et al., 1978).
4. Measurement of daily eating and smoking habits by interview (Post & Kemper, 1980).
5. Measurement of habitual physical activity: heart rate (Saris, 1977), pedometer (Verschuur & Kemper, 1980), and interview (Kemper et al., 1983 appendix).

A selection of the longitudinally measured data are presented in this article as developmental curves of the mean with standard error vs. calendar-age groups. The results of the longitudinal group are reported and discussed. The results of the control groups were reported only in cases of an existing test effect.

The longitudinal and cross-sectional data are arranged in age groups irrespective of the year of measurement and the year of birth. In this way, a developmental pattern over 6 years (from 12 years in 1976 to 17 years in 1979) were included unless there was evidence indicating the presence of a cluster or cohort effect.

Practical Problems

In the statistical analyses for interfering effects, however, different problems arose:

1. The three-factor model was quite simple. However, because the measurements were a mixture of dependent and independent observations, special computer programs had to be written to estimate and to test cluster and time-of-measurement effects. It appeared that significant effects of cluster and time-of-measurement could be caused by only two outlyers in a group of teenagers.
2. Learning effects were tested with SPSS-MANOVA (Cohen & Burns, 1976) under the assumption that the data were normally distributed. However, the univariate test for homogeneity of variances sometimes gave different results. This contradiction was possibly due to the inequality of the cell-frequencies combined with a non-normal distribution. A more robust test was not available at the available computer site.
3. For different variables, it was discovered afterwards (while a cluster effect did not exist) that the oldest and/or youngest groups were different from the others.

Strategy

The large number of variables, combined with the fact that almost all of them needed a personal treatment, makes it clear that it was impossible to solve the previously mentioned problems with standard computer programs. This led to the following strategy: The data were observed by making graphical plots of the age curves for different birth cohorts. If these showed any relevant differences, it was decided to test these differences statistically.

Results

A selection of data in which one of the interfering effects appeared are presented in the following sections.

Time-of-Measurement Effect

Pedometer week score was one of the three methods used to quantify habitual physical activity. In boys a significant time-of-measurement effect was found in the pedometer week score: Data from the 1st year of the study were relatively low in comparison with the 2nd year. This held true for all 3 birth cohorts (see continuous lines in Figure 5).

A possible explanation was a difference in climatic conditions during the measurement period (from the middle of January until the end of March). In The Netherlands, cold winter days will keep the children inactive inside their homes, unless the temperature is below freezing over a relatively long period of time. In that case, the Dutch waters freeze and become an ice-skating playground for Dutchmen of any age. The control group (hatched line in Figure 5) shows the same development.

Cohort Effects

The Dutch Personality Inventory (Bücking, Egmond, Elsenga, & Haanstra, 1975) contained five subscales, one of them measuring rigidity (Rg), that is, the need for regularity, having unalterable habits and principles, a sense of duty, and positive task appraisal. In Figure 6, a rather sharp decline existed for girls and boys ($p < .001$). The apparent rise for the girls between 16 and 17 years has to be attributed to a cohort effect. The 1964 girls-cohort had a higher average Rg score during all the years of the study. Although these girls showed a decrease in Rg score, the difference in level

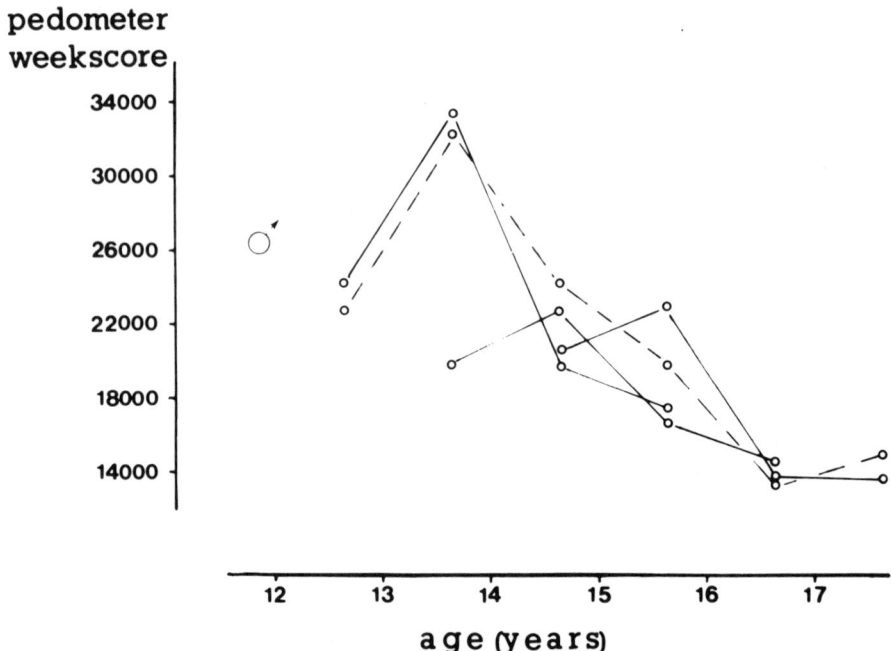

Figure 5—Time of measurement effect in the pedometer-week score of boys, illustrated by the mean scores of the 3 birth cohorts (solid lines) and the mean scores of the control groups (dotted line), vs. calendar age.

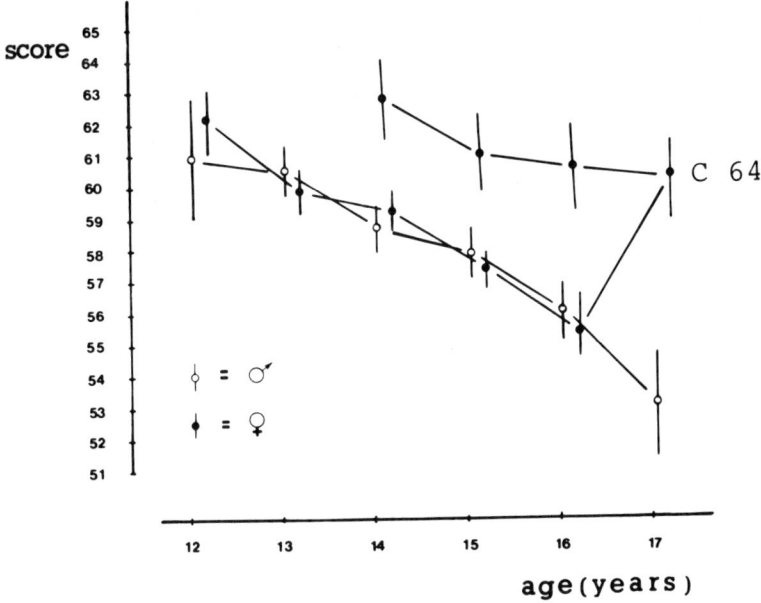

Figure 6—Average rigidity scores of girls and boys from 12 to 17 years. The girls-cohort of 1964 is taken apart.

resulted at age 17 and an apparent increase existed when their data were combined with the other cohorts.

Testing Effect

From the dietary history interview, a modified version of the one developed by Burke (1947), the intake of energy (protein, fat, and carbohydrate) of an average weekday was calculated (see Figure 7). Considering the total energy intake, the results in the longitudinal group of boys increased less compared with those of the control group and a testing effect was obvious.

An explanation could be that the repeated interview led to reporting a lower quantity and frequency of the food items than were consumed.

Drop-Outs

The Amsterdam Sociometric Scale (ASS) offered the possibility of gathering information on the social status of individual group members and the cohesion of their group. The children were asked to rate each of their classmates on a 5-point scale in terms of (a) how much they liked to cooperate in doing homework or work at school with each classmate, and (b) how much they liked to accept each classmate on a school sports team. Boys and girls do not differ from drop-outs in popularity as sports team partners. The popularity on homework partnership, however, revealed striking differences

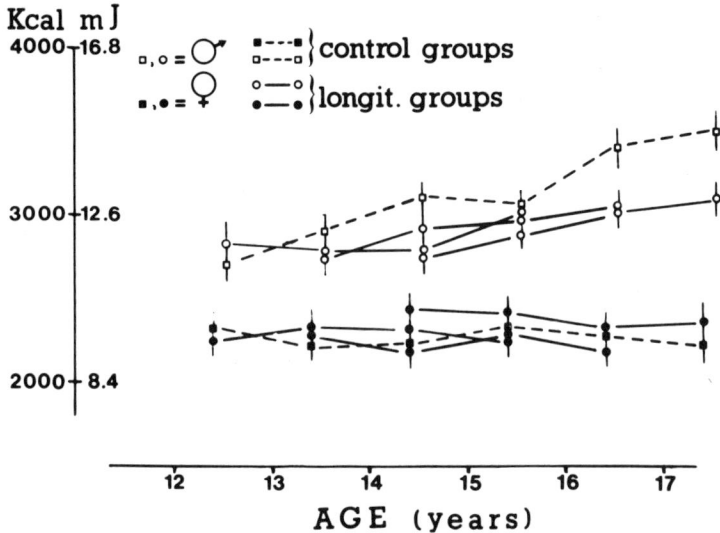

Figure 7—Developmental curves of energy intake of boys and girls of the longitudinal group and the control group. The longitudinal curves are divided into the 3 cohorts.

between pupils from the longitudinal sample and the drop-outs (see Table 1). Drop-outs were significantly less popular ($p < .0001$) than the pupils who stayed at school. Apparently, boys and girls who (have to) leave school are less popular than those who stay.

Interperiod Correlations

Figure 8 is a good example of a reliably measured variable: Height was measured 3 times a year and as a consequence 11 interperiods were available. The IPC of height in boys and girls showed a very distinct pattern. Figure 9 shows mean and standard error of systolic blood pressure (upper part) and of diastolic blood pressure (lower part) of both boys and girls. In diastolic pressure, no age trend could be established in either boys or in girls. A drawback of this variable is its low reproducibility. The test-retest

Table 1

Popularity on Homework Partnership
Mean and Standard Deviation of Longitudinal Group and of Drop-Outs

	Boys			Girls		
	n	x	sd	n	x	sd
Longitudinal group	101	48.97	9.50	131	52.47	8.85
Drop-out group	44	41.98	7.92	28	45.43	8.97

reliability was estimated on the basis of the interperiod correlation matrix of this variable in Figure 10. In girls, extrapolated to the fictitious zero-time-lag point, the reliability appeared to be between 0.70 and 0.60 and in boys even lower between 0.60 and 0.50.

This low reproducibility was also found by others (Hofman, 1983) and could be explained by the indirect method and the influence of treadmill running which was the following test.

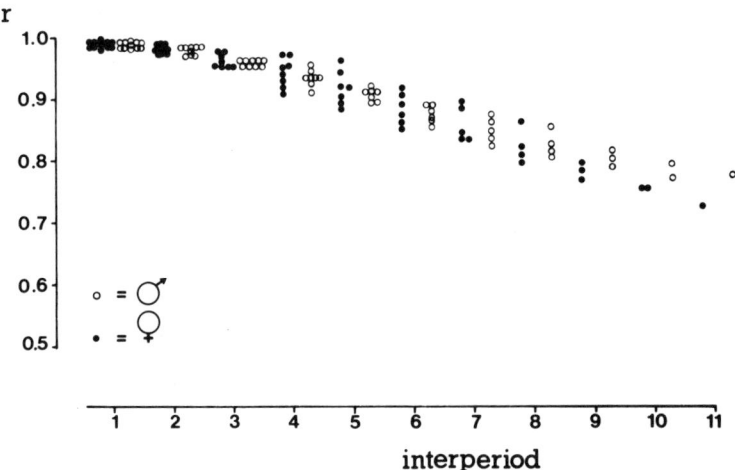

Figure 8—Interperiod correlations of height of boys and girls.

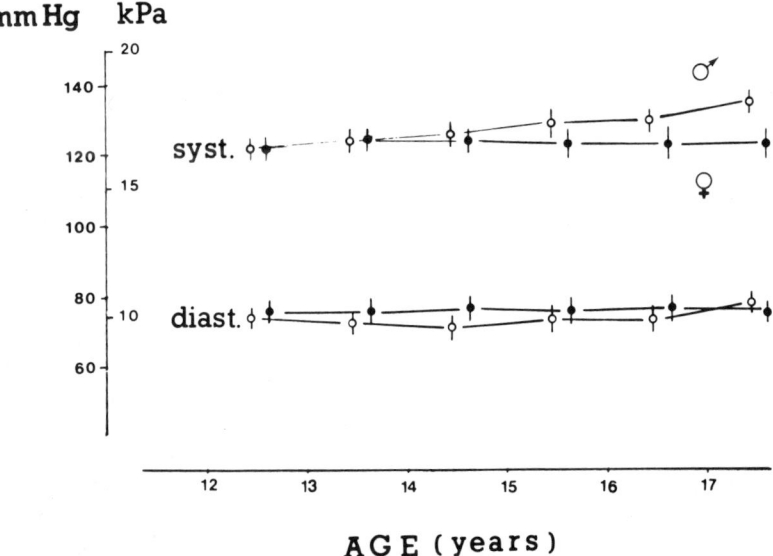

Figure 9—Mean and standard error of systolic and diastolic blood pressure of boys and girls vs. calendar age.

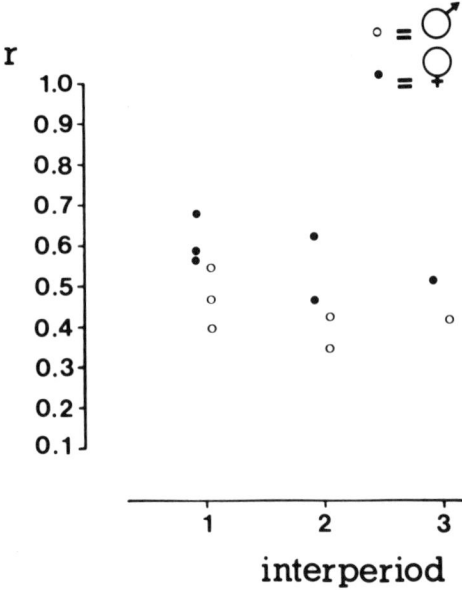

Figure 10—Interperiod correlation matrix of diastolic blood pressure of boys and girls.

Discussion

An Overview

From the results already presented, it would seem that most of the measured variables showed interfering effects. This was certainly not the case, however. In Table 2 an overview is given of the interfering effects that appeared in the measurements previously mentioned. From the 18 physical measurements, only a drop-out effect was found in hip width of boys. Physiological variables are sometimes influenced by testing effects. In three physical performance tests, the effects were sometimes negative, as in the case of the flexed arm hang and sometimes positive—for example, the arm pull and the 12-minute endurance run.

As for the psychosocial variables, 8 times out of 10, cohort effects interfered with the results. Also testing effects (in girls) were present. Because of the rather low interperiod correlation and several drop-out effects, it is recommended to use the results of the psychosocial variables with great care and to use the scores preferably on a group level. The measurements of normal daily diet and habitual physical activity were predominantly interfered with by testing and/or school effects in boys. A testing effect could be expected from the rather time-consuming interviews that required a certain motivation or habituation of the subjects when repeatedly measured. In only one case (pedometer week score) a time of measurement effect was evident. The female drop-outs differed in their total activity time and total METs (Metabolic EquivalenT) from the group which remained for the entire study.

Table 2
Overview of the Variables That Showed Interfering Effects

Number of Variables Tested on Confounding Effects		Physical 18	Physiological 20	Psychosocial 10	Style of Living 10
Time of measurement	♂				Pedometer week score
	♀				
Cohort	♂			Debilit. anxiety Homework Sport team	
	♀			Achievement motivation Facil. anxiety Social inadequacy Rigidity Homework Sport team School Attitude	
Testing	♂		Arm pull Bent arm hang 12 min endurance Resting heart rate		Energy intake Protein intake Carbohydrate Total activity time Light activity time
	♀		Arm Pull Bent arm hang Resting heart rate Total cholesterol	Social inadequacy School attitude	

Table 2 (Cont.)

Overview of the Variables That Showed Interfering Effects

Number of Variables Tested on Confounding Effects		Physical 18	Physiological 20	Psychosocial 10	Style of Living 10
IPC	♂		12 min endurance run Diastolic blood pressure	Facil. anxiety School attitude	
	♀		12 min endurance run Diastolic blood pressure	School attitude	
Drop-out	♂	Hip width	10 × 5 m sprint	Facil. anxiety Inadequacy Homework	
	♀		10 × 5 m sprint 12 min endurance run HDL cholesterol	Homework	Total activity time Total METs score

Maximal Aerobic Power

Maximal aerobic power or $\dot{V}O_2$max ($l \cdot min^{-1}$) is a physiological parameter that has very seldom been measured longitudinally (Mirwald, 1980; Saris, 1982). It is, therefore, interesting to know whether this parameter is influenced by confounding effects or not. Maximal aerobic power is a universally accepted parameter. Most of the developmental curves presented in literature are based on cross-sectional data (Åstrand, 1952; Robinson, 1938). It is interesting, therefore, to see if longitudinally measured $\dot{V}O_2$max data show interfering effects. Measurement of $\dot{V}O_2$max required a great deal of motivation of the subjects to reach their maximal performance. It was expected that repeated testing would cause either a negative effect, because the pupil was no longer willing to exercise to his/her maximum, or a positive effect as a consequence of more practice and learning.

Inspection of the data measured during the treadmill test in order to find interfering effects of $\dot{V}O_2$max did not demonstrate any significant result: The IPC (see Figure 11) showed a high reproducibility accompanied by great differences in growth between individuals. Further analyses, however, revealed that the high correlations were weight dependent (Ritmeester, Kemper, & Verschuur, 1984).

Figure 12 shows the mean and standard error of $\dot{V}O_2$max of boys and girls divided into three different cohorts. Visual inspection of these curves did not reveal any time of measurement and cohort effect. Comparison of the $\dot{V}O_2$max values with the control groups did not show any testing effects. This was contrary to the findings of Lange-

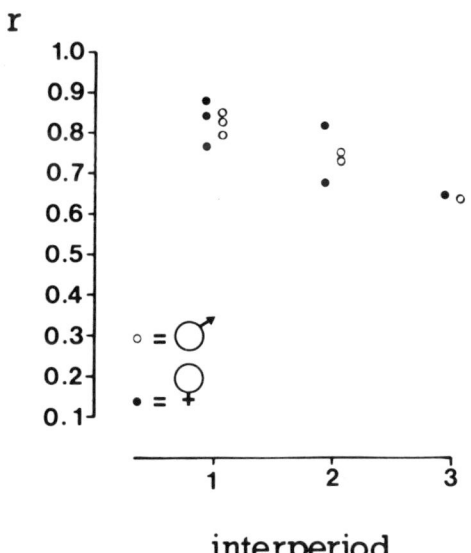

Figure 11—Interperiod correlation matrix of $\dot{V}O_2$max of boys and girls from the longitudinal group.

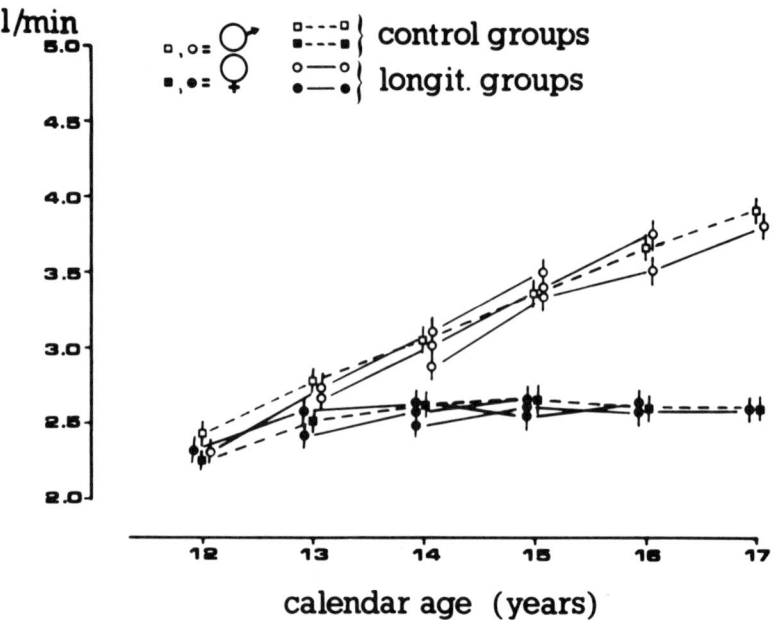

Figure 12—Developmental curves of $\dot{V}O_2$max of boys and girls of the longitudinal group and the control group. The longitudinal curves are divided into the 3 cohorts.

Andersen, Seliger, Rutenfranz, and Skobak-Kazymski (1976). They presented data of longitudinal and cross-sectional measurements on boys and girls from the ages 8 to 12 years. From their data, a positive effect in the longitudinal group in relation to the cross-sectional group existed for both boys and girls. The different ages may have contributed to this discrepancy. It can be argued that learning effects are more important at younger ages.

Conclusions

Although in principle it is possible to control for interfering effects, all available methods turned out to have serious drawbacks. This was caused by the mixture of dependent and independent data, the nonnormal distribution of most of the variables, and inequality of all frequencies.

The developmental trends in physical measurements were only slightly influenced by interfering effects. Physiological variables showed both positive (maximal arm strength) and negative (endurance strength of the arms) testing effects. Maximal aerobic power ($\dot{V}O_2$max in liter/min) showed no testing effects and high IPCs.

The age trends of psychosocial variables were influenced by time of measurement, cohort, and testing effects. Because of the rather low IPCs and drop-out effects, it seemed feasible to recommend the use of the longitudinal results with great care. The measurement of style of living was relatively seldom influenced by confounders.

References

ADAMS, R.S. (1963). Two scales for measurement attitude toward physical education. *Research Quarterly,* **34**(1), 91-94.

ÅSTRAND, P.O. (1952). *Experimental studies of physical working capacity in relation to sex and age.* Copenhagen: Munksgaard.

BAR-OR, O., & Zwiren, L.D. (1975). Maximal oxygen consumption test during arm exercise—Reliability and validity. *Journal of Applied Physiology,* **38**, 424-426.

BELL, R.Q. (1954). An experimental test of the accelerated longitudinal approach. *Child Development,* **25**, 281-286.

BÜCKING, H., Egmond, J. van, Elsenga, S., & Haanstra, F. (1975). De konstruktie van en jeugdversie van de NPV, de NPV-j (Construction of a youth version of the NPV, the NPV-j). *Heymans Bulletin* (Groningen), HB 75-190.

COHEN, E., & Burns, P. (1976). *Multivariate analysis of variance and covariance.* SPSS-Manova, Document no. 413, Rev. A, Northwestern University.

DEFARES, P.B., Kema, G.N., Praag, E. van, & Werff, J.J. van der (1970). *Syracuse Amsterdam Groningen sociometrische schaal (Syracuse Amsterdam Groningen sociometric scale).* Issue for use in research.

GARDNER, E.F., & Thompson, G.G. (1956). *Social relations and morale in small groups.* New York: Appleton-Century Crofts Inc.

GROOT, A.D. de (1968). *Bewegingsmeetkunde (Movement-mathematics).* Groningen: Wolters Noordhoff.

HERMANS, H.J.M. (1971). *Prestatiemotief en faalangst in gezin en onderwijs (Achievement motivation and fear of failure in family and education).* Amsterdam: Swets & Zeitlinger.

HOF, M.A. van 't, & Kowalski, C.J. (1979). Analysis of mixed longitudinal data-sets. In B. Prahl-Andersen et al. (Eds.), *A mixed longitudinal interdisciplinary study of growth and development* (pp. 161-172). New York: Academic Press.

HOFMAN, A. (1983). *Blood pressure in childhood. Epidemiological probes into the etiology of high blood pressure.* Unpublished doctoral dissertation, Erasmus University, Rotterdam, The Netherlands.

KEMPER, H.C.G., Poulus, A.J., & Helm, N. van der (1971). Circuit training und körpererziehung: über den einfluss einer kreis-trainung beim schulsport auf einige morphologische und funktionelle merkmale bei 12- und 13-jährige jungen (Circuit training and physical education: About the influence of circuit training in PE lessons in school on a few morphological and functional characteristics in 12- and 13-year old boys). *Medizin und Sport,* **6**, 179-184.

KEMPER, H.C.G. (1973). The influence of extra lessons in physical education in physical and mental development of 12- and 13-year old boys. *Proceedings of the Satellite Symposium of the XXV Int. Congress of Physiological Sciences: Physical Fitness,* pp. 212-216.

KEMPER, H.C.G., Dekker, H., Ootjers, G., Post, B., Ritmeester, J.W., Snel, J., Splinter, P.G., Storm-van Essen, L., & Verschuur, R. (1983). *Growth and health of teenagers. A multiple longitudinal study in Amsterdam, The Netherlands.* Unpublished manuscript.

KEMPER, H.C.G., & Hof, M.A. van 't (1978). Design of a multiple longitudinal study of growth and health of teenagers. *European Journal of Pediatrics,* **129,** 147-155.

KEMPER, H.C.G., Ras, J.G.A., Snel, J., Splinter, P.G., Tavecchio, L.W.C., & Verschuur, R. (1974). Invloed van twee lessen lichamelijke oefening per week gedurende één schooljaar op de lichamelijke en geestelijke ontwikkeling van 12- en 13-jarige jongens van de brugklassen van een school voor VWO en HAVO te Amsterdam (Influence of two lessons physical education a week during one school year to the physical and mental development of 12- and 13-year old boys of the first year of a secondary school in Amsterdam). *Thomas,* **10 & 11,** 325-370.

KEMPER, H.C.G., Verschuur, R., & Bovend'eerdt, J. (1979). The Moper fitness test, I—A practical approach to motor performance test in physical education. *Proceedings of ICPFR S.A., Journal for Research in Sport, Physical Education and Recreation,* **2**(2), 81-90.

KEMPER, H.C.G., Verschuur, R., Ras, J.G.A., Snel, J., Splinter, P.G., & Tavecchio, L.W.C. (1975). Biological age and habitual physical activity in relation to physical fitness of 12- and 13-year old schoolboys. *Journal of Pediatrics,* **119,** 169-179.

KOWALSKI, C.J., & Prahl-Andersen, B. (1979). General considerations in the design of studies of growth and development. In B. Prahl-Andersen, C.J. Kowalski, & P. Heyendael (Eds.), *A mixed longitudinal interdisciplinary study of growth and development.* New York: Academic Press.

LANGE-ANDERSEN, K., Seliger, V., Rutenfranz, J., & Skobak-Kazymski, J. (1976). Physical performance capacity of children in Norway. Part IV: The rate of growth in maximal aerobic power. *European Journal of Applied Physiology,* **35,** 49-58.

MIRWALD, R.L. (1980). Saskatchewan growth and development study. In Ostijn, Beunen, & Simons (Eds.), *Kinanthropometry II* (pp. 289-305). Baltimore: University Park Press.

POST, G.B., & Kemper, H.C.G. (1980). Kruisvraagmethode en 24-uurs navraagmethode—een onderzoek naar de reproduceerbaarheid van 2 enquête-technieken ter bepaling van de voedselconsumptie bij tieners (Cross-check method and 24-hours recall—An investigation into the reproducibility of 2 interview techniques to ascertain food intake of teenagers). *Voeding,* **41**(4), 123-129.

RAO, M.N., & Rao, C.R. (1966). Linked cross-sectional study for determining norms and growth rates—A pilot survey on Indian school-going boys. *Saykhya,* **68,** 237-258.

RITMEESTER, J.W., Kemper, H.C.G., & Verschuur, R. (1985). Is a levelling-off in oxygen uptake a prerequisite in the measurement of $\dot{V}O_2$max in teenagers. In Binkhorst, Kemper, & Saris (Eds.), *Children and exercise XI* (pp. 161-169). Champaign, IL: Human Kinetics.

ROBINSON, S. (1938). Experimental studies of physical fitness in relation to age. *Arbeitsphysiologie,* **10,** 252-323.

SARIS, W.H.M. (1982). *Aerobic power and daily physical activity in children, with special reference to methods and cardiovascular risk indicators.* Thesis K.U. Nijmegen, Meppel, Krips, Repro.

SARIS, W.J.M., Snel, P., & Binkhorst, R.A. (1977). A portable heart rate distribution recorder for studying daily physical activity. *European Journal of Applied Physiology,* **37,** 19-25.

SCHAIE, K.W. (1965). A general model for the study of development problems. *Psychologisch Bulletin,* **64,** 92-107.

SEROO, T., Storm-van Essen, L., & Kemper, H.C.G. (1982). Het meten van de voor- en achterwaartse krommingen van de rug bij tieners (Measurement of the forward-backward curvatures of the back in teenagers). *Geneeskunde en Sport,* **2**, 78-82.

SPLINTER, P.G., Tavecchio, L.W.C., Kemper, H.C.G., Ras, J.G.A., Snel, J., & Verschuur, R. (1978). On the reliability of a questionnaire to measure pupils' attitudes toward physical education. *International Journal of Physical Education,* **15**(4), 19-22.

TANNER, J.M. (1962). *Growth at adolescence.* Oxford: Blackwell.

VELING, S.H.J., & Hof, M.A. van 't (1980). Data quality control methods in longitudinal studies. In M. Ostyn, G. Beunen, & J. Simons (Eds.), *Kinanthropometry II* (pp. 436-442). International Series on Sport Sciences. Baltimore: University Park Press.

VERSCHUUR, R., & Kemper, H.C.G. (1980). Adjustments of pedometers to make them more valid in assessing running. *International Journal of Sports Medicine,* **1**, (2), 95-98.

WEINER, J.S., & Lourie, J.A. (Eds.) (1969). *IBP handbook nr. 9: Human biology: A guide to field methods.* Oxford: Blackwell.

Long-Term Studies of Physical Activity in Children—
The Trois Rivières Experience

Roy J. Shephard
University of Toronto
Toronto, Ontario,

and Université de Québec à Trois Rivières,
Quebec, Canada

Long-term studies of physical activity will be discussed in this article with particular reference to information gained in the Trois Rivières longitudinal study (Lavallée & Shephard, 1982; Shephard, 1982). Specific questions to be addressed include the impact of exercise upon physical growth and development, academic performance, and health.

Physical Growth and Development

Physical Growth

The impact of physical activity upon growth depends upon the nature of the required exercise and the age at which it is applied. The Trois Rivières study assigned cohorts of boys and girls from both an urban and a "rural-industrial" milieu to a modified curriculum which added an hour of endurance-type physical activity per day to the normal Québec primary school program from ages 6 to 11 years. The immediate growth curves were unchanged relative to preceding and succeeding cohorts who followed the standard Québecois program—one 40-minute activity period per week, taught by the normal classroom teacher.

Nevertheless, radiographs of the wrist showed a 3.6 month delay of maturation in the active group (Lavallée & Shephard, 1982), a finding confirmed by Suzuki (1970). In certain young athletes such as ballet dancers and gymnasts, very heavy training schedules have also retarded menarche (Frisch, Wyshak, & Vincent, 1980), although there is often an associated energy imbalance (Ledoux, Brisson, & Pérronet, 1982). Such results, thus, cannot be extrapolated to more normal situations where body mass and body fat are well maintained.

Table 1

Exponents Relating Various Components of Performance to Stature, as Determined Experimentally in the Trois Rivières Study

Variable	Exponent	Variable	Exponent
Maximum oxygen intake ($\ell \cdot min^{-1}$)	2.78	Sit ups (n)	1.97
Physical working capacity (W)	3.37	Flexed arm hang (s)	0.98
Vital capacity (ℓ)	2.68	Standing broad jump (m)	1.22
Handgrip force (N)	3.23	Shuttle run (s)	−0.53
Back extension force (N)	2.72	50 yard run (s)	−0.87
Leg extension force (N)	2.88	300 yard run (s)	−0.81

Note. Based on data of Shephard et al., 1980, for both experimental and control subjects; in general, the experimental program had only a minor influence on exponents.

Any delay of maturation may lead to a larger adult size in experimental than in control subjects. The investigator must then adjust physiological data for size effects, using either theoretical or experimentally determined height exponents (see Table 1).

Oxygen Transport and Physical Performance

Students enrolled in the enhanced activity program at Trois Rivières developed increases of (a) directly measured maximum oxygen intake, (b) PWC_{170}, (c) isometric muscle strength, and (d) scores for the CAHPER performance test battery relative to control subjects (see Figure 1). Because the relative size was similar to control subjects, these gains could not be attributed to dimensional factors (Shephard et al., 1980).

A number of previous authors have failed to demonstrate a training response in children. Among possible explanations are the following:

1. *Initial fitness.* Some studies have drawn volunteers from special sports camps (Cumming, Goodwin, Baggley, & Antel, 1967). In contrast, the Trois Rivières students were representative of their community with an initial fitness level below some European samples (maximum oxygen intake of 45 ml·kg^{-1}min^{-1} at 6 years) (Shephard et al., 1971).
2. *Seasonal effects.* Fitness levels may be biased by seasonal variations of sports participation, term and vacation activities, and climatic influences (Shephard et al., 1978). At Trois Rivières, this problem was avoided by carrying out annual tests within 4 weeks of each child's birthday.
3. *Observation period.* Hickson, Hagberg, Ehsani, and Holloszy (1981) have argued that in adults the halftime needed for a training response is as little as 10 days. This is true if the intensity of training is not increased, but with a well-designed progressive program, improvements of performance continue over several years. In young children, the basic skills of movement must also be learned before serious training can be undertaken. At Trois Rivières, a statistically significant advantage

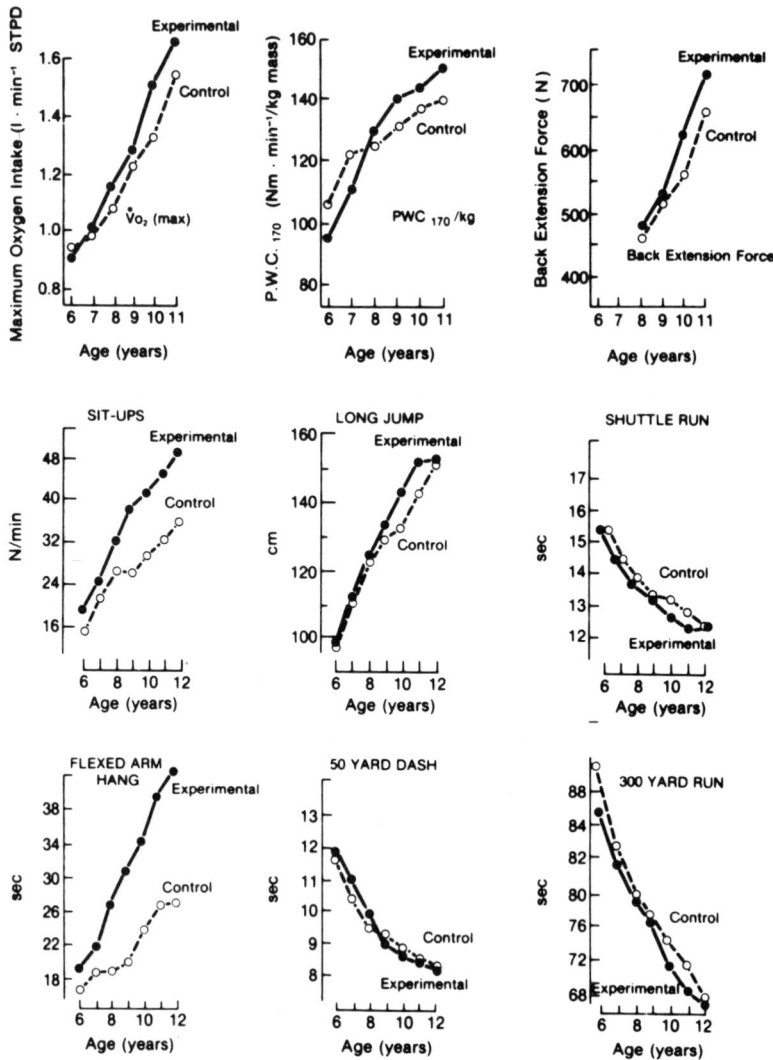

Figure 1—Influence of experimental program upon (a) directly measured maximum oxygen intake, (b) P.W.C.$_{170}$, (c) muscle strength, and (d) field performance as assessed by CAHPER test battery. Data of Shephard, Lavallée, Jéquier, LaBarre, & Rajic, 1977; reprinted with permission from R.J. Shephard. *The physiology and biochemistry of exercise.* New York: Praeger, 1982.

was not observed during the first 2 years (see Figure 1). Other studies may thus have had too short a duration to observe a response.

4. *Sample size.* The precision of most fitness tests is no more than 5 to 10% with a coefficient of variation of 7 to 14% for repeated measures. A substantial sample is thus needed to demonstrate fitness gains of 5 to 10%.

5. *Other confounding factors.* Negative results can also result from poor compliance and contamination of controls. Poor compliance is particularly likely with a leisure-

based program. At school, known amounts of activity can be required over a number of years, but leisure activity may nevertheless show a compensating reduction. At Trois Rivières, activity diaries suggested only a slight reduction of leisure activities on weekdays, but over the weekend, the experimental students were more active than controls (Shephard et al., 1980).

Control students who had brothers or sisters enrolled in the experimental program were checked. Such subjects did not differ significantly from other controls, arguing against significant contamination of our reference population.

Type and Quantity of Activity

Type of Activity

Effective activity is matched to the age of the child. Over the first 2 years, the mastery of skills and socialization were stressed. Later, there was progression to cardiovascular and muscular endurance training and, finally, instruction in team games.

It has not yet been determined whether experimental students remain more active than the controls when they become adults. While there are experimental advantages to a required school program, the obligatory nature of the activity may weaken the development of self-motivation.

Two measures suggest the Trois Rivières students viewed their required program favorably: The voluntary physical activity of experimental students exceeded that of controls on Saturdays, while 80% of the academic teachers favored the program. Further follow-up during the period of self-will is necessary, but difficult to arrange due to defections from the experiment and from physical dispersal of the students to institutions of higher learning.

Intensity of Exercise

The dose of exercise must reach the training threshold. Goode et al. (1976) demonstrated that a typical physical education class of 50 min involved the average student in only 1 to 2 min of activity at the training threshold. Nevertheless, the same authors found that a training response could be induced in both primary and secondary school children if vigorous, large muscle activity was assured for at least 6 min/weekday.

The focus of the Trois Rivières program was upon endurance-type exercise such as swimming, cross-country skiing, and games in the gymnasium with vigorous participation by the entire class. Time and motion studies and telemetry showed individual students were active for 20 to 30 min per session at a heart rate of 157 to 175 beats/min.

Mental Development

Academic Scores

School boards are often reluctant to allocate curricular time for physical activity on the grounds that academic performance will be impaired. At Trois Rivières, academic

Table 2

Influence of an Experimental Program Upon Academic Grades

Grade	Urban Milieu Exp. (% of Sample)	Control (% of Sample)	Rural-Industrial Milieu Exp. (% of Sample)	Control (% of Sample)
A	42.8	38.6	65.5	52.2
B	41.2	39.3	23.8	33.0
C, D, E, or F	16.0	22.1	10.7	14.9

Note. Based on data of Shephard, Volle, LaBarre, Jéquier, & Rajic, 1981. Significance of exp./control difference $p < .001$

instruction of the experimental students was curtailed 13 to 14%, but nevertheless higher grades were earned, both in the urban and in the rural-industrial milieu, as shown in Table 2 (Shephard, Volle, LaBarre, Jéquier, & Rajic, 1981).

Many of the teachers thought that behavior was improved by the added physical activity, but the class averages showed no objective gains except in Grade 6. Province-wide objective examinations, taken in Grade 6, confirmed teacher ratings of mathematical ability and French language, but disagreed with the teachers in showing the experimental students to have poorer scores for overall intelligence.

Psychomotor Development

The Trois Rivières study suggested an impact of added physical education upon knowledge of the physical self, including the correct perception of body dimensions, concepts of verticality, and finger recognition (see Table 3).

Table 3

Influence of Experimental Program Upon Estimation of Height and Arm Span at Distances of 2 and 4 m

Source of Variance	Height at 2 m	at 4 m	R Arm (Half-Span) at 2 m	at 4 m	L Arm (Half-Span) at 2 m	at 4 m
Exp. vs. control	16.6	12.4	21.5	16.2	30.1	14.5
Sex	n.s.	n.s.	16.7	12.0	19.1	10.1
Urban vs. rural	6.3	10.1	7.2	5.1	3.5	4.6

Note. Based upon data of Volle et al., 1981. Results are expressed as F ratios for the difference between actual and perceived dimensions.

Data Interpretation

Possible explanations of the enhanced academic performance include (a) a "halo" effect, due to teacher approval of the program, (b) a fresher and better prepared approach by academic teachers due to a shorter workday, (c) an immediate arousal of experimental students, (d) long-term improvements of body image, and (e) an accelerated psychomotor development (Curcio, Robbins, & Ela, 1971; Rigal, 1976).

From the practical point of view, one may conclude that the primary school child can sacrifice curricular time to physical development without disadvantage to academic learning.

Immediate and Long-Term Health

In Grade 1, the experimental students at Trois Rivières averaged almost 13 days of absence, compared with 10 days for control students. In subsequent years, the absence rate for both groups dropped to about 4 days per year. Thus, these data gave no evidence that additional physical activity protects against acute disease (Shephard, 1982).

Active teenagers and adults have a reduced chance of developing such coronary risk factors as cigarette smoking, hypertension, and an adverse lipid profile (Shephard, 1982). However, there is as yet no evidence that daily exercise in primary school will induce this pattern of behavior as an adult; this remains an important topic for future investigation.

Summary

The potential for enhancing physical and mental development through regular daily classroom activity is reviewed with specific reference to the controlled trial undertaken at Trois Rivières. It has been shown that endurance activity of the type possible in a primary school setting leads to an increase of aerobic power, muscular strength, and physical performance without any immediate effect upon body dimensions. While time is easily "lost" in classroom activity programs, a nominal hour of such instruction is sufficient to develop fitness if sustained over a period of several years. The allocation of curricular time is well justified because psychomotor development is enhanced, and perhaps for this reason, marks for a number of academic subjects are improved. There is little immediate effect upon the health of the children concerned, and a more extended study is needed to determine whether an enhanced primary program will encourage a healthy lifestyle as an adult.

Acknowledgment

The work discussed has been undertaken in collaboration with Dr. Hugues Lavallée and investigators associated with the Dept. of Health Sciences, University of Québec at Trois Rivières (R. LaBarre, J.C. Jéquier, M. Volle, & M. Rajic).

References

CUMMING, G.R., Goodwin, A., Baggley, G., & Antel, J. (1967). Repeated measurements of aerobic capacity during a week of intensive training at a youths' track camp. *Canadian Journal of Physiology and Pharmacology,* **45**, 805-811.

CURCIO, F., Robbins, O., & Ela, S.S. (1971). The role of body parts and readiness in acquisition of number conservation. *Child Development,* **42**, 1641-1646.

FRISCH, R.E., Wyshak, G., & Vincent, L. (1980). Delayed menarche and amenorrhea in ballet dancers. *New England Journal of Medicine,* **303**, 17-19.

GOODE, R.C., Virgin, A., Romet, T.T., Duffin, J., Crawford, P., Pallandi, T., & Woch, Z. (1976). Effect of a short period of physical activity in adolescent boys and girls. *Canadian Journal of Applied Sports Science,* **I**, 241-250.

HICKSON, R.C., Hagberg, J.M., Ehsani, A.A., & Holloszy, J.O. (1981). Time course of the adaptive responses of aerobic power and heart rate to training. *Medicine and Science in Sports,* **13**, 17-20.

LAVALLÈE, H., & Shephard, R.J. (1982). *International symposium on growth and development.* Trois Rivières: Université a Trois Rivières.

LEDOUX, M., Brisson, G., & Perronet, F. (1982). Nutritional status of adolescent female gymnasts. *Medicine and Science in Sports,* **14**, 145.

RIGAL, R.A. (1976). Influence de l'évolution des composantes du développement psychomoteur sur le rendement en mathématiques chez des enfants de 6 à 9 ans (Influence of the evolution of components of psychomotor development on the mathematical ability of children aged 6 to 9 years). *Enfance,* **29**, 346-355.

SHEPHARD, R.J. (1982). *Physical activity and growth.* Chicago: Year Book.

SHEPHARD, R.J., Jéquier, J.C., Lavallée, H., LaBarre, R., Rajic, M., & Beaucage, C. (1980). Habitual physical activity—Effects of sex, milieu, season and required activity. *Journal of Sports Medicine & Physical Fitness,* **20**, 55-66.

SHEPHARD, R.J., Lavallée, H., Jéquier, J.C., LaBarre, R., Rajic, M., & Beaucage, C. (1978). Seasonal differences in aerobic power. In R.J. Shephard & H. Lavallée (Eds.), *Physical fitness assessment—Principles, practice, and application* (pp. 194-210). Springfield, IL: C.C. Thomas.

SHEPHARD, R.J., Lavallée, H., Jéquier, J.C., LaBarre, R., Volle, M., & Rajic, M. (1977). Un programme complémentaire d'éducation physique. Etude préliminaire de l'expérience pratiquée dans le district de Trois Rivières (A program of additional physical education. Preliminary study of an experiment in the Trois Rivières region). In J.R. LaCour (Ed.), *Facteurs limitant l'endurance humaine. Les techniques d'amélioration de la performance (Factors limiting human endurance. Methods of improving performance)* (pp. 43-54). Université de St. Etienne, France.

SHEPHARD, R.J., Lavallée, H., LaBarre, R., Jéquier, J.C., Volle, M., & Rajic, M. (1980). On the basis of data standardization in pre-pubescent children. In M. Ostyn et al. (Eds.), *Kinanthropometry II* (pp. 360-370). Basel: Karger A.G.

SHEPHARD, R.J., Volle, M., Lavallée, H., LaBarre, R., Jéquier, J.C., & Rajic, M. (1984). Required physical activity and academic grades—A controlled study. In J. Ilmarinen (Ed.), *Proceedings of 10th pediatric work physiology symposium,* Joutsa, Finland, 1981. Berlin: Springer Verlag.

SUZUKI, S. (1970). Experimental studies on factors in growth. *Social Research in Child Development,* **35**, 6-11.

VOLLE, M., Tisal, H., LaBarre, R., Lavallée, H., Shephard, R.J., Jéquier, J.C., & Rajic, M. (1984). Required physical activity and psychomotor development of primary school children. In J. Ilmarinen (Ed.), *Proceedings of 10th pediatric work physiology symposium,* Joutsa, Finland, June, 1981. Berlin: Springer Verlag.

Changes in Lung Function, Ball-Handling Skills, and Performance Measures During Adolescence in Normal School Boys

David A. Brodie
University of Liverpool
Liverpool, England

This study is part of a more substantial project involving 88 variables measured sequentially over 5 years with a group of normal school boys. The purpose of the project was to provide data on aspects of growth and on the relationships among the many variables. Of particular general interest is the aspect of biological aging compared with chronological age, but the present article will mainly be concerned with the latter because most comparative data are presented in terms of chronological age.

The majority of published data in children has been collected cross-sectionally, so the following longitudinal data may provide useful supportive information for the trends already observed. This is particularly so, as the age range of the study includes the peak height changes during adolescent growth.

Materials and Methods

Subjects

The 39 subjects comprised an entire year group of normal boys in a middle school in Leeds, England. They were members of the same class and were involved in the same pattern of school activities. The socio-economic classification of the boys' parents closely matched the normal distribution for the United Kingdom. Informed consent was obtained from the boys, their parents, the educational authorities and the hospital ethical committees. The study commenced before the boys had achieved puberty at a mean starting age of 10.9 (SD = ± 0.26) years, and it continued for 5 years.

Lung Function

Forced vital capacity (FVC), forced expiratory volume in 1 second (FEV_1), forced expiratory ratio ($FEV_1\%$) and forced mid-expiratory flow (FMF) were measured annually using a single-breath dry spirometer (Vitalograph Ltd.).

Height

Height was measured with a wall-mounted stadiometer to the nearest completed millimeter. Maximum extension of the spine was achieved by gentle upward pressure under the jaw and occiput.

Ball-Handling Skills

The tasks chosen to represent aspects of motor development were the following four main categories of ball-handling skills:

1. Throwing a ball for accuracy (i.e., aiming)
2. Hitting a ball for accuracy with an instrument (e.g., bat or racket) held in the hands (i.e., striking)
3. Receiving a ball (i.e., catching)
4. Transporting a ball using an instrument (e.g., hockey or lacrosse stick) held in the hands (i.e., dribbling)

The measurement procedure was as follows:

Aiming. The task involved an underarm throw, using a standard tennis ball, over a distance of 6.1 m (20 ft) from a restraining line to the center of a target placed horizontally on the ground. The target consisted of concentric circles of radii 15.2 cm (6 in.), 30.4 cm (12 in.), 45.6 cm (18 in.), 60.8 cm (24 in.) and 77.5 cm (32 in.), representing scores of 5, 4, 3, 2, and 1 points, respectively.

After 6 practice trials, subjects received 2 blocks of 10 recorded trials with concurrent verbal and visual knowledge of results. Test reliability (split/half) was $r = .56$, ($p < .001$).

Striking. Subjects were required to drop a tennis ball from the nonpreferred hand onto the ground behind the 6.1 m (20 ft) restraining line and hit the rebound at the target with a paddle-tennis bat held in the preferred hand. All the conditions with respect to the target, scoring system, and the number of trials were the same as those of the aiming task. Test reliability (split/half) was $r = .55$ ($p < .001$).

Catching. Subjects using the preferred hand attempted to catch a tennis ball propelled over a distance of 6.1 m (20 ft). The balls were projected at 10-s intervals by a Castle "Stroke Master" into a 15 × 25 cm high rectangular area between the shoulder and the top of the head. Each subject received 6 practice trials before 2 blocks of 15 recorded trials. Test reliability (split/half) was $r = .62$, ($p < .001$).

Dribbling. A hockey stick held with both hands was used to dribble a tennis ball in and out of 4 skittles placed in a line, 4 m apart. The task included the return journey carried out in a similar manner. Subjects were not permitted to touch the ball with the feet or hands, and if the experimenter decided that the control of the ball was lost (i.e., the ball could not be reached with the stick), the trial was restarted.

The recorded score was the time taken to complete the course from the command "Go," when the ball was stationary on the Start/Finish line, to when the ball was seen to cross the line on the return. Subjects received 2 practice trials followed by 3 recorded trials. Test reliability (split/half) was $r = .54$, ($p < .001$).

Performance Measures

The seven-item AAHPER Youth Fitness Test was administered annually. A cricket ball throw was substituted for the softball throw, as this was considered more appropriate for British schoolboys. The seven items were

1. pull-ups (maximum number),
2. sit-ups (maximum number with 100 as a limit),
3. shuttle run (best time of 2 trials),
4. standing broad jump (best of 3 trials),
5. 50-yard dash (time for 1 trial),
6. cricket throw (best of 3 throws), and
7. 600-yard run-walk (time for 1 trial).

The procedure followed was as is specified in the AAHPER Test Manual (AAHPER, 1965).

Results

The values for each year of the study are presented in Table 1. The lung function and performance values were compared with a selection of studies from the literature (Baldwin, 1928; Beaudry, 1967; Bjure, 1963; Cherniack, 1962; Cook & Hamann, 1961; Dugdale & Moeri, 1968; Engstrom, Karlberg, & Kraepelien, 1956; Godfrey, Kamburoff, & Mairn, 1970; Hellieson, Cook, Friedland, & Agathon, 1958; Lunn, 1965; Lyons, Tanner, & Picco, 1960; Morse, Schultz, & Cassels, 1952; Strang, 1959; Yoshizaqa, 1971).

The general criteria for including a certain set of values for comparison were as follows:

1. The data covered a wide range of childhood development.
2. The number of subjects had to be stated in the literature.
3. A description of the type of population had to be stated with a reasonable certainty that the subjects were normal.
4. The experimental method had to be stated so that only data obtained by similar techniques were compared.
5. The data had to be related to some standard value of growth and development so that comparison with other studies was easily facilitated.
6. The evaluation of the results had to conform with some accepted statistical techniques. This was waived if the raw data were available.

Although the changes during childhood have been correlated with many anthropometric measurements, height was chosen as the principal parameter in the following consideration of the data. Where a study had presented multiple correlations with various bodily measurements including height, the results were considered using height alone by taking the 50th percentile age and weight values corresponding to the given standing height. The standard measurements used for this conversion were taken from Scott (1959).

Table 1

Means (Standard Deviations) for Each Year of Measurement of Lung Function, Age, Height, Ball-Handling Skills and Performance Measures

Measure	1st	2nd	3rd	4th	5th
Forced vital capacity (l)	2.33(0.33)	2.75(0.34)	2.99(0.49)	3.53(0.59)	4.19(0.75)
Forced expiratory vol. in 1 s. (l)	1.93(0.33)	2.38(0.28)	2.58(0.39)	2.99(0.51)	3.58(0.68)
FEV₁.FVC (%)	85.5 (6.5)	86.8 (5.8)	86.8 (5.5)	84.9 (6.3)	85.7 (6.1)
FMF (l. s^{-1})	2.31(0.57)	2.42(0.56)	2.68(0.67)	2.85(0.78)	3.43(0.97)
Age (years)	10.86(0.26)	11.92(0.26)	12.87(0.26)	13.84(0.26)	14.86(0.26)
Height (cm)	141.6 (5.0)	146.4 (5.5)	151.0 (6.4)	159.6 (7.4)	166.6 (7.4)
Ball-handling skills					
Aiming (score)	26.3 (6.4)	27.6 (5.7)	29.6 (5.4)	31.8 (4.9)	31.4 (4.9)
Striking (score)	9.3 (4.1)	10.9 (4.9)	14.8 (5.8)	17.7 (5.1)	16.8 (4.7)
Catching (n)	5.9 (4.3)	8.6 (3.6)	11.4 (3.0)	12.1 (2.9)	12.9 (2.4)
Dribbling (s)	20.7 (3.9)	16.6 (3.8)	14.4 (2.8)	13.1 (2.5)	11.5 (1.4)
Pull-ups (n)	2.2 (1.8)	2.1 (1.8)	2.9 (2.9)	4.6 (3.8)	5.1 (3.7)
Sit-ups (n)	46.5 (30.8)	47.3 (26.4)	53.2 (29.8)	65.8 (29.0)	75.6 (23.7)
Shuttle run (s)	11.3 (0.6)	11.6 (0.7)	11.3 (0.9)	11.0 (0.8)	10.7 (0.7)
Standing long jump (m)	1.54(0.14)	1.41(0.19)	1.65(0.15)	1.84(0.21)	1.97(0.21)
50-yard sprint (s)	8.37(0.49)	8.34(0.54)	8.55(0.87)	8.15(0.73)	7.41(0.76)
Cricketball throw (m)	26.1 (4.7)	29.5 (4.7)	37.0 (5.5)	38.5 (6.8)	43. 6(7.6)
600-yard run-walk (in)	2.20(0.35)	2.10(0.23)	2.02(0.28)	1.94(0.32)	2.15(0.21)

When the data were presented in the form of equations, the measures were computed at arbitrarily chosen standing heights and plotted on rectangular coordinates as a function of height in centimeters. When data were reported as means and standard deviations at specific standing heights, the mean value for every 10 cm of height from 110 to 170 cm were plotted on rectangular coordinates.

Lung Function

The major aspect of these results was that although there may be significant differences between authors at specific heights, the general pattern of the results among the authors was quite consistent. It was not possible to assess which authors' data were most trustworthy; thus composite values have been produced with a set of precision limits representative of the data. These composite values are shown in Table 2 compared to the equivalent height values from the present study.

Ball-Handling Skills

The scores in the catching task showed significant improvement ($p < .01$) up to the age of 12.9 years, increasing from 39% to a 76% success rate. Beyond this point, which approached the asymptote level, relatively small gains were recorded.

The aiming and striking tasks involved projecting the ball under the same stimulus conditions of target size and distance. Both produced the same pattern of consistent gains up to the age of 13.9 years, followed by a slight decrement. It was, however, only in the striking task that significant changes were noted, and then only between the ages of 11.9 to 13.8 years.

The annual improvements in dribbling were significant at each stage.

Performance Measures

A consistent increase in the values as the boys grew older was observed for the measures of sit-ups and cricketball throw only. Other measures showed the occasional

Table 2

Composite Lung Function Values From the Literature in Comparison With the Present Study

Measure	Values acording to height (cm), mean (standard deviation)			
	140	150	160	170
FVC (1) Composite	2.35(0.15)	2.85(0.20)	3.40(0.25)	4.00(0.40)
FVC (1) Present study	2.15(0.33)	2.85(0.45)	3.50(0.58)	4.05(0.70)
FEV_1(1) Composite	2.20(0.20)	2.65(0.20)	3.25(0.25)	3.80(0.30)
FEV_1(1) Present study	1.85(0.33)	2.50(0.39)	2.95(0.50)	3.50(0.65)
FMF (1 sec^{-1}) Composite	2.15(0.35)	2.70(0.37)	3.25(0.40)	3.60(0.42)
FMF (1 sec^{-1}) Present study	2.25(0.57)	2.55(0.67)	2.85(0.78)	3.20(0.97)

year which did not follow the expected pattern: for example, the 1976 values for the measures of pull-ups, shuttle runs, and standing long jump; the 1977 values for 50-yard spring; the 1979 value for 600-yard run. The measurement techniques remained identical throughout the 5 years, so this is an unlikely cause of any discrepancy.

Discussion

The results in Table 2 indicate that the 50th percentile of the composite values were always within the 95% confidence limits of the present study. This suggested that although differences were readily observed between individual lung function studies, the general trend was a reasonable similarity between results. This is particularly useful when comparing a longitudinal study such as the present one with the majority of the studies in the literature which are cross-sectional. The associated difficulties in the collection of longitudinal data do not appear to produce results which differ markedly from the more easily obtained cross-sectional values.

A useful method of considering growth is to examine the annual incremental change. This has the advantage of indicating rate of change and is used to obtain peak height changes which is a valuable anthropometric marker during adolescence. The subjects' heights were measured 3 times per year, so it was relatively easy to obtain the mean peak height changes. The peak value for this group occurred at about 13.3 years. The annual change for the lung function measures produced different peaks with the largest increment occurring at age 15 years. This was the last data point measured, so it is possible that an even greater increment occurred during the following year. Previous work (Brodie, 1972) has shown that at about the age of 15, the peak changes occur for the measures FEV_1, FVC, and FMF. These earlier results were based on cross-sectional data, so the present longitudinal data confirms the time lag of approximately 2 years between the maximum growth rate of stature and lung function. This may reflect the tendency of boys to increase their thoracic dimensions somewhat after this rapid increase in stature. The delay in the peak velocity curve for FMF cannot be explained in this way and is more likely to be a consequence of the respiratory musculature reaching its peak velocity for strength at the same time.

The lung function indices reported in this study would seem to be less important during physical activity in normal children than the efficiency of gaseous exchange. However, there may be certain activities of an intensive, dynamic nature when lung power, as indicated by FEV_1, may become an important performance correlate. In such cases, it is important for the physical educator, coach, and sport scientist to appreciate that there is a clear delay between the peak changes in stature and lung function. This should influence the expectations, training programs, and coaching of growing boys accordingly.

In maturational terms, skill in catching is acquired comparatively late but fairly rapidly and with relatively little practice. It also appears to be easily transferable within a wide range of stimulus-response situations.

The absence of any significant changes at successive stages in aiming was due to the large variance within the group. The perpetual-motor requirements of the aiming and striking tasks appeared to demand accurate judgments of distance and kinesthetic sensitivity with a refined sense of coincident timing in the act of striking or releasing the ball. The little evidence available indicates that these abilities are normally more fully developed at a later age, and that they are very largely task-specific (Fleishman & Rich, 1963; Gibson, 1963; Morris, 1974; Weibe, 1975).

The dribbling task involved the coordination of running with ball control and represented a broad category of transporting skills which included the use of the feet and hands. The scores indicated a fairly rapid and continuous rate of skill acquisition which was not associated consistently with the other ball-handling skills.

The observations that emerged from these results confirmed the limitations of such a narrow test battery in predicting either the generalized rate of learning or final performance level in ball-handling tasks.

The performance results indicated a complex interplay of maturation and performance. The individual changes in strength and power to body weight ratios may account for the decreased values in the measures of pull-ups, shuttle run, and standing long jump during the 2nd year of the study. The increased time for the 600-yard run during the last year could possibly have been attributed to a lack of motivation as the boys grew older, although the value of oxygen uptake, measured separately, did suggest a relative decrease in aerobic capacity per kilogram body weight. The present data were similar to other works (A.A.H.P.E.R., 1965; Campbell & Tucker, 1967; C.A.H.P.E.R., 1966; Ellis, Carron, & Baily, 1975; Espenschade, 1960; Hunsicker & Reiff, 1977; Jones, 1949; Rarick, Widdop, & Broadhead, 1970; Ruskin, 1978) although the majority of the published data is cross-sectional reported longitudinally.

The most striking differences in the present, true longitudinal study are the measures of 50-yard sprint and 600-yard run/walk. The 50-yard sprint times are slower than the other published studies, which would suggest a poorer anaerobic capacity in the present population. The 600-yard run/walk times, on the other hand, were generally faster which would indicate a comparatively better developed aerobic system. In all the other measures, the values from this study were very similar to the data presented elsewhere. This suggests that few differences exist between children of other nationalities in these items of motor fitness. It also illustrated that no major discrepancies in the trends occur between longitudinal and cross-sectional data for these measures.

References

AMERICAN Association of Health, Physical Education and Recreation. (1965). *Youth Fitness Test Manual* (Rev. Ed.). Washington, D.C.: American Association for Health, Physical Education and Recreation.

BALDWIN, B.T. (1928). Breathing capacity according to height and age of American-born boys and girls of school age. *American Journal of Physical Anthropology,* **12**, 257-67.

BEAUDRY, P.H., Wise, M.B., & Seely, J.E. (1967). Respiratory gas exchange at rest and during exercise in normal and asthmatic children. *American Review of Respiratory Diseases,* **94**, 248-254.

BJURE, J. (1963). Spirometric studies in normal subjects. IV. Ventilatory capacities in healthy children 7-17 years of age. *Acta Paediatrica,* **52**, 232-240.

BRODIE, D.A. (1972). The relationship of pulmonary measurements to selected indices of physical performance, anthropometry and academic achievement within a schoolboy population. Unpublished M.Sc. thesis, University of Loughborough.

CAMPBELL, W.R., & Tucker, N.M. (1967). *An introduction to tests and measurement in physical education,* London: Bell & Son.

CANADIAN Association for Health, Physical Education and Recreation. (1966). *Fitness-performance test manual.* Ottawa: C.A.H.P.E.R.

CHERNIACK, R.M. (1962). Ventilatory function in normal children. *Canadian Medical Association Journal,* **87**, 80-1.

COOK, C.D., & Hamann, J.F. (1961). Relation of lung volumes to height in healthy persons between the ages of 5 and 38 years. *Journal of Pediatrics,* **59**, 710-14.

DAVIES, M.J.R., & Garbe, D.R. (1965). Criteria of measuring techniques for standardized tests of lung volume and respiratory capacity. *World Medical Electronics,* **3**, 187-254.

DREW, C.D.M., & Hughes, D.T.D. (1969). Characteristics of the Vitalograph spirometer. *Thorax,* **24**, 703-6.

DUGDALE, A.E., & Moeri, M. (1968). Normal values of forced vital capacity, forced expiratory volume and peak flow rate in children. *Diseases of Childhood,* **43**, 229-234.

ELLIS, J.D., Carron, A.V., & Baily, D.A. (1975). Physical performance in boys from 10 through 16 years. *Human Biology,* **47**(3), 263-281.

ENGSTROM, I, Karlberg, P., & Kraepelien, S. (1956). Respiratory studies in children. 1. Lung volumes in healthy children 6-14 years of age. *Acta Paediatrica,* **45**, 277.

ESPENSCHADE, A.S. (1960). Motor development. W.R. Johnson (Ed.), *Science and medicine of exercise and sports* (pp. 419-439). New York: Harper and Row Publishers.

FLEISHMAN, A.E., & Rich, S. (1963). Role of kinesthetic and spatial-visual abilities in perceptual-motor learning, *Journal of Experimental Psychology,* **66**, 6-11.

GIBSON, E.J. (1973). Perceptual Development. In H.W. Stevenson, J. Kgan, & C. Spiker, (Eds.), *Child psychology,* (pp. 145-195). Chicago: University of Chicago Press.

GODFREY, S., Kamburoff, P.L., & Nairn, J.R. (1970). Spirometry, lung volumes and airway resistance in normal children aged 5 to 18 years. *British Journal of Diseases of the Chest,* **64**, 15-24.

HELLIESEN, P.J., Cook, C.D., Friedland, L., & Agathon, S. (1958). Studies of respiratory physiology in children. 1. Mechanics of respiration and lung volumes in 85 normal children 5 to 17 years of age. *Pediatrics,* **22**, 80-93.

HUNSICKER, P., & Reiff, G. (1977). Youth fitness report: 1958-1965-1975. *Journal of Physical Education and Recreation,* **48**, 32.

JONES, H.E. (1949). *Motor performance and growth.* Berkeley: University of California Press.

LUNN J.E. (1965). Respiratory measurements of 3556 Sheffield school-children. *Brit. J. Pre. Soc. Med.,* **19**, 115-22.

LYONS, H.A., Tanner, R.W., & Picco, T. (1960). Pulmonary function studies in children. *American Journal of Diseases of Childhood,* **100**, 196-207.

MORRIS, P.R. (1974). *Perceptual-motor abilities related to performance and learning in ball-handling skills.* Unpublished M.Ed. thesis, University of Newcastle on Tyne.

MORSE, M., Schultz, F.W., & Cassels, D.E. (1952). The lung volume and its subdivisions in normal boys 10-17 years of age. *Journal of Clinical Investigations,* **31**, 380-91.

RARICK, G.L., Widdop, J.H., & Broadhead, G.D. (1970). The physical fitness and motor performance of educable mentally retarded children. *Exceptional Children,* **36,** 509-519.

RUSKIN, H. (1978). Physical performances of school children in Israel. In R.J. Shepherd & H. Lavallee (Eds.), *Physical fitness assessment* (pp. 273-320). Springfield IL: Charles C. Thomas.

SCOTT, J.A. (1959). Report on the heights and weights of school pupils in the County of London in 1959. *London County Council.*

STRANG, L.B. (1959). The ventilatory capacity of normal children. *Thorax,* **14,** 305-310.

WEIBE, V.R. (1954). A study of tests of kinesthesis. *Research Quarterly,* **25,** 220-230.

YOSHIZAWA, S. (1971). Aerobic work capacity of Japanese adolescents of the rural district. *Japanese Research Journal of Physical Education,* **15**(3), 21-32.

Acknowledgments

The author wishes to acknowledge the assistance of his colleagues, P.R. Morris, P.J. Atkinson, L. Burkinshaw, and J.M.H. Bucker, who all made a substantial contribution to the project.

Organization and Learning of Movements

Jan J. Denier van der Gon and Marianne H. Vincken
Utrecht State University, Utrecht, The Netherlands

Over the last decades countless studies have been devoted to the human motor system, and recently quite a few excellent reviews have appeared (Grillner, 1975; Keele, 1981; McCloskey, 1981; Schmidt, 1981; Stein, 1974). This contribution will be confined to an outline of the motor system and its organization as referred to by these review articles. In addition, attention will be focused upon a few rather arbitrarily chosen recent developments that concern the organization and learning of movements.

First, a hierarchically structured tentative scheme of the motor system will be presented. That the higher levels of this scheme are ill-defined from a neurophysiological point of view will be evident. The current knowledge of these elements is derived mainly from psychological and psychophysical experiments and from a general knowledge of control systems. Although neuroanatomical and neurophysiological knowledge of the brain is growing fast and, in general, corroborates the views presented, it is unlikely that in the near future the higher motor functions will be completely understood in terms of their neurophysiological substratum.

A little more detailed knowledge is available of the lower, more peripheral, parts of the motor system, although the current insight into what is exactly going on, for example, in the spinal cord is rather poor. Furthermore, a thorough functional analysis of this part is not possible without insight into the other parts of the motor system. The motor system can only be understood in its entirety when it is considered with all its interconnections.

The Overall Organization of the Motor System

Internal Representation

Meaningful motor activities are necessarily based upon an organism's awareness of its surroundings. Ultimately, therefore, motor functions should be studied in interrelation with perceptive functions. The higher motor functions are controlled from an internal representation of the surroundings of the organism in relationship to the organism itself. Numerous sense organs contribute to the internal representation (see Figure 1).

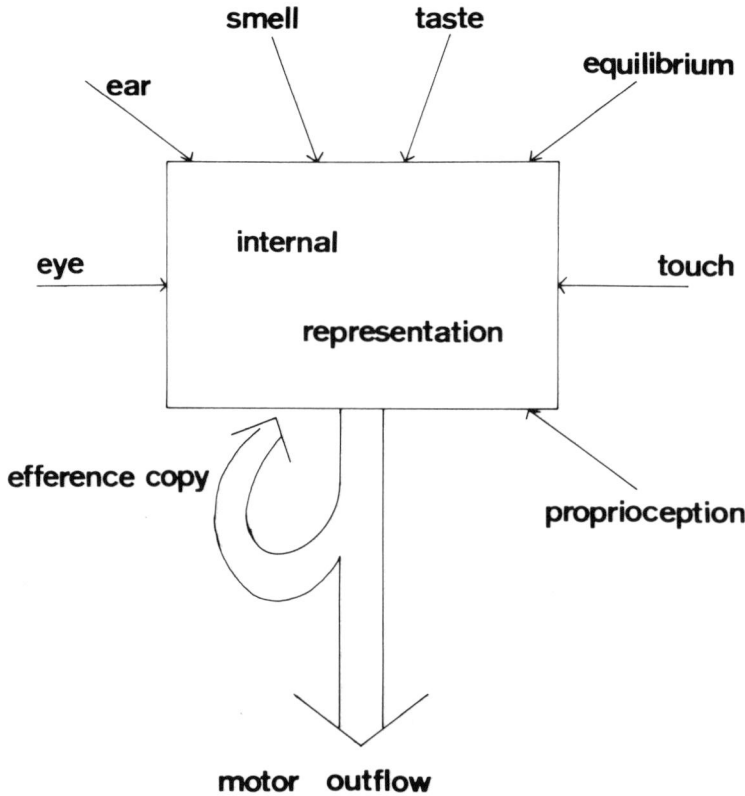

Figure 1—Many perceptive channels contribute to the internal representation of the surroundings. An important input channel contains a copy of the efferent motor outflow. The internal representation is updated by this outflow. The sensory inflow is also correlated with the exploring motor activities of the organism. Perception is mainly an active process.

The internal representation is certainly not merely a "photograph" of the surroundings, continuously adapting to what is going on. In addition, it comprises all kinds of expectancies concerning what will happen during the next moment and also what the effect of "voluntary" actions of the organism will be (Sommerhoff, 1974). In this way, anticipatory and goal-directed activities may be selected and put into effect. There are indications that the internal representation is also updated directly by its own output (efference copies, Holst & Mittelstaedt, 1950). When an activation pattern for the execution of a movement is initiated, this activation pattern is fed back and the consequences are incorporated into the internal representation (McCloskey, Colebatch, Potter, & Burke, 1983). As long as no conflicting evidence reaches the internal representation from other sources, this updated internal representation is the starting point for further planning. Although the framework or hardware used to construct internal representations is inborn, it appears that the ability to construct effective internal representations is basically a learning process to which both sensory perception and motor activities contribute. In a certain phase of their development, animals that are deprived of the possibility to explore and improve these sensory and motor activities in combination with each other show lasting motor disabilities (Held & Hein, 1963). Perception on its own probably is mainly an active explorative function in which motor activity is essential. The discussion on this subject is not yet closed.

The Movement Effector System

Movements are effected by muscles. The smallest functional units are the motor units consisting of a single motoneurone together with the muscle fibers that it innervates. Such a unit is highly nonlinear in its behavior. If the stimulation of a motoneurone exceeds a certain recruitment threshold, it starts firing directly with a rather high frequency. Increase of the level of stimulation may further increase the firing frequency. The overall transfer properties of a motor unit from stimulation to force generation are rather poor, from the point of view of a control engineer (see Figure 2).

However, many motor units act in parallel and recruitment thresholds, and twitch forces of motor units of a muscle appear to be jointly distributed in such a way that a muscle as a whole, including its motoneurones, is an easily manageable force-generating unit.

Intermediate Levels

The internal representation may activate a "movement generator" that produces motor patterns or programs that may be sent to the motor effector system (see Figure 3).

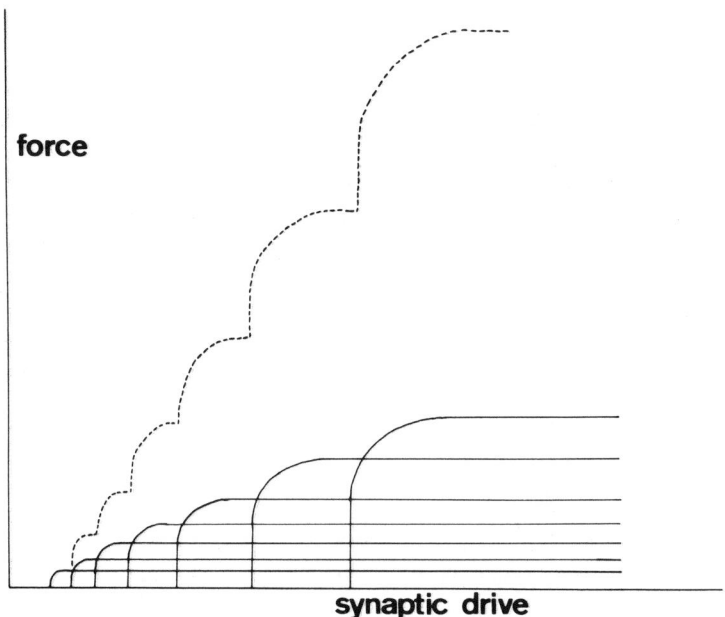

Figure 2—Motor units (—) show highly nonlinear properties. Motor units of a muscle act in parallel and their forces add. The muscle as a whole (---) shows rather good control properties as a result of the joint distribution of the recruitment thresholds and sizes of the motor units.

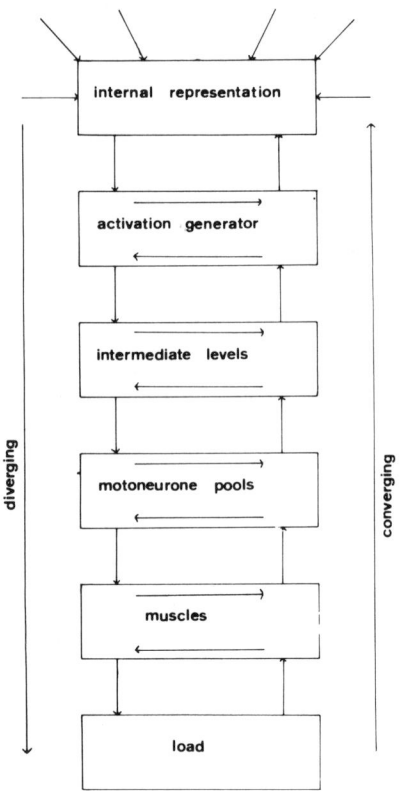

Figure 3—The motor control system is hierarchically structured. Movements that are planned by the internal representation give rise to contractions of a large number of muscle fibers. The activity of numerous sense organs are jointly interpreted. The level interactions are controllable, resulting in a highly versatile system. Horizontal arrows indicate interactions between ascending and descending signals.

Fast goal-directed arm movements give rise to two separate bursts of activity in the agonist muscles, and a single burst appears between them from the antagonist muscles (Wadman, Denier van der Gon, Geuze, & Mol, 1979). The first burst of agonist activity accelerates the arm; the antagonist burst decelerates it; and, finally, the second burst of agonist activity contributes to a rapid stop and a stabilization of the arm. The duration of the first burst of activity is a main determinant of movement distance.

In experiments in which a subject has to react to incoming visual information by flexing or extending the arm, it takes about 150 to 250 ms (reaction time) before such an electromyographic pattern is elicited (Gielen, van den Heuvel, and Denier van der Gon, 1983; Keele & Posner, 1968). A number of electromyographic responses can also be elicited by a forced displacement of a limb. The response pattern depends on the instruction given to the subject, but, in general, three different responses can be distinguished. First is a short burst of activity after some 20 ms—a short latency reflex. Next is a burst after some 50 ms. This activity is often referred to as medium latency reflex (Jaeger, Agarwal, & Gottlieb, 1982). It is not known which parts of the central nervous system contribute to this reflex, but because of its plasticity, it is likely that higher levels are involved. Still, the actual reflex loop is probably limited to the spinal cord. Finally, after some 100 ms, a complete pattern of activity similar to that of a goal-directed movement emerges. Because of the latencies involved, it is likely that this long latency reflex is a triggered reaction of the movement pattern generator and not a voluntary reaction (Crago, Houk, & Hasan, 1976).

There has been much debate on the functional significance of these reflexes. They most probably artificially reflect a number of control loops that in themselves are not very effective in controlling movements. They may control system variables and contribute to position and stiffness control of a limb, load compensation, and the like. Going from top to bottom in Figure 3, planned activity becomes more specific and diverges, resulting in activations of selected sets of motoneurones. This transformation is stepwise. Somewhere in between, use is made of elementary motor patterns that produce simple and stereotyped movements such as withdrawal and scratching movements, stride patterns, and so on. The higher levels merely activate and modify these basic patterns. In the reverse direction, signals originating from sense organs in the skin, muscles, tendons, and joints merge stepwise into patterns that may elicit those elementary movements and, finally, also contribute to the internal representation.

The Organization of Movement

Directional Organization of Movement

A voluntary motor act is effected by a number of muscles that are activated with certain intensities during certain periods. The force developed by a single muscle depends

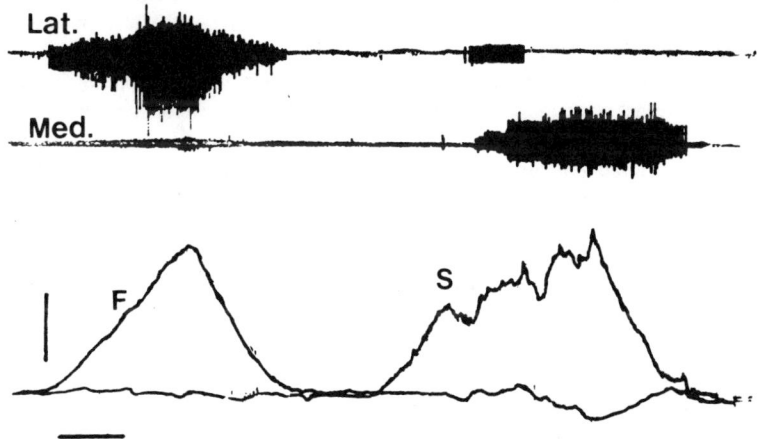

Figure 4—Motor unit activity recorded in the biceps muscle with the help of thin wire electrodes. Laterally located motor units are recruited when a flexion force (F) is exerted, and medially located motor units are recruited when the subject is supinating (S).

on the number of activated motor units and on their firing frequencies. In general, the motor units of a muscle are recruited in a fixed order. From research on the biceps brachii, a multifunctional muscle contributing to flexion, supination, and exorotation of the forearm, it appears that this principle may be task-related (see Figure 4) (Haar Romeny ter, Gielen, & Denier van der Gon, 1982).

Medially located muscle units are only recruited when flexion is performed. The most laterally located units are recruited when supination and exorotation is performed while the other units respond to all tasks. So it appears that three homogeneous and clearly different groups of muscle units are present in this muscle (Haar Romeny ter, Denier van der Gon & Gielen, 1984). This suggests three nonoverlapping groups of motoneurones in the motoneurone pool of that muscle, each related to a different task or principal movement direction and with its own recruitment order. An arbitrary movement direction may be composed of such principal directions so that the muscles or parts of muscles involved in the movement are activated synchronously (Soechting & Lacquani, 1983; Wadman, Denier van der Gon, & Derksen, 1980). Many questions still must be answered; for example, how the different sets of motoneurons are mapped on the motoneurones pools in the spinal cord and how the dependency on posture of the principal direction is taken into account. Furthermore, a mapping of higher centers of the CNS on these sets of motoneurones must be such that elementary movements may be elicited by activating those centers. Certainly, it has been shown that stimulation of single sites in the brain can cause completely coordinated movements.

Open-Loop Versus Closed-Loop Control

An interesting discussion ongoing for several decades is whether movements are open-loop (programmed) or closed-loop (feedback) controlled. Because arguments favor both theories makes it probable that they are not mutually exclusive. It has been shown that the first part of a fast goal-directed movement is programmed because an unexpected mechanical blocking of the movement does not disturb the muscle activation pattern (Wadman, Denier van der Gon, Geuze, & Mol, 1979). Eventually, all movements are feedback controlled, albeit delayed.

In agreement with the hierarchical structure of the motor system, it appears that control loops are present at a number of levels. If a limb making a movement meets resistance, muscle shortening is slowed down, resulting in higher muscle forces in conformity with the Hill force-velocity relationship of the muscle. In addition to this immediate effect, short, medium, and long latency reflexes may assist the movement. These loops are inactive if the movement is executed according to the preplan. Prior to the movement, sensory responses that are to be expected are also generated by the internal representation. If the actual responses match the expected ones, the movement is considered to be carried out in conformity with the intended one.

The control signals are not only generated by numerous sense organs and transmitted by afferent nerves to the higher control levels, but, as previously mentioned, it is likely that the central nervous system also evaluates the generated motor action by immediately estimating the effects to be expected from these activities. The use of such efference copies may give rise to rather early movement corrections or adjustment of the internal representation. For instance, if a subject has to quickly track a target that jumps once or twice, and the first movement has been too small, the next one following within 100 ms has to be so large that the second target position is reached (see Figure 5) (Gielen, unpublished results).

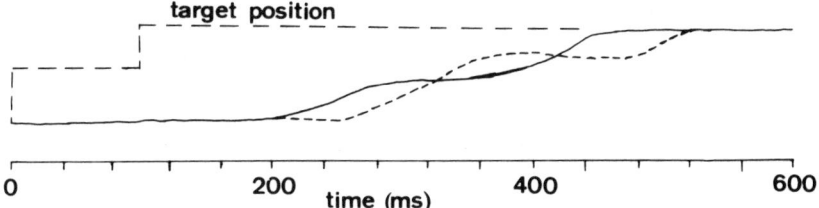

Figure 5—Position recordings in a tracking task in which the target jumped twice. The solid line and the dashed line indicate two different responses to the stimulus. The first step is too small (—) or too large (---). These deviations are corrected by adapting the size of the response to the second step. The latencies involved are considered to be too small for the correction to be based upon sensory perception. The correction is thought to arrive from efference copy signals that update the internal representation immediately.

What Muscle Variables Does the Central Nervous System Control?

The question of the muscle variables controlled by the nervous system has been raised (Stein, 1982) and many researchers in motor control have made comments. The question is of interest because it directly relates the performance of the central nervous system to its output and thus to measurable variables. Attention is paid to force, position, velocity, acceleration, stiffness, and so on. Arguments in favor of almost every variable are presented. This suggests that the central nervous system does not control just one variable, but controls a movement or other motor performance in all its aspects. If, for instance, the motor system primarily controls positions by using position feedback with a high gain (the actual feedback loops, incidentally, have a too low gain for this purpose), then objects to be grasped might easily be damaged. A combined control of position and force certainly has advantages.

In the last two decades, a number of interesting studies have been devoted to stiffness and control of stiffness of muscles and limbs (Nichols & Houk, 1976). Stiffness may be defined as the ratio of imposed forces to induced displacement. Stiffness is an important variable in motor control. It plays a role in, for instance, absorbing shocks, (partial) correcting for misjudged loads, smoothing of movements, and so on. Part of the stiffness results from intrinsic muscle properties. Muscle force is thought to be generated by crossbridges that link myosin and actin filaments in muscle. These crossbridges have elastic properties. Many parallel crossbridges implying a large muscle force due to many activated motor units result in a stiff muscle. Thus, simultaneous contraction of mutually antagonistic muscles results in a stiff limb. This stiffness, however, is only maintained over a short range of muscle stretch because crossbridges break as a result of large stretches.

An important contribution to apparent muscle stiffness and limb stiffness is made by reflexly generated counter forces (Vincken, Gielen, & Denier van der Gon, 1983). As soon as a muscle is stretched, stretch sensitive sensors are activated that give rise to such forces. (For a review, see Prochazka, 1981.) Because the gain of the reflex loops involved is controllable, stiffness can also be controlled. Stiffness control is to be seen as an element in motor control. If a movement is carried out, it appears that stiffness changes in conformity with the requirements of the movement. Moreover, it appears that the changes in stiffness before and after the movement are reproducible and time-locked to the movement (Wieneke & Denier van der Gon, 1974; Vincken,

Gielen & Denier van der Gon, 1984). Thus, stiffness is controlled by the same motor program that controls the movement. Stiffness changes with the movement; for example, limb stiffness after a slow movement is less than after a fast movement. This implies that stiffness control is part of the motor program for a movement.

Motor Skill and Learning

Movements should be evaluated in relation to the appointed motor task. The required accuracy and velocity as well as the load play a role in this evaluation. Skilled movements may often have a number of features in common. They may be carried out rapidly and smoothly, suggesting little feedback corrections and the running of a perfect motor program. Stiffness is as low as permitted, meaning little cocontraction of muscles and minimum fatigue. Muscles that take no part in the movement, directly or indirectly, are relaxed. Moreover, the subject's attention is not directed to the movement pattern but focused on the goal to be achieved. It is as if the subconscious levels automatically generate the movement program. These features come to the fore if one studies the performance of artists in painting and drawing or in playing musical instruments (e.g.,

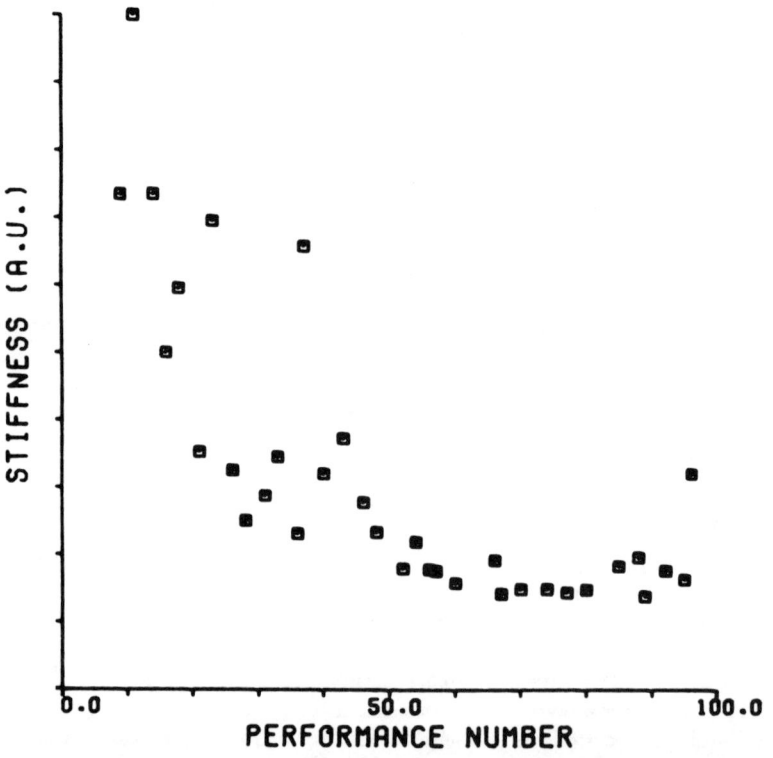

Figure 6. Stiffness (expressed in arbitrary units) measured as the inverse of the deviation resulting from a force disturbance while practicing a complicated movement.

see Denier van der Gon, 1979). The features mentioned may be used as cues in a learning process. If, for instance, a subject is instructed to imitate a complex movement, the first movement of a series will be slow and hesitating while limb stiffness is often high. During the learning process, the movement becomes smoother and is speeded up. Limb stiffness may go down as is shown in Figure 6.

The variation in stiffness as shown in Figure 6 is to be attributed to changes in the apparent gain of the reflex loops. γ-static and γ-dynamic control may be involved. Coactivation of α and γ systems may reflect the fact that stiffness control is part of control of movements. The relation between the activations of both systems, however, is not fixed. Voluntary changes of stiffness are possible, and in a learning process, a change in the relation between movement velocity and stiffness takes place (Vincken & Denier van der Gon, 1985).

References

CRAGO, P.E., Houk, J.C., & Hasan, Z. (1976). Regulatory actions of the stretch reflex. *Journal of Neurophysiology,* **39**(5), 925-935.

DENIER VAN DER GON, J.J. (1979). Spontaneity in motor expression and the art of playing the spinal c(h)ord. In H.L.C. Jaffe, J. Storm van Leeuwen, & L.H.v.d. Tweel (Eds.), *Authentication in the visual arts.* Amsterdam: BM Israel BV.

GIELEN, C.C.A.M., van den Heuvel, P.J.M., & Denier van der Gon, J.J. (1984). Modification of muscle activation patterns during fast goal-directed arm movements. *Journal of Motor Behavior,* **16**(1), 2-19.

GRILLNER, S. (1975). Locomotion in vertebrates: Central mechanisms and reflex interaction. *Physiological Review,* **55**, 247-303.

HAAR ROMENY, B.M. ter, Gielen, C.C.A.M., Denier van der Gon, J.J. (1982). Changes in recruitment order of motor units in the human biceps muscle. *Experimental Neurology,* **78**, 360-368.

HAAR ROMENY, B.M. ter, Denier van der Gon, J.J. & Gielen, C.C.A.M. (1984). Relation between location of a motor unit in the human biceps brachii and its critical firing levels for different tasks. *Experimental Neurology,* **85**, 631-650.

HELD, R., & Hein, A. (1963). Movement produced stimulation in the development of visually guided behavior. *Journal of Comparative Physiology and Psychology,* **56**, 872-876.

HOLST, E. von, & Mittelstadt, H. (1950). Das Reafferenzprinzip. Wechselwirkungen zwischen Zentralnervensystem und Peripherie. *Naturwissenschaften,* **37**, 464-478.

JAEGER, R.J., Gottlieb, G.L., & Agarwal, G.C. (1982). Myoelectric responses at flexors and extensors of human wrists to step torque perturbations. *Journal of Neurophysiology,* **48**, 388-402.

KEELE, S.W. (1981). Behavioral analysis of movement. In V.B. Brooks (Ed.), *Handbook of Physiology* (pp. 1391-1414).

KEELE, S.W., & Posner, M.I. (1968). Processing of visual feedback in rapid movements. *Journal of Experimental Psychology,* **77**, 155-158.

McCLOSKEY, D.I. (1981). Corrolary discharges: Motor commands and perception. IN V.B. Brooks (Ed.), *Handbook of Physiology* (pp. 1414-1447).

McCLOSKEY, D.I., Colebatch, J.G., Potter, E.K., & Burke, D. (1983). Judgments about onset of rapid voluntary movements in man. *Journal of Neurophysiology,* **49**(4), 851-863.

NICHOLS, T.R., & Houk, J.C. (1976). Improvement in linearity and regulation of stiffness that results from actions of stretch reflex. *Journal of Neurophysiology,* **39**, 119-142.

PROCHAZKA, A. (1981). Muscle spindle function during normal movement. In R. Porter (Ed.), *Handbook of neurophysiology IV,* **25**, Baltimore: University Park Press.

SCHMIDT, R.A. (1981). *Motor control and learning.* Champaign, IL: Human Kinetics Publishers.

SOECHTING, J.F., & Lacquaniti, F. (1983). Modification of trajectory of a pointing movement in response to a change in target location. *Journal of Neurophysiology,* **49**(2), 548-564.

SOMMERHOFF, G. (1974). *The logic of the living brain.* New York: J. Wiley and Sons Ltd.

STEIN, R.B. (1974). Peripheral control of movement. *Physiological Reviews,* **54**, 215-243.

STEIN, R.B. (1982). What muscle variables does the nervous system control in limb movements? *The Behavioral and Brain Sciences,* **5**, 535-577.

VINCKEN, M.H., Gielen, C.C.A.M., & Denier van der Gon, J.J. (1983). Intrinsic and afferent components in apparent muscle stiffness in man. *Neuroscience,* **9**, 529-534.

VINCKEN, M.H., Gielen, C.C.A.M. & Denier van der Gon, J.J. (1984). Stiffness control after fast goal-directed arm movements. *Human Movement Science,* **3**, 269-280.

VINCKEN, M.H. & Denier van der Gon, J.J. (1985). Stiffness as a control variable in motor performance. *Human Movement Science,* (in press).

WADMAN, W.J., Denier van der Gon, J.J., & Derksen, R.J.D. (1980). Muscle activation patterns for fast goal directed arm movements. *Journal of Human Movement Studies,* **6**, 19-37.

WADMAN, W.J., Denier van der Gon, J.J., Geuze, R., & Mol, R.H. (1979). Control of fast goal-directed arm movements. *Journal of Human Movement Studies,* **5**, 3-17.

WIENEKE, G.H., & Denier van der Gon, J.J. (1974). Variations in the output of the human motor system. *Kybernetic,* **15**, 159-178.

Motor Performance as Related to Somatotype in Adolescent Boys

Gaston Beunen, Albrecht Claessens, Michel Ostyn, Roland Renson, Jan Simons, and Dirk Van Gerven
Katholieke Universiteit Leuven, Leuven, Belgium

At the extremes of performance, somatotype is fairly closely related to physical performance. To be successful in international competition, athletes should have (or should try to acquire) the appropriate somatotype that is characteristic of those who are already successful (Carter, 1981; Carter, Aubry, & Sleet, 1982). Examination of data on younger athletes, 12 to 18 years old, shows that the successful ones have somatotypes quite similar to those of the outstanding older athletes (Carter, 1980). The relationship between somatotype and fitness components such as strength, speed, flexibility, endurance, and balance are less well investigated, especially in general populations of growing children.

The studies conducted so far seem to indicate that mesomorphy is positively associated with performance, and endomorphy is negatively associated with performance with the exception of static or isometric strength. Ectomorphy shows either none or a slight positive association (Beunen, Ostyn, Renson, Swalus, & Van Gerven, 1977; Carter, 1980; Štěpnička, 1976). The aims of this study are twofold: (a) to analyze the age-specific relationships between physical performance characteristics and the somatotype components, and the three components together; and (b) to investigate the changes with age of these relationships.

Methods

Sample

The data were from a mixed longitudinal study of the physical fitness of a representative sample of Belgian school boys aged 12 to 19 years (Ostyn, Simons, Beunen, Renson, & Van Gerven, 1980). The testing program started in 1969 and ended in 1974. Each year between 2500 and 4500 boys of one secondary school grade were tested, beginning with the 1st grade. A total of 21,052 examinations were made. A stratified sample of schools was randomly selected, taking into account the following factors:

(a) language group: French or Flemish speaking; (b) type of schooling: vocational, technical schooling, or humanities; (c) school affiliation: private (Catholic) or state schools; and (d) geographical distribution of the school population by province.

In each school a random sample of classes was selected and all the boys in each class were examined. The same schools were studied throughout, which resulted in a combined longitudinal and cross-sectional study.

For the present study a cohort of 210 boys was selected. All boys were born in 1955-1956, followed during 6 years between 1969 and 1974, and measured at exact yearly intervals.

Measurements

For the motor ability components, a valid and reliable battery of tests was selected for boys of these age levels (Simons et al., 1969). For each factor, the test with the highest factor loading and test-retest reliability was chosen. Somatotype ratings were carried out by 3 different observers. The correspondence of their ratings was as reported in the literature (for endomorphy and ectomorphy, the correlations within and between observers varied between $r = .80$ and $r = .98$, and for mesomorphy between $r = .75$ and $r = .94$). All ratings were carried out according to a modification of Sheldon's method (Sheldon, Dupertuis, & McDermott, 1954) and agreed closely with the 1940 anthropometric-anthroposcopic technique (Sheldon, Stevens, & Tucker, 1940) and with the atlas technique (Sheldon et al., 1954) as was shown by Claessens et al. (1980).

Statistical Analysis

Stepwise multiple regression equations were derived with the 3 somatotype components as the independent variables for all the motor ability tests and the pulse recovery test (Nie, Hull, Jenkins, Steinbrenner, & Bent, 1975). The order of entry of the equations was determined by the partial correlation coefficients and no a priori order was fixed. To obtain the proportion of the variance accounted for by each of the independent variables, the product of the partial beta coefficient by the zero-order correlation (βxr) was calculated (Guilford, 1965).

Results

For each chronological age level, the coefficients of determination (R^2) and the explained variance (βxr) by each of the 3 somatotype components separately are given in Tables 1 and 2.

Static strength (arm pull) exhibited a moderately high correlation with somatotype components. The explained variance ranged between 16% and 34% and reached a maximum for 16-year-old boys (see Table 1). Mesomorphy and endomorphy were both positively correlated with static strength, although mesomorphy explained the largest portion of the variance in test results (between 13% and 31%).

The somatotype components, mainly mesomorphy, explained between 5% and 13% of the variance in explosive strength (vertical jump). The explained variance remained fairly similar between 13 and 18 years.

Table 1

Explained Variance[a] in Strength Test Results Accounted for by Somatotype Components

Dependent Variable	Independent Variable	Age Category (years)					
		13	14	15	16	17	18
Static strength	Endom.	17	3	12	5	6	2
(Arm pull)	Mesom.	13	13	31	29	26	26
	Ectom.	7*	—	13*	—	—	—
	R^2	24	16	30	34	32	28
Explosive strength	Endom.	—	5*	3*	—	—	—
(Vertical jump)	Mesom.	4	—	12	11	10	13
	Ectom.	6	—	2	—	1	—
	R^2	11	5	11	11	11	13
Functional strength	Endom.	21*	13*	14*	12*	9*	10*
(Bent arm hang)	Mesom.	5	6	7	6	3	—
	Ectom.	—	—	—	—	—	—
	R^2	26	19	21	18	12	10
Trunk strength	Endom.	12*	—	—	—	—	—
(Leg lifts)	Mesom.	—	9	10	22	11	14
	Ectom.	1*	—	—	—	—	7
	R^2	13	9	10	22	11	21
	N	155	166	165	170	163	139

[a]Explained variance in percentage (βxr)
R^2 = coefficient of determination in percentage
N = number of subjects
* = negative zero-order correlation
— = partial regression coefficient not significantly different from zero ($\alpha = 0.05$)

For functional strength (bent arm hang) between 10% and 26% of the variance was accounted for by the combined effects of endomorphy and mesomorphy. The coefficients of determination decreased somewhat with age. Endomorphy explained, by far, the largest part of the variance, but higher values of endomorphy were associated with lower results on the bent arm hang test.

Trunk strength generally showed a lower association (9% to 13%) with somatotype components, although at 16 and 18 years 22% and 21% of the variance was accounted for by the somatotype components. Except at 13 and 18 years, mesomorphy was the only component which contributed significantly to the explained variance.

Also flexibility (sit and reach) correlated rather moderately with somatotype and no age trend was seen (between 9% and 11% of the variance was explained). Mesomorphy was once more the only component which contributed significantly to the total explained variance (see Table 2).

For running speed 4% to 8% of the variance in test results was explained by the somatotype. No clear age trend was found and mesomorphy was the most important predictor at nearly all age levels.

Table 2

Explained Variance[a] in Flexibility and Speed Test Results Accounted for by Somatotype Components

Dependent Variable	Independent Variable	Age Category (years)					
		13	14	15	16	17	18
Flexibility	Endom.	—	—	—	—	—	—
(Sit and reach)	Mesom.	11	10	10	10	9	11
	Ectom.	—	—	—	—	—	—
	R^2	11	10	10	10	9	11
Running speed	Endom.	—	5*	—	—	5*	—
(Shuttle run)	Mesom.	4	—	8	4	3	—
	Ectom.	—	—	—	—	—	—
	R^2	4	5	8	4	7	—
Speed of limb movement	Endom.	—	—	—	—	—	—
(Plate tapping)	Mesom.	—	3	3	4	—	—
	Ectom.	—	—	—	—	—	—
	R^2	—	3	3	4	—	—
	N	155	166	165	170	163	139

[a]Explained variance (βxr) in percentage
R^2 = coefficient of determination in percentage
N = number of subjects
* = negative zero-order coefficient
— = R^2 or partial regression coefficient not significantly different from zero ($\alpha = 0.05$)

Also for speed of limb movement, mesomorphy was the only significant predictor. Between 14 and 16 years, only 3% to 4% of the total variance was accounted for. Eye-hand coordination (stick balance) was not correlated with somatotype. Furthermore, neither pulse rate at rest nor pulse rate after the 1-min step test was correlated with somatotype. Only at one or two age levels, 2% to 6% of the variance in pulse frequency was accounted for by one of the somatotype components.

Discussion

Generally speaking, the results reported herein confirm the previous findings (Beunen et al., 1977; Carter, 1980; Štěpnička, 1976). Somatotype is not associated with factors such as eye-hand coordination (stick balance) and speed of limb movement (plate tapping), or with pulse rate at rest or with pulse recovery after a 1-min step test. Low associations (explained variance ranged between 4% and 11%) were found for flexibility (sit and reach) and for running speed (shuttle run), whereas for explosive strength (vertical jump), and trunk strength (leg lifts) between 5% and 22% of the variance was accounted for by somatotype components. Functional strength (bent arm hang) and especially static strength (arm pull) were fairly highly correlated with somatotype components (10% to 34% of variance explained).

For most fitness factors, the associations between the test results and the somatotype components remain fairly stable, except for static strength for which a maximal correlation is reached at 16 years and for functional strength for which the correlations decrease with age.

Mesomorphy is by far the most important predictor for nearly all motor items at each age level. Higher levels of mesomorphy are always associated with better performance for groups. Endomorphy was positively correlated with static strength (arm pull), and negatively with functional strength (bent arm hang). For the other tests, no correlations or slightly negative correlations were found at some age levels. Ectomorphy correlated slightly positive with explosive strength (vertical jump) and trunk strength (leg lifts), slightly negative with static strength (arm pull), and showed no relationship with all the other fitness components.

It was not surprising that somatotype was not related to eye-hand coordination and speed of limb movement, because one would not expect that such characteristics are related to body build or body shape. One would anticipate a negative relationship between pulse recovery and endomorphy. However, it should be mentioned that a 1-min step test is of insufficient duration to adequately load the cardiovascular system. Also the positive associations between mesomorphy and most motor items were not surprising. Mesomorphy was a reflection of athletic build, and those with a high muscular mass tend to load high on the mesomorphy component (Beunen & Van Hellemont, 1980). Consequently, a higher mesomorphy would be expected to be associated with a better performance. Ectomorphy does not contribute significantly to the prediction, which may be due to the fact that the 3 somatotype components are not independent (Claessens et al., 1980), and that in predicting motor performance the information given by the ectomorphy component is already included in the information given by mesomorphy and/or endomorphy.

From the above it appears that for a general population of adolescent boys, somatotype components, especially mesomorphy and to a lesser extent endomorphy, are fairly highly correlated with some motor fitness components such as static strength and functional strength, and show a low to moderate relationship with trunk strength, explosive strength, flexibility, and running speed. The explained variance is, however, not high enough to predict individual performances, which points to the fact that motor fitness components are fairly independent factors. However, several of the multiple correlations are high enough to separate poor, average, and good performers from each other. Whatever the criticisms against the somatotype methods presently used may be, the findings reported herein together with those reported by others (Carter, 1980, 1981; Carter et al., 1982; Štepnička, 1976) indicate the validity and utility of the somatotype concept, for it helps to understand more about the physical performance capacities of youngsters and adults.

References

BEUNEN, G., Ostyn, M., Renson, R., Simons, J., Swalus, P., & Van Gerven, D. (1977). Somatotype and physical fitness of 14 year old boys. In H. Lavallée & R.J. Shephard (Eds.), *Frontiers of activity and child health* (pp. 115-123). Québec: Editions du Pélican.

BEUNEN, G., & Van Hellemont, A. (1980). Body structure and somatotype in physical education students. *Anthropologiai Közlemények* (Budapest), **24**, 15-21.

CARTER, J.E.L. (1980). The contributions of somatotyping to kinanthropometry. In M. Ostyn, G. Beunen, & J. Simons (Eds.), *Kinanthropometry II* (pp. 409-422). Baltimore: University Park Press.

CARTER, J.E.L. (1981). Somatotypes of female athletes. In J. Borms, M. Hebbelinck, & A. Venerando (Eds.), *The female athlete. A socio-psychological and kinanthropometric approach. Medicine and Sport,* **15**, 85-116.

CARTER, J.E.L., Aubry, S.P., & Sleet, D.A. (1982). Somatotype of Montreal Olympic Athletes. In J.E.L. Carter (Ed.), *Physical structure of Olympic athletes, Part I: The Montreal Olympic Games anthropological project. Medicine and Sport,* **16**, 53-80.

CLAESSENS, A., Beunen, G., Simons, J., Swalus, P., Ostyn, M., Renson, R., & Van Gerven, D. (1980). A modification of Sheldon's anthroposcopic somatotype technique. *Anthropologiai Közlemények* (Budapest), **24**, 45-54.

GUILFORD, J.P. (1965). *Fundamental statistics in psychology and education* (4th ed.). New York: McGraw-Hill.

NIE, N.H., Hull, C.H., Jenkins, J.G., Steinbrenner, K., & Bent, D.H. (1975). *Statistical package for the social sciences.* New York: McGraw-Hill.

OSTYN, M., Simons, J., Beunen, G., Renson, R., & Van Gerven, D. (1980). *Somatic and motor development of Belgian secondary school boys. Norms and standards.* Leuven: Leuven University Press.

SHELDON, W.H., Dupertuis, C.W., & McDermott, E. (1954). *Atlas of men. A guide for somatotyping adult male at all ages.* New York: Harper and Brothers.

SHELDON, W.H., Stevens, S.S., & Tucker, W.B. (1940). *The varieties of human physique. An introduction to constitutional psychology.* New York: Harper and Brothers.

SIMONS, J., Beunen, G., Ostyn, M., Renson, R., Swalus, P., Van Gerven, D., & Willems, E.J. (1969). Construction d'une batterie de tests d'aptitude motrice pour garçons de 12 à 19 ans par la méthode d'analyse factorielle (Construction of a motor fitness test for 12 to 19 year old boys by factor analysis). *Kinanthropologie,* **1**, 323-362.

STEPNICKA, J. (1976). (Somatotype, body posture, motor level and motor activity of youth.) *Acta Universitatis Carolinae Gymnica,* **12**. 1-93.

Physical Performance Capacity and Specific Skills in Young Soccer Players

Jacques Vrijens and Christiaan Van Cauter
State University of Ghent, Belgium

In modern soccer, a team game with many different aspects, physical performance capacity is of major importance in the determination of the performance level. Youth competition for 9- to 10-year-old boys already exists. Because matches for youth and adults are played on similar-sized fields, the performances of the youth teams are influenced by the physical development and motor fitness of the players.

During growth, puberty in particular, large differences in physical development have been observed. Most authors agree there is a close relationship between skeletal age, body dimensions, and physical performance (Beunen, Ostyn, Renson, Simons, & Van Gerven, 1978; Beunen et al., 1974; Bouckaert, Van Uytvanck, & Vrijens, 1974; Hebbelinck & Borms, 1978; Hollmann & Bouchard, 1970; Kusnecova, 1974). Components of motor fitness such as muscular strength, cardiovascular endurance, and even speed, are somewhat influenced by skeletal maturation. This relationship is not so obvious for skills such as flexibility, agility, or more specific motor skills. Some authors have even claimed that specific skills are related to chronological age as the result of a learning effect (Balsevitch, 1970; Fisher, 1975). Most of the studies in this area have so far been limited to puberty-aged groups, and are restricted to components of general motor fitness. In this research, attention was focused on the preadolescent age group. Specifically, the relationship between biological age, somatic development, and general motor performance was investigated, as well as the relationship to specific soccer skills in order to better understand youth performance.

Methods

Young soccer players (N = 66) aged 10 to 13 years were used as subjects in this study. They all had been members of a regional soccer team for at least 1 year. The following anthropometric measurements were taken: height, weight, and circumferences of the upper arm, thigh, and calf.

Breadth development was evaluated by measuring the humerus and femur width and shoulder and hip diameters. Body fat was assessed from measurements of skinfold thickness according to the method described by Parizkova (1977). Biological age was determined by measuring skeletal age from x-rays of the hand and wrist according to the method of Tanner, Whitehouse, Marshall, Healy, and Goldstein (1975). Static strength of the major muscle groups was measured with a Hettinger apparatus (Vrijens, 1978). General endurance capacity was assessed by a standard progressive bicycle ergometer test with two 5-min stages. Physical working capacity 170 was calculated by extrapolation. Specific endurance capacity was evaluated by means of a 6-min run on a standard circuit (Bovend'eert et al., 1980).

Data on the specific soccer skills of the subjects were obtained with the following tests: (a) a dribble-test, (b) a test for the evaluation of kicking capacity, (c) a soccer bounce drill, and (d) a test to evaluate ball control and precision.

Results and Discussion

The most important anthropometric data are presented in Table 1. The coefficient of variation for skeletal age in this age group was 10%. This value was considerably lower than during puberty.

The most important anthropometric data have been compared with norms of Belgian children published by Hebbelinck and Borms (1978) for the same age group (see Table 2). Only slight differences were found between the groups, which indicates that the sample in the present study was representative. The higher body fat content in this group was probably the result of differences in measuring technique.

The relationships between skeletal age and chronological age as criteria of biological development with body dimensions are shown in Figure 1. Correlation coefficients of anthropometric variables with skeletal age varied from .40 to .70 and were considerably higher than the correlations with chronological age, which ranged from .12 to .43. In prepubescence, the influence of skeletal maturation on somatic development is marked.

Table 1

Anthropometric Characteristics of Subjects

Characteristics (N = 66)	$\bar{X}$	±	SD	V%[a]
Chronological age (yrs)	11 yrs 3 mos		0.8	7.3
Skeletal age (yrs)	11 yrs 5 mos		1.1	10.0
Height (cm)	144.3		6.3	4.4
Weight (kg)	34.7		5.0	14.4
Fat (%)	18.2		3.7	20.3
Arm circumference (cm)	20.5		1.4	6.8
Thigh circumference (cm)	42.4		2.8	6.6
Biacromial diameter (cm)	31.2		1.7	5.4
Biiliac diameter (cm)	21.7		1.2	5.5

[a]V is the coefficient of variation.

Table 2

Anthropometric Variables—Comparative Data

	Vrijens & Van Cauter (1983) (N = 66)	Hebbelinck & Borms (1976) (N = 478)
Chronological age (yrs)	11 yrs 2 mos	11 yrs 0 mos
Height (cm)	144.3	141.5
Weight (kg)	34.7	33.8
Fat (%)	18.2	16.5

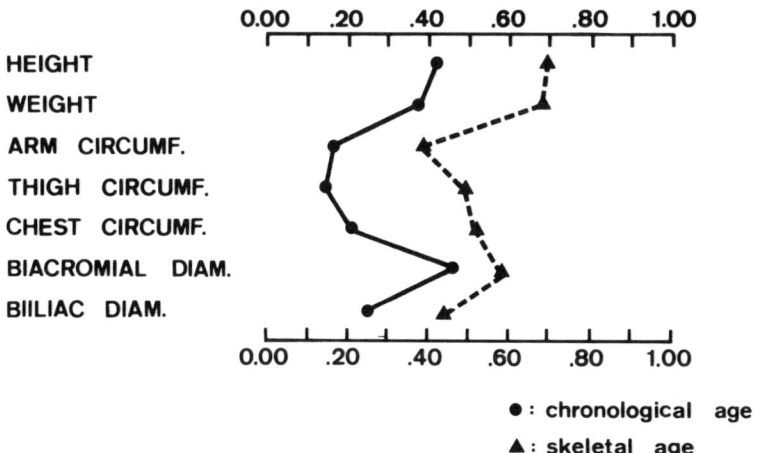

Figure 1—The relationship between chronological and skeletal age on selected anthropometric variables.

The results of strength measurements and endurance capacity indices are grouped in Table 3. The sum of isometric strength scores for the six muscle groups examined in this study did not differ from the results from untrained boys of the same age group (Vrijens, 1978).

For the evaluation of general endurance capacity, the results were compared with those of Hebbelinck and Borms for the same age group. Scores for physical working capacity of the boys in this study (74 W) corresponded to the average level of 78 W for this same age group as reported by Hebbelinck and Borms (1978).

Attention was also focused on the relationship between strength or endurance capacity and skeletal maturation in prepubescence. These results are shown in Figure 2. Only slight differences were found between the correlations of chronological age and skeletal age with respect to maximal isometric muscular strength. Correlation coefficients were .49 and .56, respectively. Explosive strength, however, was more closely related to

Table 3

Strength Scores and Endurance Capacity Indices

N = 66	X̄	± SD	V%
Isometric strength (kg) (Sum of scores)	165.9	25.3	15.2
Explosive leg strength (cm)	41.1	4.7	11.4
PWC 170 (W)	73.9	17.3	23.4
6 min endurance run (m)	1286.2	113.4	8.8

skeletal age. This result was not in agreement with the observed close relationship during puberty. Previous studies found that differences in strength between advanced and retarded boys were marked in the age group, from 13 to 17 years (Beunen, 1974). No differences in relationship between skeletal and chronological age were found with respect to general and specific endurance capacity. This finding is also in contradiction to the results for the adolescent age group. In a previous study (Hollmann & Bouchard, 1970), a positive relationship was found between skeletal maturation and physical working capacity 170, or maximal oxygen intake.

The last and probably most important aspect of this study was the evaluation of the specific soccer skills. The average results of the group are shown in Table 4.

For the first three tests an almost normal distribution (coefficient of variation varying between 10 and 20%) was found. For the bounce drill, however, there were large individual differences up to 50%. The reliability of the specific skill tests was examined by a test-retest procedure.

The soccer bounce test was a highly reliable test (r = .975). The other tests can also be considered as reliable (r ranging from .84 to .89) with the exception of the dribble-test (r = .724).

The influence of biological age on the specific motor abilities of soccer players is shown in Figure 3. In contrast to body dimensions, no significant relationship between

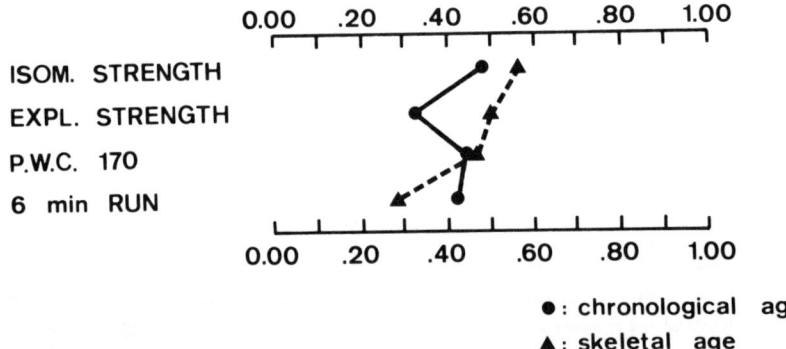

Figure 2—The relationship between chronological and skeletal age on strength and endurance capacities.

Table 4

Soccer Skills

N = 66	X̄	± SD	V%
Dribble (n)	33.1	5.3	10.0
Kicking capacity (n)	22.7	4.9	20.0
Ball control and precision (n)	10.3	1.6	10.0
Soccer bounce (n)	56.0	30.5	50.0

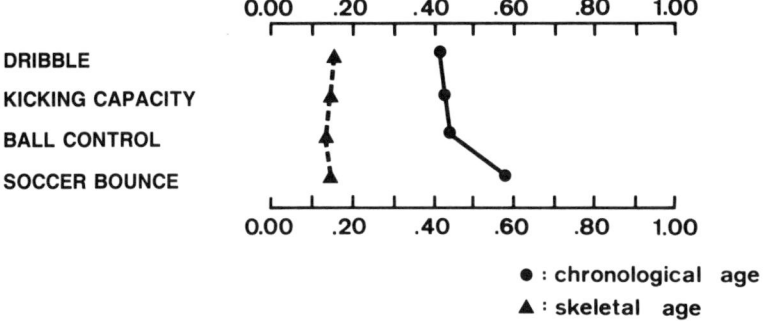

● : chronological age
▲ : skeletal age

Figure 3—The relationship between chronological and skeletal age on selected soccer skills.

any of the tests and skeletal age was found. With chronological age, however, the coefficients of correlation varied from .42 to .57 and were highly significant. This confirms the theory of some authors who suggest that the development of specific motor skills is the result of a neuromuscular learning process (Balsevitch, 1970; Fisher, 1975).

Another method to evaluate the influence of biological age on the different aspects of the somatic development and performance capacity is the comparative study of different maturity groups. Therefore, the total group was divided into three subgroups. The first was composed of boys with a retarded maturity (skeletal age 1 year or more below chronological age). The second group was composed of those boys who had an advanced skeletal maturity (skeletal age 1 year or more above chronological age). In the third group, the difference between skeletal age and chronological age was less than 3 months. The mean values of anthropometric characteristics of each of the three groups are summarized in Table 5.

Differences between retarded boys and the other groups were significant at the .05 level for height, weight, and shoulder width. On the other hand, no differences were found between average and advanced boys.

Retarded boys obtained lower results for maximal isometric strength, explosive strength, and endurance capacity. Differences, however, were not statistically significant. Also no significant differences were found between the average and advanced boys.

As already indicated by the correlation coefficients, no differences in specific soccer skills were found among the group in soccer skill test scores. The results were almost identical (see Table 6).

Table 5

Anthropometric Data of Three Maturity Groups[a]

	Retarded $\bar{X}$ n = 8	Average $\bar{X}$ n = 13	Advanced $\bar{X}$ n = 15	F-test
Height (cm)	139.3	147.5	148.7	< .01
Weight (kg)	31.7	36.0	36.5	< .05
Fat (%)	17.5	17.8	18.0	n.s.
Arm circumference (cm)	20.2	20.3	20.7	n.s.
Thigh circumference (cm)	41.1	42.5	43.2	n.s.
Biacromial diameter (cm)	29.9	31.6	31.7	< .05
Biiliac diameter (cm)	21.0	22.0	22.0	n.s.

[a]Values underlined are significantly different from each other ($p \leq .05$).

Table 6

Soccer Skill Scores of Three Maturity Groups

	Retarded $\bar{X}$ n = 8	Average $\bar{X}$ n = 13	Advanced $\bar{X}$ n = 15	
Dribble (n)	33.0	32.9	32.2	n.s.
Kicking capacity (n)	23.1	22.5	24.2	n.s.
Ball control (n)	10.4	10.7	10.6	n.s.
Soccer bounce (n)	59.0	57.3	64.3	n.s.

Finally, a signaletic profile was constructed for the three groups. The profile of the retarded boys was shifted to the left for somatic development and for the basic components of physical performance. For some of these parameters, the difference was statistically significant (see Figure 4). For the 6-min run and the soccer skills, no significant differences were found among the three groups.

Conclusions

From the results, the following conclusions can be drawn:

In the prepubescent age group, it seems that there is a relationship between skeletal

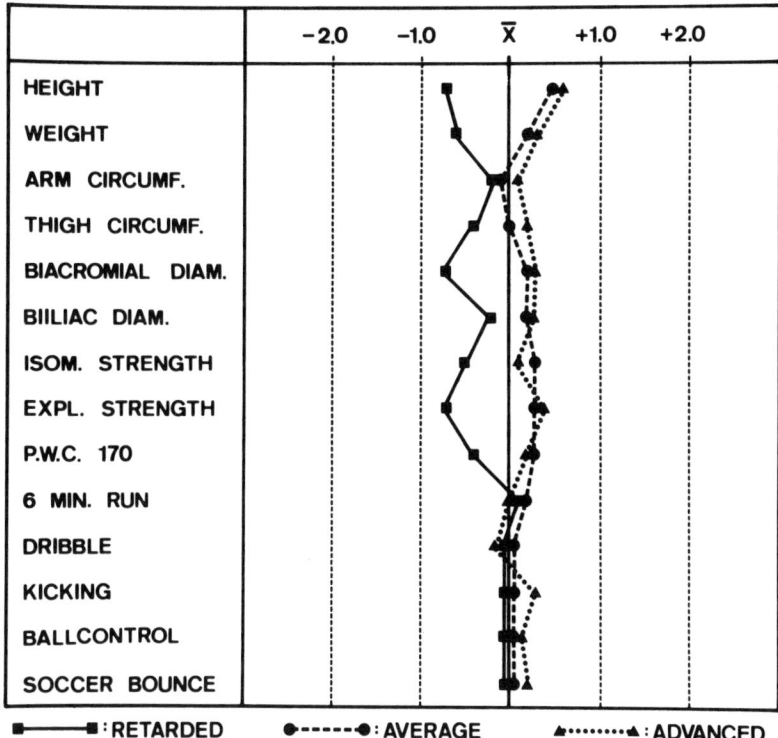

Figure 4—Signaletic profile of three maturity groups of young soccer players.

age and body dimensions. This relationship, however, is less obvious than during the adolescent age period.

General motor performance is also influenced by skeletal maturation, but no distinct differences were found with respect to chronological age.

No relationships between skeletal age and specific motor skills were found. Specific soccer skills are influenced by differences in chronological age. This suggests that specific motor performance must be seen as a neuromuscular learning process.

References

BALSEVITCH, V. (1970). Wann soll die Ausbildung im Lauf einsetzen (When is training in running supposed to begin?). *Leibeserziehung*, **19**, 77.

BEUNEN, G., Ostyn, M., Renson, R., Simons, J., Van Gerven, D. (1978a). Motor performance as related to age and maturation. In R.J. Shephard and H. Lavallee (Eds.), *Physical Fitness Assessment, Principles, Practice and Applications* (pp. 229-237). Springfield, IL: Thomas.

BEUNEN, G., Ostyn, M., Renson, R., Simons, J., Swalus, P., & VanGerven, D. (1974). Skeletal maturation and physical fitness of 12 to 15 year old boys. *Acta Paediatrica Belgica*, **28** (Supplement), 221-232.

BOUCKAERT, J., Van Uytvanck, P., & Vrijens, J. (1974). Anthropometrical data, muscle strength, physiological and selected motor ability factors of 11 year old boys. *Acta Paediatrica Belgica,* **28** (Supplement), 60-67.

BOVEND'EERT, J.H.F., Bernink, M.S.E., Van Hyfte, T., Ritmeester, J.W., Kemper, H.C.G., & Verschuur, R. (1980). *De Moper Fitness Test.* Haarlem: De Vriesebach.

FISHER, D. (1975). Zur Entwicklung biomechanischer Untersuchungsmethoden der Bewegungsanalyse des Laufer (The development of biomechanical methods for investigations of runners). *Sportarzt und Sportmedizin,* **26**, 11.

HEBBELINCK, M., & Borms, J. (1978). *Körperliches Wachstum und Leistungsfähigkeit bei Schulkindern (Bodily growth and performance capabilities of school children).* Leipzig: Barth.

HOLLMANN, W., & Bouchard, C. (1970). Untersuchungen über die Beziehungen zwischen chronologischem und biologischem Alter zu Spirometrischem Messgröszen, Herzvolumen, anthropometrischem Daten und skeletmuskelkraft bei 8-18 jährigen Jungen (Investigation of the relationship between chronological and biological age to large spirometric measures, heat volume, anthropometric data and skeletal muscle strength in 8- to 18-year-old youth). *Z. Kreislaufforschung,* **59**, 170-176.

KUSNECOVA, S. (1974). Zur Dynamik von körperlicher und Sportlicher Leistungsentwicklung im Schulalter (The dynamics of bodily and sport performance development during school ages). *Theorie und Praxis der Körperkultur,* **23**, Beiheft 1.

MAES, M. (1978). Het lichamelijk prestatievermogen bij jongens en meisjes in de prepuberteit. Unpublished doctoral dissertation, HILO, University of Ghent.

PARIZKOVA, J. (1977). *Body fat and physical fitness.* The Hague: Nyhoff.

TANNER, J.M., Whitehouse, R.H., Marshall, W.A., Healy, M.J.R., & Goldstein, H. (1975). *Assessment of skeletal maturity and prediction of adult height (TW 2 method).* London: Academic Press.

VRIJENS, J. (1978). Muscle strength development in the pre- and post-pubescent age. *Medicine and Sport,* **11**, 152-158.

Body Composition, Strength, and Motor Performance in Undernourished Boys

Robert M. Malina and Bertis B. Little
University of Texas, Austin, Texas, U.S.A.

Studies of well-nourished children indicate a significant effect of lean body mass and body fat on physical performance which is independent of the influences of stature and body weight (Boileau & Lohman, 1977; Malina, 1975). Chronic undernutrition is associated with reduced body size and changes in body composition (Barac-Nieto, Spurr, Lotero, & Maksud, 1978; Cheek, Habicht, Berall, & Holt, 1977; Metcoff, 1967; Spurr, Barac-Nieto, & Maksud, 1978; Viteri, 1971; Waterlow, Cravioto, & Stephen, 1960). The relationships of body composition and physical performance may thus be altered in chronically undernourished individuals. This question is considered in a sample of school-age boys who were born and raised, and who currently live under conditions of chronic mild-to-moderate undernutrition. School-age children in communities with chronic malnutrition can be viewed as somewhat special. They are the survivors of an early childhood characterized by intense nutritional and infectious disease stress, which takes a significant toll in the preschool population.

Methods

In 1978, the growth, strength, and motor performance of school children, 6 through 15 years of age, in a rural Zapotec-speaking community in the Valley of Oaxaca in southern Mexico were surveyed (Malina, Selby, Buschang, & Aronson, 1980). It was a subsistence agricultural village with about 1,700 inhabitants in 1978. Lifestyle in the community was typical of traditional middle-American communities: that is, largely endogamous, and small farmers working tiny plots of individually owned land. The village did not have a doctor.

The nutritional status of the community was at best marginal. Estimated caloric, protein, vitamin, and mineral intakes (Amdurer, 1978) were considerably lower than recommended levels for Mexico (Hernandez, Chávez, & Bourges, 1974). The marginal nutritional status was reflected in high crude death rates and especially high infant mortality, estimated at 152/1000 live births in the 1970s. This rate was about three times that for all of Mexico. The marginal nutritional circumstances were also reflected in the statures and weights of school children who were small relative to reference data for Mexico (Ramos-Galván, 1975). Furthermore, there was no change in the growth status of the school population from 1968 to 1978 (Malina, Selby, Buschang, & Aronson, 1980), and evidence from adult stature and the age of menarche indicated virtually no secular change in size and sexual maturity of individuals from Zapotec-speaking communities in the Valley of Oaxaca over the past 80 years or so (Malina, Selby, Buschang, Aronson, & Wilkinson, 1983). These conditions were apparently representative of the relatively poor nutritional status which characterized the rural south of Mexico, including the state of Oaxaca (Pérez Hidalgo, Chávez, & Madrigal, 1970, 1973).

The sample included 126 boys, 9 through 15 years of age. However, 89% of the sample were 9 through 12 years of age. The measures of strength (right and left grip) were taken with a Stoelting adjustable dynamometer. Measures of motor performance included a 35-yard dash, the standing long jump, and the softball throw for distance. These items were selected because of their suitability for field research conditions and the availability of comparable data for well-nourished children. Within day reliabilities, calculated on the basis of the first versus second trial and the best versus the second best trial, yielded generally acceptable levels of reliability for comparable age groups and test methods.

The age range of the sample was limited by that of the sample used to develop an equation for the prediction of body density. Given the population or sample specific nature of body composition prediction equations, and possible ethnic or racial variation, an equation was developed for the prediction of body density in a sample of 95 lower socioeconomic status Mexican-American boys, 9 through 14 years of age (Zavaleta & Malina, 1982). Measurement procedures and technical errors of measurement were comparable in both studies. The latter were smaller than those in the United States Health Examination Survey (Johnston, Hamill, & Lemeshow, 1972). The equation included age and four skinfolds and was as follows:

$$\text{Density (gm/cc)} = 1.0882 - .0012 \text{ Triceps} - .0005 \text{ Suprailiac} - .0011 \text{ Midaxillary} - .0003 \text{ Age} + .0004 \text{ Subscapular},$$

where $R = .69$, $R^2 = .47$, and $SEE = .0092$. The standard error of estimate was within the range of those reported for preadolescent and adolescent boys, .0075 to .0100 gm/cc (Lohman, 1981).

The average of two estimates of percentage body fat for each boy, using the formulae of Siri (1956) and Brožek, Grande, Anderson, & Keys (1963), was used to estimate relative fatness as in the study of Mexican-American boys. Relative fatness was also used to estimate lean body mass (LBM) and fat mass in kilograms for each boy. Correlation and stepwise regression procedures were used in the analysis.

Results

Descriptive statistics for the stature, weight, skinfolds, body composition, and physical performance of Zapotec boys are shown in Table 1. The available comparative data for Mexican-American boys are also included in the table. Zapotec boys, as expected because of their marginal nutritional status, have absolutely less lean body mass, fat mass, and strength, reflecting their smaller body size. However, they also have slight-

Table 1

Comparison of Anthropometric, Body Composition, and Performance Characteristics of Zapotec and Mexican-American Boys

Variable	Zapotec (n = 126) M	SD	Mexican-American[a] (n = 95) M	SD
Age (yrs)	10.9	1.5	11.9	1.8
Stature (cm)	128.5	8.6	141.0	11.3
Weight (kg)	27.6	5.4	36.0	9.0
Skinfolds:				
Triceps (mm)	6.7	1.6	8.4	3.2
Subscapular (mm)	5.2	0.9	7.3	2.7
Midaxillary (mm)	3.9	0.8	6.3	3.1
Suprailiac (mm)	5.9	1.8	8.1	4.8
Density (gm/cc)	1.072	0.003	1.067	0.012
Fat (%)	12.1	1.3	14.1	5.2
LBM (kg)	24.3	4.5	30.7	7.2
FM (kg)	3.3	0.9	5.3	2.9
Right grip (kg)	15.8	3.8	22.5	6.9
Left grip (kg)	15.0	4.3		
Dash (sec)	6.7	0.4		
Jump (cm)	124.0	14.5		
Throw (m)	24.3	6.4		

[a]Adapted from Zavaleta & Malina (1982).

ly less strength (right grip) per unit body weight (0.57 kg/kg) and per unit lean body mass (0.65 kg/kg) than the better nourished Mexican-American boys (0.63 kg/kg and 0.73 kg/kg, respectively). The motor performance of Zapotecs was also less than that of better nourished children.

Zero-order correlations between age, body composition, and physical performance are shown in Table 2. All correlations were significant except those between percentage body fat and the dash and jump. Given the significant relationship between age and performance, first-order partial correlations between body composition and performance, controlling for the effects of age, are shown in Table 3. These correlations were considerably lower than the zero-order correlations. Lean body mass, fat mass, and percentage body fat were significantly related to grip strength, while lean body mass and fat mass were significantly related to the distance throw. Only lean body mass was related to the jump, while none of the body composition estimates were related to the dash after the effects of age were statistically controlled.

Stepwise regression was used to further examine the relationship between body composition and performance. Regressions of age and absolute body composition on performance and of age and relative body composition on performance were done separately. Variables were entered into the regression in a free-weighted order; that is, the variable accounting for the most variance was entered first. Addition of subsequent

Table 2

Zero-Order Correlations Between Age, Estimated Body Composition, and Performance in Zapotec Boys

	Age	Lean Body Mass	Fat Mass	Percentage Fat
Right grip	.74	.80	.74	.35
Left grip	.75	.83	.76	.32
Dash[a]	.53	.50	.36	(.04)
Jump	.61	.64	.49	(.07)
Throw	.74	.83	.72	.26

Note. Correlations in parentheses are not significant ($p < .05$).
[a]Signs of all correlations for the dash were inverted because a lower time reflects a better performance.

Table 3

First-Order Correlations Between Estimated Body Composition and Performance in Zapotec Boys, Controlling for the Effects of Age

	Lean Body Mass	Fat Mass	Percentage Fat
Right grip	.49	.44	.22
Left grip	.58	.47	.17
Dash[a]	(.12)	(−.04)	(.14)
Jump	.32	(.08)	(−.13)
Throw	.58	.40	(.09)

Note. Correlations in parentheses are not significant ($p < .05$).
[a]Signs of all correlations for the dash were inverted because a lower time reflects a better performance.

variables depended on their ability to account for a significant amount of the outstanding variance.

Results of the regression analysis are summarized in Table 4. Absolute lean body mass and age contributed significantly to the prediction of performance in all five items. Fat mass contributed significantly and negatively only to running and jumping performance. In contrast, when age and relative body composition were regressed on performance, age was the more important predictor. Percentage lean body mass contributed significantly only to right grip strength, but the beta was negative.

Table 4

Unstandardized Beta Coefficients for the Regression of Estimated Body Composition and Age on Performance of Zapotec Boys

A. Absolute Body Composition

Performance Variable	Lean Body Mass	Age	Fat Mass	Constant (Intercept)	R	R²
Right grip	.36	.68	(.62)	−2.54	.81	.66
Left grip	.58	.61	(.19)	−6.46	.84	.70
Dash[a]	.048	.097	−.176	−8.298	.57	.32
Jump	2.72	2.25	−7.22	57.80	.69	.47
Throw	1.09	0.81	(−.89)	−8.00	.83	.70

B. Relative Body Composition

Performance Variable	Percentage Lean Body Mass	Age	Constant (Intercept)	R	R²
Right grip	−45.14	1.71	36.91	.75	.56
Left grip	(−36.73)	2.00	25.50	.75	.56
Dash[a]	(3.72)	0.15	−11.54	.54	.29
Jump	(125.31)	6.02	−51.77	.61	.38
Throw	(−22.72)	2.99	11.73	.73	.54

Note. Coefficients in parentheses are not significant ($p < .05$).
[a]Signs of the coefficients for the dash were inverted because a lower time reflects a better performance.

Discussion

Changes in body composition wth a moderate degree of malnutrition are primarily related to a reduction in lean body mass, primarily muscle mass (Barac-Nieto, Spurr, Latero, & Maksud, 1978). The reduced lean body mass in Zapotec boys was probably the result of the cumulative effects of daily nutritional deficiencies. Muscle tissue is the major component of lean body mass. It is comprised largely of protein, and a daily deficiency in protein intake would likely limit the growth of this primary tissue component of lean body mass. Estimated intakes of calories and proteins among school children 6 to 14 years of age in the Zapotec community were approximately only 58% and 63%, respectively, of the daily recommended intakes for Mexico (Amdurer, 1978).

Relationships between absolute body composition and physical performance of Zapotec boys were generally similar to those for well-nourished boys. Ismail, Christian, and Kessler (1963), for example, reported correlations of .56, .57, and .63 between absolute lean body mass and the 50-yard dash (sign inverted as indicated in Table 2), the standing long jump, and the ball throw for distance, respectively, in 81 boys, 10 through 12 years of age. Slaughter, Lohman, and Misner (1977) reported correlations of .57 and .65 between absolute lean body mass and the 50-yard dash (sign inverted) and standing long jump, respectively, in 68 boys, 7 through 12 years of age. The correlations for absolute lean body mass in these two studies were virtually identical for those observed in undernourished Zapotec boys, .50, .64, and .83 for the dash, jump, and throw, respectively (see Table 2).

In contrast, relationships between relative body composition and performance were different in Zapotec boys compared to well-nourished boys. Percentage body fat was positively related to grip strength in Zapotec boys but was not related to running and jumping performance (see Tables 2 and 3). Among well-nourished boys, relative fatness exerts a negative influence, especially on events requiring the displacement of body weight. Slaughter, Lohman, and Misner (1977), for example, reported correlations of .37 for the dash; that is, a high percentage of fat was related to high times or poorer performances, and −.44 for the jump in boys 7 through 12 years of age. Because relative fatness is the inverse of relative lean body mass, the correlations reported by Ismail, Christian, and Kessler (1963) indicate the same relationships. Correlations between percentage body fat and the dash, jump, and throw were, respectively, .55, −.44, and −.16 in boys 10 through 12 years of age.

Results of the regression analysis were consistent with the correlational studies. The beta coefficients for absolute lean body mass were significant and positive for all performance items (see Table 4). The coefficients for absolute fat mass were significant and negative for the dash and jump, thus emphasizing the negative influence of fatness on performances involving the displacement of the body mass even in undernourished boys. This was in contrast to the lack of significant effects of relative fatness on such performances.

The results suggested that a higher percentage of body fat is indicative of relatively better nutritional status in undernourished boys from this subsistence agricultural community. Estimated absolute and relative fatness were related to an absolutely larger lean body mass ($r = .90$ and $.37$, respectively, $p \leq .01$) in these boys. Thus, relative fatness is an indication of a larger lean body mass and is a good predictor of static strength in undernourished samples. This influence is consistent with the negative beta coefficients observed for relative lean body mass in the regression analysis (see Table 4). However, relative fatness does not contribute significantly to predicting motor performance.

Absolute lean body mass was positively related to static strength in undernourished (see Tables 2 and 3) and well-nourished boys (Malina, 1975). The correlation between grip strength and lean body mass in Zapotec boys ($r = .74$) was, however, slightly lower than that observed in better-nourished Mexican-American boys ($r = .91$, Zavaleta & Malina, 1982) and Anglo boys ($r = .91$, Forbes, 1965) of a similar age. Chronic protein-energy undernutrition is associated with reduced muscle fiber size and energy metabolism (Malina, 1978), and such changes may underlie the reduced correlation between lean body mass and grip strength in mild-to-moderately undernourished Zapotec boys.

Conclusion

Changes in body composition under conditions of mild-to-moderate undernutrition do not alter the relationship between lean body mass and performance compared to well-nourished children. However, relationships between fatness and performance are changed. The lack of an influence of relative fatness on performances involving the displacement of body mass in these moderately undernourished boys may be suggestive of a threshold level above which an excessive percentage of fatness exerts a negative influence on performance.

Acknowledgments

This research was supported in part by the Institute of Latin American Studies of the University of Texas at Austin, by National Science Foundation grant BNS 78-10642, and by funds granted to the Institute of Latin American Studies by the Andrew W. Mellon Foundation.

References

AMDURER, L.R.K. (1978). Nutrition in a Zapotec-speaking rural community, Oaxaca, Mexico. Unpublished master's thesis, University of Texas, Austin.

BARAC-NIETO, M., Spurr, G.B., Lotero, G.B., & Maksud, M.G. (1978). Body composition in chronic undernutrition. *American Journal of Clinical Nutrition, 31*, 23-40.

BOILEAU, R.A., & Lohman, T.G. (1977). The measurement of human physique and its effect on physical performance. *Orthopedic Clinics of North America, 8*, 563-581.

BROŽEK, J., Grande, F., Anderson, J.T., & Keys, A. (1963). Densitometric analysis of body composition: Revision of some quantitative assumptions. *Annals of the New York Academy of Sciences, 110*, 113-140.

CHEEK, D.B., Habicht, J.-P., Berall, J., & Holt, A.B. (1977). Protein-calorie malnutrition and the significance of cell mass relative to body length. *American Journal of Clinical Nutrition, 30*, 851-860.

FORBES, G.B. (1965). Toward a new dimension in human growth. *Pediatrics, 36*, 825-835.

HERNANDEZ, M., Chávez, A., & Bourges, H. (1974). Valor nutritivo de los alimentos Mexicanos. Tablas de uso practico (Nutrient value of Mexican foods: Tables for practical use) (6th ed.). Mexico: Instituto Nacional de la Nutricion, Publicacion L-12.

ISMAIL, A.H., Christian, J.E., & Kessler, W.V. (1963). Body composition relative to motor aptitude for preadolescent boys. *Research Quarterly, 34*, 462-470.

JOHNSTON, F.E., Hamill, P.V.V., & Lemeshow, S. (1972). Skinfold thickness of children 6 to 11 years, United States. *Vital and Health Statistics*, Series 11, No. 120.

LOHMAN, T.G. (1981). Skinfolds and body density and their relation to body fatness: A review. *Human Biology, 53*, 181-225.

MALINA, R.M. (1975). Anthropometric correlates of strength and motor performance. *Exercise and Sport Sciences Reviews, 3*, 249-274.

MALINA, R.M. (1978). Growth of muscle tissue and muscle mass. In F. Falkner & J.M. Tanner (Eds.), *Human growth. Volume 2. Postnatal growth* (pp. 273-294). New York: Plenum.

MALINA, R.M., Selby, H.A., Buschang, P.H., & Aronson, W.L. (1980). Growth status of schoolchildren in a rural Zapotec community in the Valley of Oaxaca, Mexico, in 1968 and 1978. *Annals of Human Biology, 7*, 367-374.

MALINA, R.M., Selby, H.A., Buschang, P.H., Aronson, W.L., & Wilkinson, R.G. (1983). Adult stature and age at menarche in Zapotec-speaking communities in the Valley of Oaxaca, Mexico, in a secular perspective. *American Journal of Physical Anthropology,* **60**, 437-449.

METCOFF, J. (1967). Biochemical effects of protein-calorie malnutrition in man. *Annual Review of Medicine,* **18**, 377-422.

PÉREZ HIDALGO, C., Chávez, A., & Madrigal, H. (1970). Recopilación sobre el consumo de nutrientes en diferentes zonas de México. I. Consumo calórico-proteico (Comparison of the consumption of nutrients in different zones of Mexico. I. Consumption of calories and proteins). *Archivos Latinoamericanos de Nutricion,* **20**, 367-381.

PÉREZ HIDALGO, C., Chávez, A., & Madrigal, N.S.P.H. (1973). Recopilación sobre el consumo de nutrientes en diferentes zonas de México. II. Consumo de vitaminas y minerales (Comparison of the consumption of nutrients in different zones of Mexico: I. Consumption of vitamins and minerals). *Archivos Latinoamericanos de Nutricion,* **23**, 293-304.

RAMOS-GALVÁN, R. (1975). Somatometria pediatrica estudio semilongitudinal en niños de la ciudad de México (A mixed longitudinal study of pediatric somatometry in children of Mexico City). *Archivos Investigación Medica,* **6** (supplement 1), 83-396.

SIRI, W.E. (1956). The gross composition of the body. *Advances in Biological and Medical Physics,* **4**, 239-280.

SLAUGHTER, M.H., Lohman, T.G., & Misner, J.E. (1977). Relationship of somatotype and body composition to physical performance in 7- to 12-year-old boys. *Research Quarterly,* **48**, 159-168.

SPURR, G.B., Barac-Nieto, M., & Maksud, M.G. (1978). Childhood undernutrition: Implications for adult work capacity and productivity. In L.J. Folinsbee, J.A. Wagner, J.F. Borgia, B.L. Drinkwater, J.A. Gliner, & J.F. Bedi (Eds.), *Environmental stress: Individual human adaptations* (pp. 165-181). New York: Academic Press.

VITERI, F.E. (1971). Considerations on the effect of nutrition on the body composition and physical working capacity of young Guatemalan adults. In N.S. Scrimshaw & A.M. Altschul (Eds.), *Amino acid fortification of protein foods* (pp. 350-375). Cambridge, MA: MIT Press.

WATERLOW, J.C., Cravioto, J., & Stephen, J.M. (1960). Protein malnutrition in man. *Advances in Protein Chemistry,* **15**, 131-238.

ZAVALETA, A.N., & Malina, R.M. (1982). Growth and body composition of Mexican-American boys 9 through 14 years of age. *American Journal of Physical Anthropology,* **57**, 261-271.

Somatotype and Motor Function Changes in Children

Ivan Szmodis, Tamas Szabo, Zsuzsa Temesi, and Maria Rendi
Központi Sportiskola
Budapest, Hungary

Information is scarce on body size and proportional development, and on the functional and motor characteristics of children attending the lower form of primary school in Hungary. This period of a child's life is generally recognized to be the one in which a foundation should be established for the development of motor skills.

The main objective of this study was to follow the progress of development of this group of children by a longitudinal series of measurements. Another aspect of interest was to gain procedural experience with certain motor ability tests at this age.

Material and Methods

Children in the first grades of physical education classes in six schools in Budapest were observed begining in the second semester of the 1977 academic year. Measurements were repeated every half for a total of seven measurement sessions. The last session occurred during the second semester of 1980 when the children, finishing the fourth grade, prepared to enter the upper form of primary school. At this time, the children were to choose their preferred sport and to undergo regular training.

Of the initial sample of 97 girls and 64 boys (school classes were included as observational units), the records were complete for 59 girls and 38 boys.

Body dimensions were measured conforming to IBP recommendations (Weiner & Lourie, 1969) by the research group. Of the 27 total dimensions obtained, the present article provides data on the stature, body mass, components of the Heath-Carter anthropometric somatotype (Carter, 1975), and the indices of the Conrad growth type (Conrad, 1963). The ages of the subjects were expressed in decimal years and children were grouped in age intervals of full years $\pm$ 0.50 year. This corresponded roughly to the mean age of each grade of school.

Of the 14-test battery, 11 scores were taken by the physical education teachers and 3 (bilateral hand and foot tapping, and 12-min run-walk) scores were taken by the research group. Of these measures, performances in the 2 $\times$ 15 m shuttle run, ball-dribble run (5 obstacles, total distance about 30 m), and 12-min run-walk distance are discussed in this article.

Data on physique and performance were averaged over the schools and plotted against age to obtain developmental curves of the means for both sexes separately.

Results and Discussion

Somatotype components and Conrad indices found for the respective half years are presented in Table 1. Developmental curves for body mass and stature are shown in Figure 1, and for the dribble skill, shuttle run, and 12-min run-walk in Figures 2 through 4, respectively.

In comparison with a recent representative study of body size in Hungary (Mészáros & Mohácsi, 1983) both the boys and the girls of the physical education classes were slightly taller and heavier by an amount corresponding to about a half year's growth. Despite the fact that they retained this difference from healthy urban school-child population until the end of observation, large within-group variance did not warrant a conclusion that they differed significantly from their peers. The development of stature as well as of body mass was almost completely linear in both sexes (see Figure 1). Developmental curves for the boys and the girls coincided very closely during the years of investigation.

Hungary is one of several countries where a growing number of schools have special classes for children, talented in motor abilities and skills, who get expert, and somewhat concentrated education in physical activity and sports. In these schools physical education instruction is given by teachers who are better qualified than those in the lower primary school, and more physical education and sports classes per week are provided as well.

Table 1

Changes in the Physical Indices for Boys (B) and Girls (G)

Age (years)		Endo-morphy B	G	Meso-morphy B	G	Ecto-morphy B	G	Metric i. B	G	Plastic i. B	G
7.0	M	2.29	2.94	4.49	4.05	2.77	2.94	−1.06	−1.74	59.8	58.6
	s	1.62	1.06	0.80	1.05	1.01	0.93	0.21	0.22	3.5	2.7
7.5	M	2.79	3.41	4.49	3.96	3.01	3.23	−1.06	−1.75	62.4	61.1
	s	1.71	1.09	0.76	0.69	1.10	0.96	0.24	0.21	3.7	2.8
8.0	M	3.03	3.88	4.44	3.90	3.19	3.28	−1.02	−1.66	64.0	62.7
	s	1.81	1.23	0.73	0.65	1.13	0.89	0.27	0.23	3.6	2.9
8.5	M	3.01	3.96	4.33	3.73	3.25	3.37	−1.01	−1.68	64.6	63.5
	s	1.81	1.30	0.83	0.72	1.07	1.00	0.28	0.24	3.8	3.0
9.0	M	2.33	3.23	4.31	3.70	3.51	3.71	−1.10	−1.74	66.4	64.9
	s	1.55	1.23	0.86	0.88	1.14	1.14	0.29	0.25	4.0	3.0
9.5	M	3.21	3.73	4.34	3.82	3.49	3.61	−1.12	−1.68	68.1	67.0
	s	1.98	1.46	0.89	0.80	1.25	1.10	0.30	0.28	4.2	3.4
10.0	M	3.03	3.80	4.42	3.72	3.51	3.73	−1.11	−1.65	69.2	68.4
	s	2.02	1.51	0.92	1.62	1.30	1.06	0.32	0.28	4.3	3.7

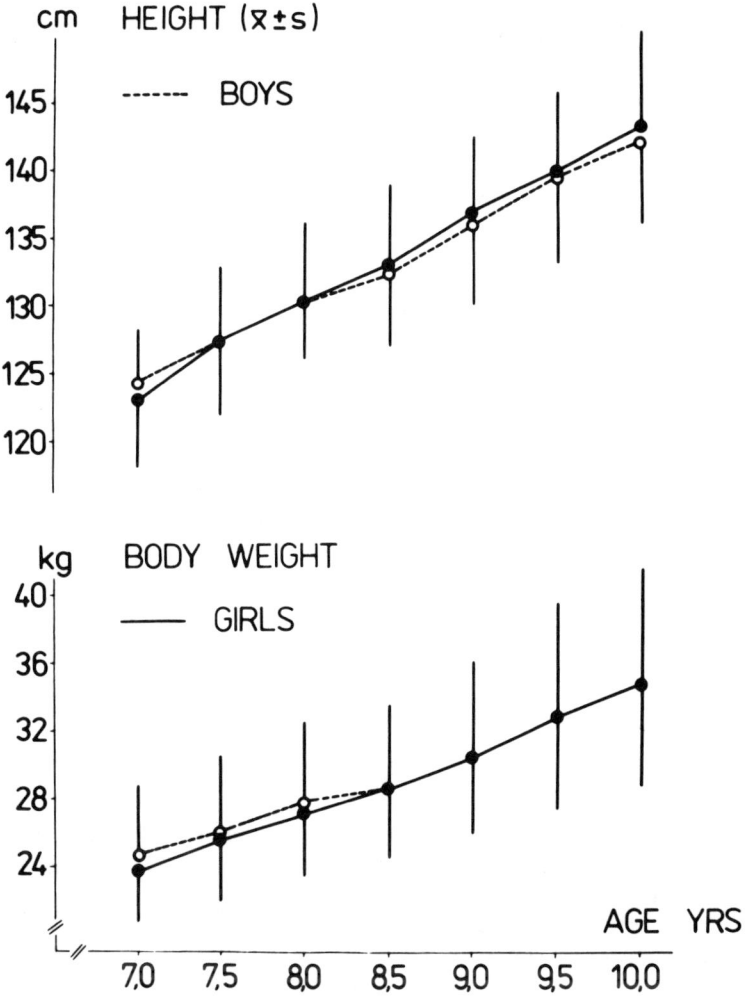

Figure 1—Developmental curves for stature and body mass, means, and standard deviations. Open circles denote boys; full circles denote girls.

The need persists to find children displaying signs of motor talent and showing under careful training fast motor development in the later years with the promise of achieving national and/or international levels of sports competition. However, in recruiting would-be pupils from regional kindergartens to these special physical education classes, it was suspected that the physical education teachers might be biased and select early developers. The obtained data did not support this suspicion, however, because the subjects did not differ statistically from the average urban population. On the other hand, this slightly advanced general development and growth status appeared a satisfactory basis on which to build.

Around 9 years of age, the first component of somatotype (endomorphy) showed a decrease of body fat in both sexes (see Table 1). At this age, body mass continued

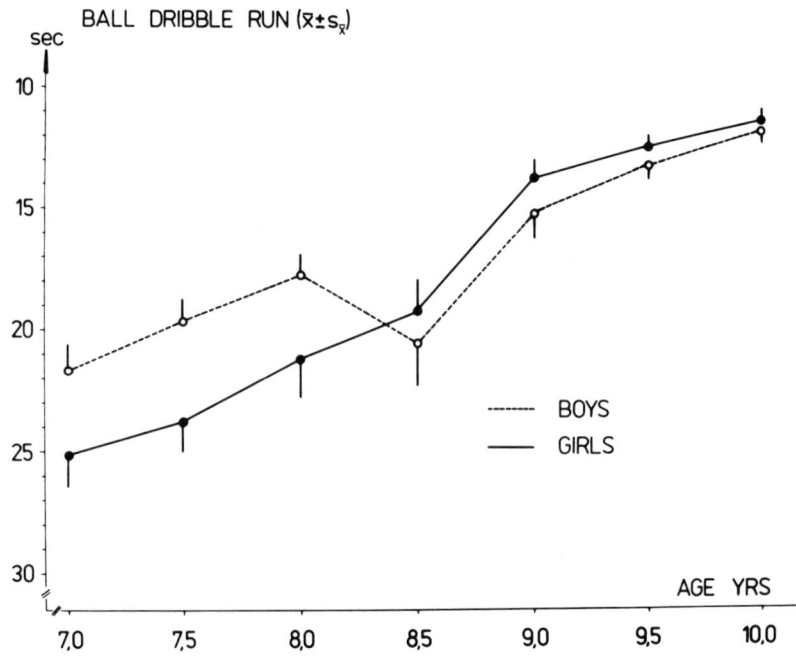

Figure 2—Performance in the ball-dribble run, means and standard errors. Symbols as in Figure 1.

its steady increase, and the lower score in endomorphy seemed to represent a gain in active muscle tissue. This assumption could not be supported by analyzing the second (mesomorphy) component. Instead, it was the third component (ectomorphy) that showed higher scores at this time. Accordingly, this observation was regarded as representing a transitory change in body proportions as well as in body composition in the sample. The observation is in contrast with a diagram of Parízková (1973) in which body fat was shown to decrease between 10 and 11 years of age. As control classes were not investigated in the present study, further research is necessary before a conclusion can be drawn.

Mesomorphy changed very little in the boys and in the girls decreased slightly, but rather steadily. When plotted on a somatochart, both the boys and the girls resided in the region of balanced mesomorphy. The girls were within the central hexagon and the boys a little above it. Ectomorphy scores gradually increased each year. Variability in the somatotype components was large, mostly exceeding one unit, in the first and third components.

As a whole, the group means of somatotype for the respective ages changed very little. Intragroup variability, however, evidenced considerable heterogeneity in the sample, which was also reflected by the large standard deviations of stature and body mass.

The means for Conrad's metric index substantiated again that these children belonged to the normal population (Mészáros, Szmodis, Mohácsi, & Frenkl, 1981). Growth trends were as usual, leptomorphy slightly increasing with age in the boys and remaining higher in the girls during the period of study. Conrad's plastic index proved its value in demonstrating subtle changes in growth tempo that were less apparent from the mean curves of either body size or somatotype. When used in the extended Conrad somatoplot, this feature of the plastic index (Szmodis, Mészáros, & Szabo, 1976) in certain respects resembles the rate of growth diagrams, but is superior to those by allowing proportional conclusions as well.

As expected, motor performance of the boys was slightly better than that of the girls at all ages. It was a surprise to note, therefore, that the curve for ball dribbling (see Figure 2) showed a cross-over between 8 and 8.5 years of age. Even when the scores at 8.5 years were disregarded and the overall trend only was considered, the boys showed a slower rate of improvement in this respect. This stands in sharp contrast to performance in the 2 × 15 m shuttle run in which the boys were consistently better (see Figure 3).

Performance in the 12-min run-walk was another unexpected finding (see Figure 4). These performances improved very little during the observation period; improvement in 3½ years hardly exceeded intraindividual variability, interindividual variation was considerable, as well. Despite the fact that endurance training was not emphasized either in the ordinary or the special classes of the lower form of general school, it was assumed beforehand that a higher rate of progress in this performance would exist.

The question of whether the ability tests administered were suitable for this age group was a point of special interest in the study. It could be said that these three tests were useful and did not raise methodological problems. Though not reported here, it should be mentioned that of the ability tests employed in this study, the ones requiring arm strength or a combination of strength and skill proved inadequate for this age group.

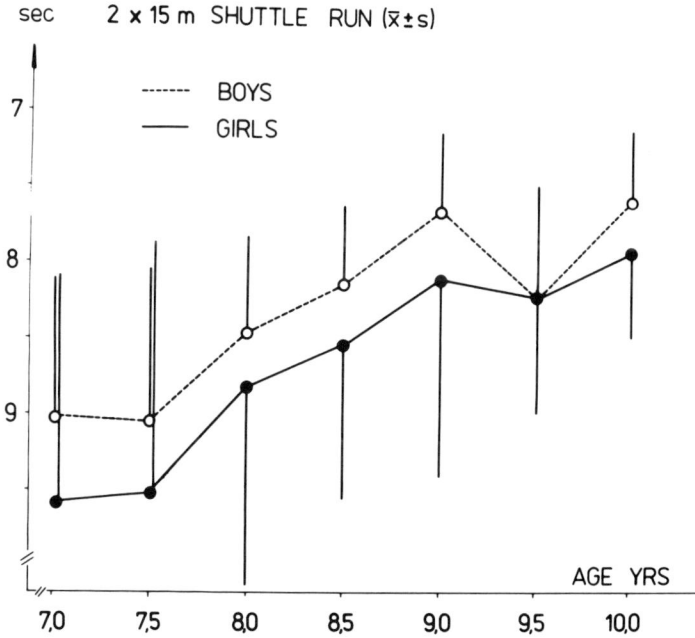

Figure 3—Performance in the 2 × 15 m shuttle run. Symbols as in Figure 1.

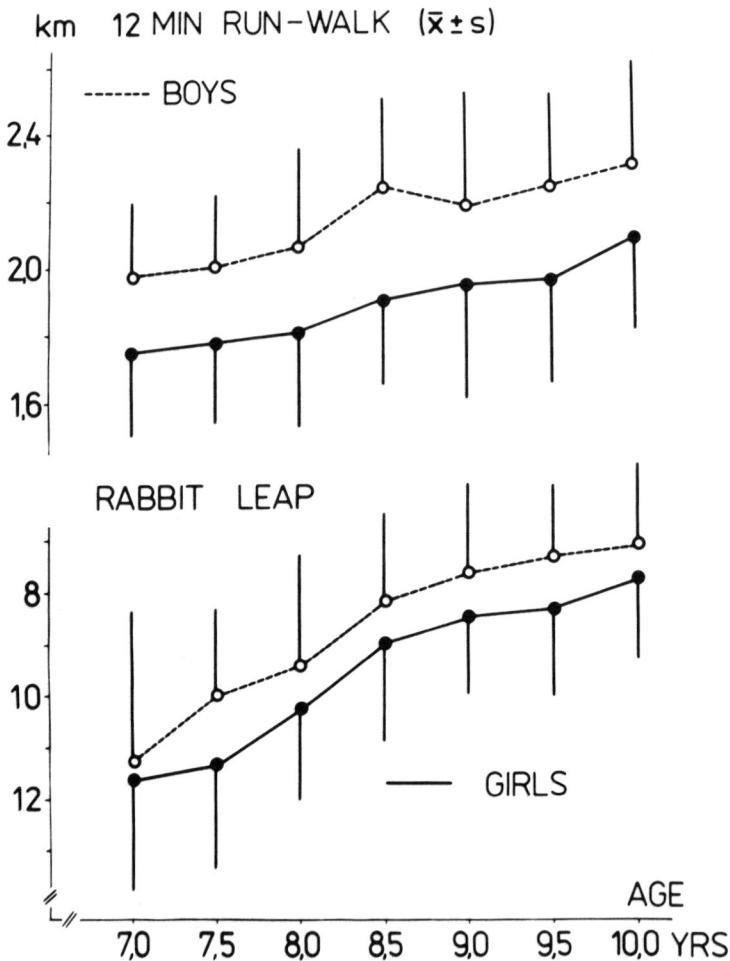

Figure 4—Performance in 12-min run-walk and rabbit leap, means and standard deviations. Symbols as in Figure 1.

Thus, it may be concluded that this sample of pupils attending classes with a special physical education curriculum showed a favorable state of development at the start of the lower form of the general school; they grew and physically developed steadily during the next three years. Because sampling was restricted to only six schools and to the special classes, it would be untimely to generalize the findings. Age-dependent rate of improvement in the endurance run was moderate corresponding to healthy standards.

References

CARTER, J.E.L. (1975). *The Heath-Carter somatotype method.* San Diego: The author's publication.

CONRAD, K. (1963). *Der Konstitutionstypus*. 2. Aufl. Berlin: Springer-Verlag.

MÉSZÁROS, J., & Mohácsi, J. (1983). A biológiai fejlettség és a felnőtt testmagasság meghatározása a városi fiatalok fejlődésmenete alapján (The assessment of biological development and adult stature on the basis of the growth curves of Hungarian urban youth). Unpublished doctoral thesis, Hungarian University of Physical Education, Budapest.

MÉSZÁROS, J., Szmodis, I., Mohácsi, J., & Frenkl, R. (1981). A nemzedéki változás és a gyermekkori fejlődés kérdései az 197o-os években végzett keresztmetszoti vizsgálat alapján (Secular trend and child development in a cross-sectional study of the seventies. In Hungarian, abstract in English). *Biologia*, **29**, 163-198.

PARÍZKOVÁ, J. (1973). Body composition and exercise during growth and development. In G.L. Rarick (Ed.) *Physical activity. Human growth and development* (p. 98). New York: Academic Press.

SZMODIS, I., Mészáros, J., & Szabó, T. (1976). Alkati és müködési mutatók kapcso- lata gyermek-, serdülő- és ifjúkorban (Relationships of indices of physique and function in children, adolescents and youths. In Hungarian, abstract in English). *Testneveles es Sportegeszsegugyi Szemle*, **17**, 255-272.

WEINER, J.S., Lourie, J.A. (Eds.) (1969). *Human Biology. A guide to field methods*. IBP Handbook No. 9. Oxford: Blackwell.

The Influence of Exercise and Training on the Locomotor System of Children: A Longitudinal Study of Adolescent Tennis Players

Hans M. Sommer
University of Heidelberg
Heidelberg, Federal Republic of Germany

The demand for high-performance and top-performance training in adolescents, especially in technically very sophisticated kinds of sport, is based on the empirical knowledge that complex locomotor sequences can be learned only up to an age of 14 years. Besides a necessary sport aptitude, this demand is an important precondition for later possible top performance. However, it also entails substantial stress (in particular, mechanical stress) which cannot always be calculated with certainty on the growing postural and locomotor apparatus. Hypotheses on the functional adaptability of the locomotor apparatus were postulated in the last century by Wolff (1982) and Roux (1895). In particular, in "Theory on the Influence of Mechanical Stimuli on the Differentiation of the Supporting Tissue," Pauwels (1960) was able to provide a generally valid formulation of the causes of this functional adaptation. On the other hand, there is no prospective statement with regard to very high stress (e.g., in high-performance and top-performance sport) with regard to the functional adaptation expected (a) on the basis of existing movement sequences, and (b) in order to avoid overstress reactions.

Importantly these questions can decide whether an athlete in high-performance and top-performance sport can be brought to a peak performance without appreciable interruption by overstressing and injury pauses and whether he or she pays for his or her high-performance sport with a "sport invalidity." These questions can be posed not only for the adult, but also for the adolescent athlete. On the one hand, it can be assumed that the tissue of the growing postural and locomotor apparatus possesses better possibilities for adaptation. On the other hand, constantly changing force-load conditions due to growth must result in factors disturbing the locomotor sequence.

Materials and Method

In a multidisciplinary longitudinal investigation carried out over 5 years, a total of 50 top adolescent players, 14 girls and 36 boys of the National German Tennis Association, underwent a clinical orthopedic and radiological examination every year. The muscular and ligamentaneous stabilization and ranges of movement were examined, taking into account individual variations and pathology of the skeleton and comparing the ideal biomechanical properties of the locomotor apparatus of one side of the body with the other.

A radiological examination of the spine was conducted once in order to verify its postural situation. X-rays of both hands, forearms, and elbows were taken nearly every year. The diameters and lengths of the long bones were measured as far as possible. These data were compared with the opposite side. The densities of the bones were also estimated. Thus, relative data were used in addition to overstress reactions in the past or present to arrive at a conclusion (Eichel, 1981; Huppertz, 1982; Krahl, Sommer, & Correll, 1981).

Results

On the playing arm side, the shoulder girdle, arm, and hand displayed unequivocal adaptation reactions of the connective and supporting tissue. There was muscle hypertrophy (see Figure 1), increase of firmness of connective tissue (see Figure 2), and a thickening of the various long bones (see Figure 3). The processess of adaptation became more marked with increasing age and training duration, and always occurred on the side of the playing arm, independently of sex. The positive consequence of this adaptation was the more favorable stress on broader bones and very much better muscle and capsule ligament movement in the elbow joint and wrist compared to the opposite side. The increased development of the musculature stabilizing the shoulder joint with tendency to shortening of the pectoral muscle compared to a relatively weak rhomboid muscle had a less positive effect (see Figure 4).

A muscular disequilibrium was evident which led to restriction of movement of the shoulder joint and was a factor disturbing the back-swing movement in tennis. Avoiding movements resulted in hyperextension and supination both in the elbow joint and in the wrist. Above all, in hyperextensibility of the elbow joint on the playing arm side, the preconditions for osteochondrosis in the region of the capitulum humeri arose (e.g., in an extreme top-spin) (see Figure 5). Overstressing symptoms in the sense of a radial humoral epicondylopathy on the left side could be similarly explained by compensatory movements.

The posture and form of the spine were determined by the hypertrophy of the back musculature on the side of the playing arm and asymmetry resulting from this, irrespective of age and sex (see Figure 4). The slight C-shaped large-arch ending of the spine to the side accompanying this (see Figure 6) had no pathological value according to our experience so far. On the other hand, the imbalance of the back musculature almost generally led to poor mobility of the thoracic and lumbar spine. A shortening of the lumbar vertebral column extensor musculature (see Figures 7 & 8) with simultaneous weakness of the abdominal musculature was observed frequently. In our opinion, this low mobility only rarely occasioned overstressing reactions.

Tennis is a running sport. Special attention, therefore, must be devoted to the pelvic girdle and the lower limbs. As in the vertebral column, we also observed a relatively low mobility in the upper limbs. The hypertrophy and shortenig of the iliopsoas muscle and the adductor musculature were the cause of this. On the other hand, the gluteal

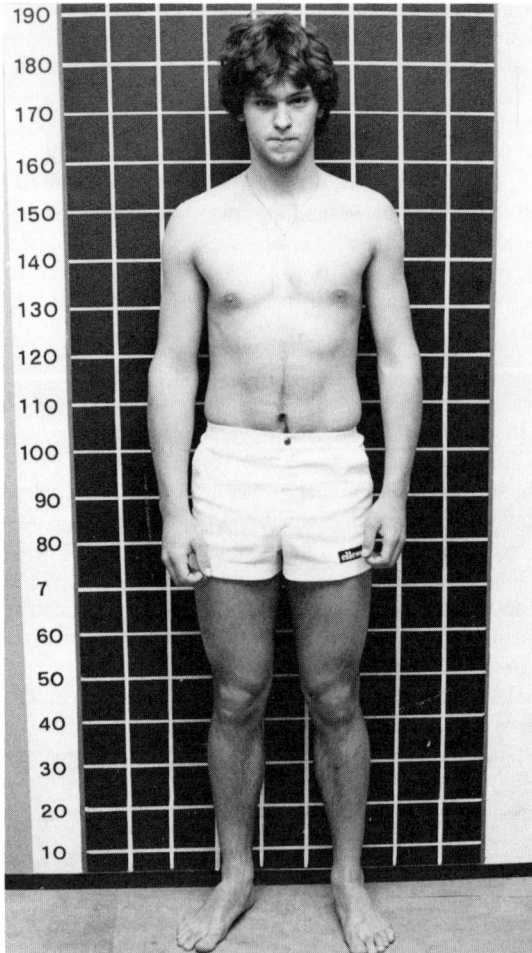

Figure 1—Right-hander with hypertrophied arm musculature on the right side.

and ischiocrural muscles were less well trained. Thus there was a ventral tilting of the pelvis and an unsatisfactory stabilization of the hip joint in splaying and rotatory movements. This in turn was a cause for a deviation of the knee joint to a valgus-internal rotation position (see Figure 7). It explains the frequent overstressing symptoms and the susceptibility of the lower limb to injuries: Insertion tendinoses were experienced in the region of the greater trochanter as the result of an unfavorable lever situation for the gluteal musculature. Insertion tendinoses of the upper leg adductor musculature resulted from the shortening tendency of these muscles. Strains of the ischiocrural muscles resulted from their relative shortening with simultaneously reduced hyperextensibility of the hip joint because of the shortening of the iliopsoas muscle.

At the knee joint, there was a muscular imbalance in favor of the vastus medialis muscle and thus to a shearing strain in the region of the femoral patellar arthrodial

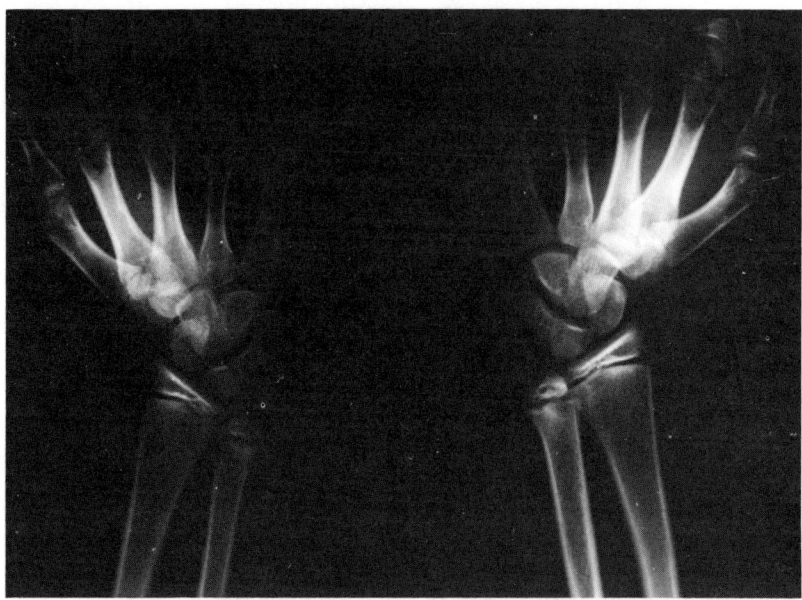

Figure 2—Left-hander with relative restriction of movement of the left wrist.

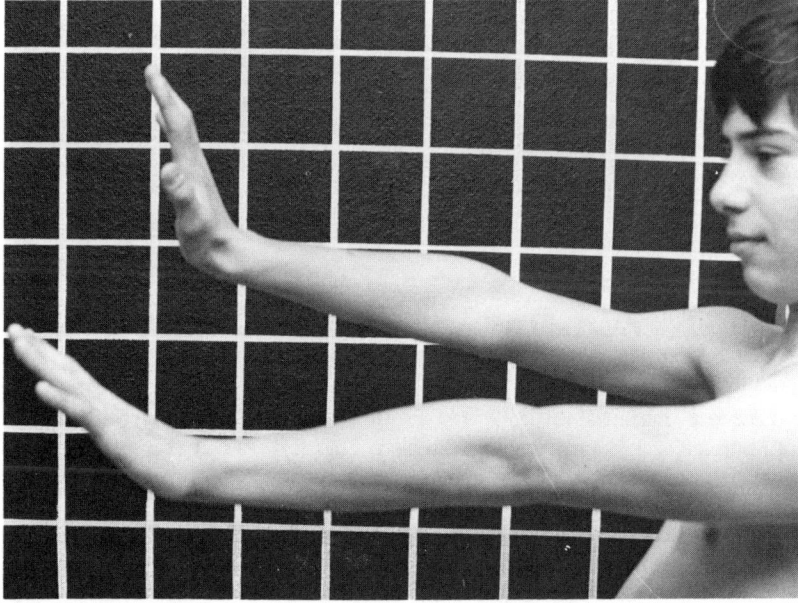

Figure 3—Right-hander with increased growth in thickness of the radius, ulna and metacarpals, above all II and III.

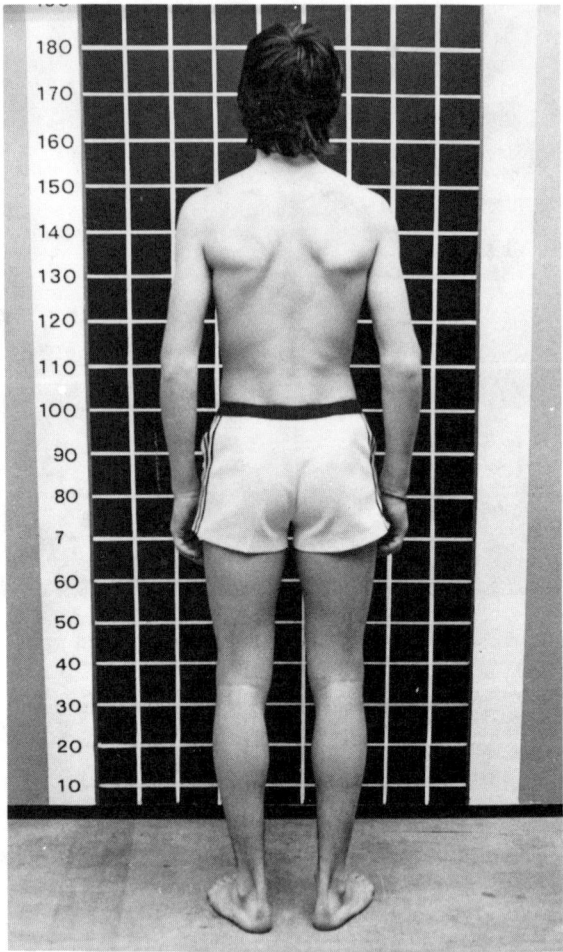

Figure 4—Back of a right-hander with an inadequate shoulder blade stabilization, strengthened back musculature on the right side, asymmetrical trapezius-rhombus.

bed due to the functional valgization (see Figure 9). Retropatellar loading pain, patellar tip syndrome, states of irritation in the region of the medial ventral capsular ligament apparatus, and compression pain in the lateral knee joint compartment resulted (see Figure 10).

A poor lateral foot stabilization favored the "functional valgus position of the knee joint" in the loading phase. If the peroneal muscles were too weak in order to ensure a plantigrade contact of the middle and forefoot region with the ground, danger of a supination distortion resulted from this slight supination (see Figure 11). In the standing phase, with flexion of the knee joint and dorsal flexion of the ankle, a fall of the longitudinal arch (because of the unfavorable action angle of the posterior tibial muscle in the supination position) with inadequate medial support of the foot was registered.

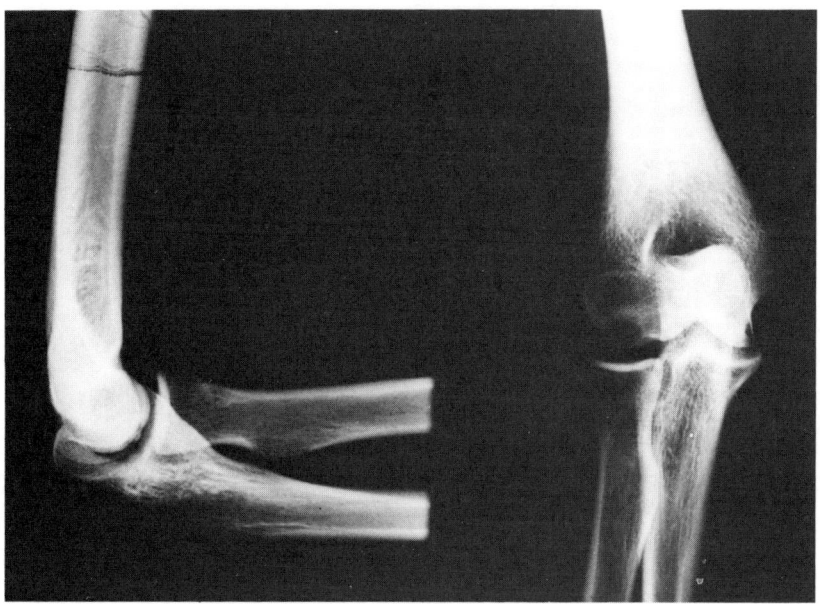

Figure 5—Right-hander with osteochondral necrosis in the region of the right head of the humerus.

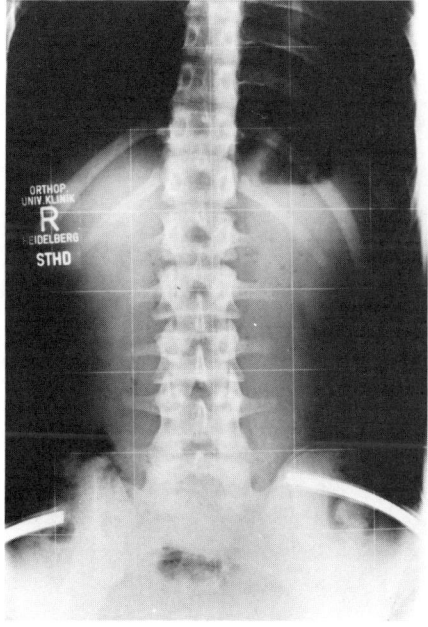

Figure 6—C-shaped right convex lateral distortion.

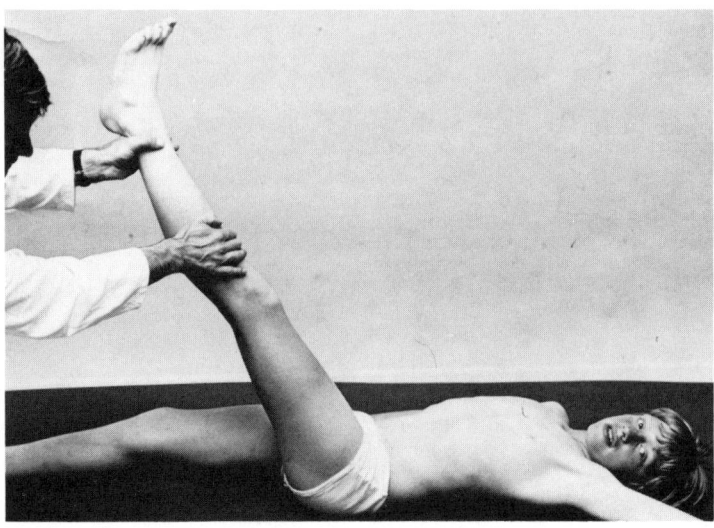

Figure 7—Pseudolasègue with shortening of the iliopsoas muscle.

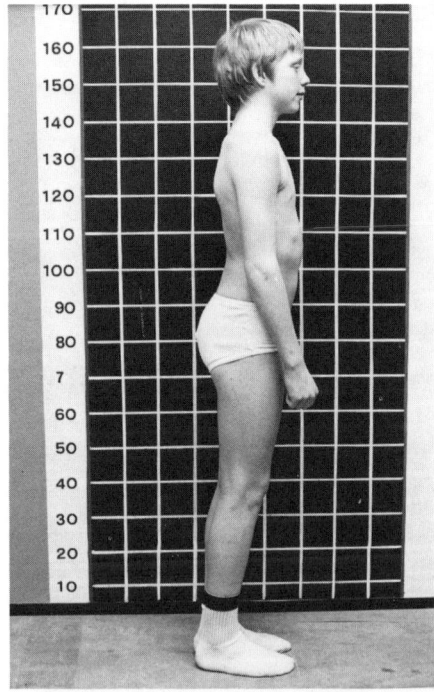

Figure 8—Hyperlordosis with ventral tilting of the pelvis in shortened iliopsoas muscle, relatively weak abdominal musculature, and buttock musculature.

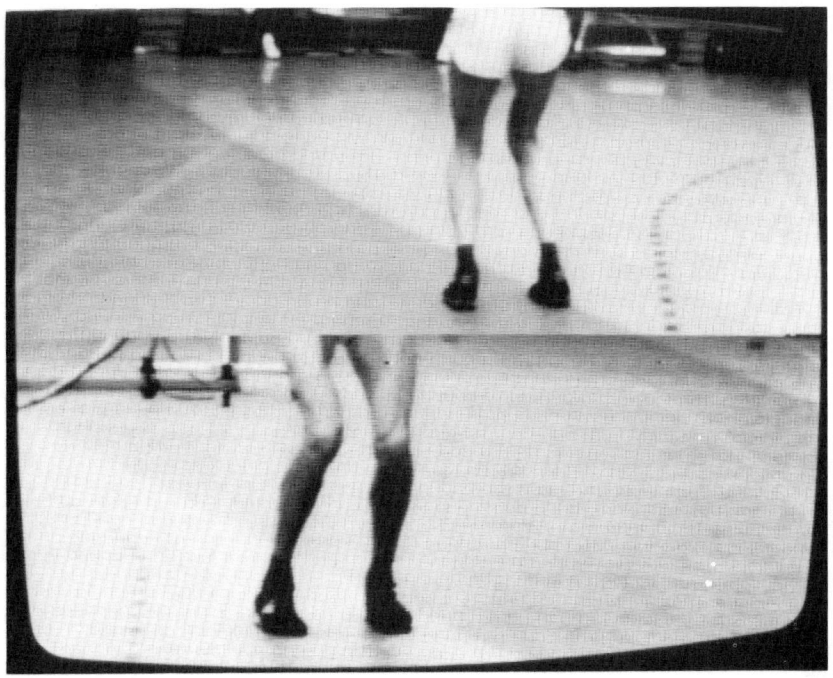

Figure 9—Phase of preparation for jump.

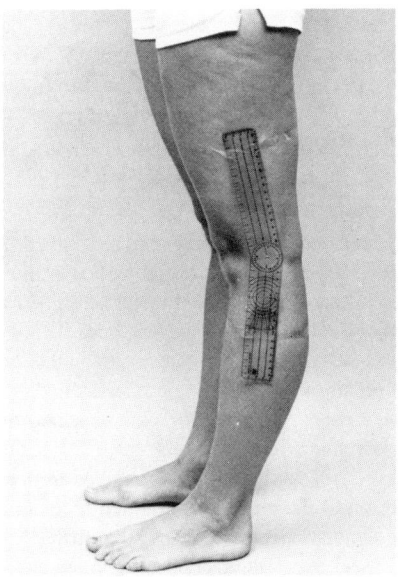

Figure 10—Recurvatum of the knee joint.

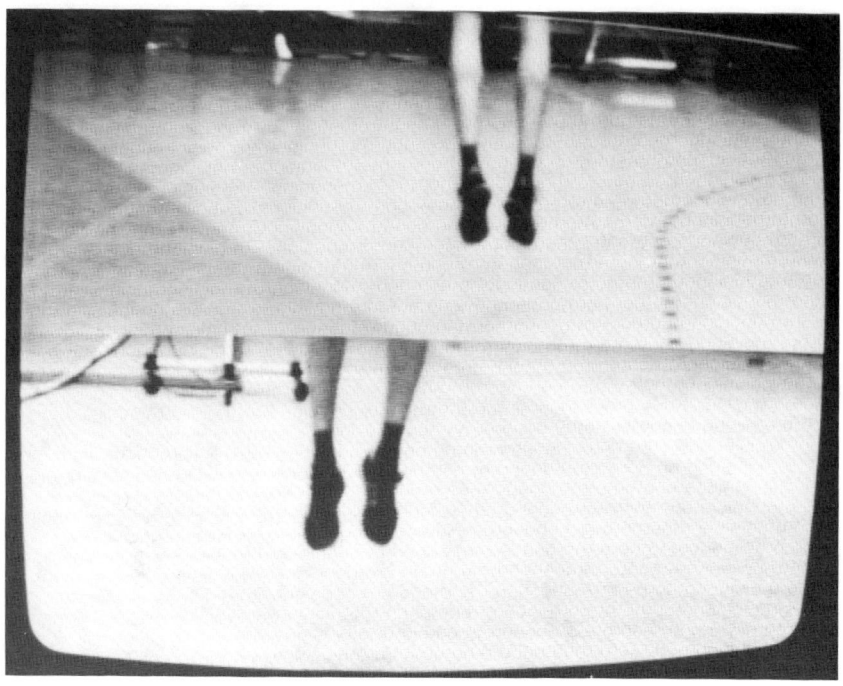

Figure 11—Flight phase in an extensor jump just before landing.

For this reason, the feet were then in slight external rotation and simultaneous internal rotation occurred at the knee and hip joints (see Figure 9). Overstressing reactions of the capsular ligament apparatus and tendopathies of the Achilles tendons resulted.

Discussion

As was expected, in some cases appreciable adaptation reactions of all connective and supporting tissue were observed. However, in particular, functional criteria revealed appreciable disturbing elements, although these test subjects were highly talented members of the National German Tennis Association. This evident discrepancy led to the insight that it was less the absolute stress parameters which decided on stress and overstressing, but rather their relative values, which resulted from a more or less optimized locomotor sequence. It was not the passive supporting elements, the bone, the cartilage, and also the tendons and ligaments which decided on stress and overstressing, but the equilibrium of the musculature. This resulted from a meaningful synergistic and reciprocal innervation of the entire postural and locomotor apparatus, as can be logically and perfectly demonstrated by reflexes after birth (Vojta, 1971). It is seriously disturbed when a vertical standing position is assumed and unfavorable force-load conditions arise, on the one hand, due to growth and, on the other hand, due to training. In both cases a susceptibility of disorders arises logically, not in the flexion phase of a movement, but in the extension phase.

This observation can be made not only in the adolescent, but also in the adult athlete. It can be demonstrated, also, in phases of convalescence, for example, from limb injuries. Logically, it occurs as the result of lever conditions which are always favored on the flexor side and which can be explained by the phylogenetic and postural development of man. This observation also means that sport (especially high-performance and top-performance) training must be concentrated on avoiding muscular asymmetry by particularly taking into account the extensor capacity of the movement sequence. The "stretching work" for the shortened musculature which is usually mentioned may not be emphasized, but, on the contrary, the intensified training of the muscles responsible for a maximum stretching is present. In addition, it must be required that in principle not simply one member of a chain is trained, but, meaningfully, an entire functional chain without deviant movement in maximum stretch must be exercised.

With such training criteria, exact movements in optimal muscular joint control would also result in a corresponding capsuloligament control, which was detected in the region of the wrist on the side of the playing arm in this study. These optimal movement sequences would reduce to a minimum particular lateral deviation movements in the region of the knee joints and in the region of the ankles, thus preventing hyperextensibility reactions in this region. The balanced musculature and the loading appropriate to the axis also entails a smooth (i.e., optimized) movement sequence with full utilization of the bony levers and maximum efficiency.

Such conditions in adolescent high-performance and top-performance athletes might possibly also be a reason for not starting a tennis-specific, one-sided training at an early age of 8 to 10 years, but only with conclusion of growth after these optimal motor preconditions mentioned above have been created in a broad sporting training program. With some certainty, even complicated movement sequences could be learned within a very short time and transformed into peak performance with maximum motivation. For this reason, there is no reason for not building upon this broad base in adolescent high-performance sport, especially since individual absolute peak performances should only be expected in adulthood. For the aforementioned reasons, overstressing reactions can be calculated better in the adult postural and locomotor apparatus and thus can be more readily avoided.

Conclusion

These results suggest that adaptive reactions following the present training procedures may be insufficient because they lead to muscular asymmetry and imbalance with an increase of overstress reactions and decrease in performances. Perfect locomotor sequences and muscular balance must be postulated. They should be helpful in avoiding overstress reactions and decreased performances.

References

EICHEL, H.W. (1981). *Reaktionsformen des Knochenskeletts bei einseitiger sportlicher Belastung im Wachstumsalter (Adaption reaction of the skeleton of adolescents after a one-sided training).* Unpublished dissertation, Universität Heidelberg.

HUPPERTZ, R. (1982). *Die einseitig belastete Hand jugendlicher Tennissportler—eine röntgenologische Querschnittsuntersuchung (The one-sided stressed hand of adolescent high per-*

formance tennis players—A radiological cross sectional investigation). Unpublished dissertation, Universität Heidelberg.

KRAHL, H., Sommer, H.M., & Correll, J. (1981). Hochleistungssport im Wachstumsalter—Reaktionsformen am Haltungs—und Bewegungsapparat (High performance sport in adolescent adaption reaction of the postural and locomotor apparatus). In H. Rickert *Sport an der Grenze menschlicher Leistrungsfähigkeit* (pp. 99-103). Berlin: Springer Verlag.

PAUWELS, F. (1960). Eine neue Theorie über den Einfluß mechanischer Reize auf die Differenzierung der Stützgewebe (A new theory of the influence of mechanical stimuli of the differentiation of the supporting tissues). *Z. Anat. Enwickl.-Gesch,* **121**, 478.

ROUX, W. (1895). *Gesammelte Abhandlungen über die Entwicklungsmechanik der Organismen I und II (A summary of the development of organism as a result of mechanical stimulation).* Leipzig: Engelmann.

VOJTA, V. (1971). Normale Entwicklung des Kindes von der Geburt bis zum Alter von 3 Jahren (Normal development of a child up to an age of 3 years). In *Allgemeine Entwicklungsneurologie*, Avicenum, Prag, 222.

WOLFF, J. (1892). *Das Gesetz der Transformation der Knochen (The law of the transformation of the bones).* Berlin: Hirschwald.

A Longitudinal Study of the Locomotor System in Trained Children

Jirina Mačková
Postgraduate Medical Institute, Salmovská, Praha

Jan Javůrek, Milos Máček and Jan Vávra
Faculty of Pediatrics, Praha

Several thousands of children selected with respect to their abilities in sports were prepared in different sport centers during extra school time. The purpose of this study was to recognize the effect of this long-term training. Several indexes of growth values, development, and circulation were recorded. After 4 years of work, coupled with previous experience (Javurek, 1982; Steinbrück, 1980) it was postulated that the locomotor system is the most sensitive indicator of possible overload and pathological movement patterns.

Material and Methods

This article reflects data collected from 2,244 trained boys from 8 sports (basketball n = 362, handball n = 503, volleyball n = 253, tennis n = 196, swimming n = 88, skiing n = 359, cycling n = 338, sport gymnastics n = 145). The ages of these males were between 12 and 17 years, with some exceptions in the swimmers, who were between 10 and 14 years of age, and in gymnasts, 7 to 12 years old. The total time spent in training was 8 to 12 hr/week, not including participation in competition. The pediatrician's opinion during the selection was fundamentally on the choice of the boys. At the beginning of training, all boys were without deviations from the healthy state. All subjects were followed up by a pediatrician and supervised by a specialist in sport medicine. All tests were carried out by 60 well-trained medical doctors in the use of these methods before participating in the project. The children were measured by using standardized methods each year during the same month. For comparison, the values of untrained male children were obtained for 60 boys who were between 8 and 16 years.

Using Janda's (1979) functional tests, relative shortening or weaknesses of different muscle groups were evaluated. The purpose of these tests was to evaluate the passive excursion of the joints, which may be limited by the shortened tonic muscles.

From the clinical point of view, two muscle systems should be evaluated. According to electromyographical observations, the system with predominantly tonic or postural function showed a tendency to develop muscle tightness, hypertonia, and shortening. The following muscles of this system were evaluated in this study: rectus femoris, iliopsoas, tensor fasciae latae, the hamstrings, levator scapulae, and pectoralis.

The other system with predominantly phasic function showed tendencies toward hypotonia, inhibition, and weakening. The following muscles belong to this system: glutei, vasti, abdominal muscles, and deep flexors of the neck.

Results

For simplification, the sum of all deviations in 4 years for all subjects in different sport categories is presented in this section.

The hamstrings were shortened in 70% of the untrained boys. In boys trained in different kinds of sports, this percentage was lower, between 10 and 60% except for the gymnasts (see Figure 1).

The hip flexors (iliopsoas, r. femoris, and tensor fasciae latae) were shortened in 60% of the untrained boys. In the trained, these muscles were shortened in only 10 to 35% of the sample (see Figure 2).

The trunk erectors were shortened in 23% of the untrained. In the sport center groups, this condition existed for a lower percentage except for tennis and handball participants (see Figure 3).

The shortening of the previously mentioned groups of postural muscles was accompanied mainly by a weakening of the local phasic muscles, which are the gluteus maximus and abdominal muscles. This imbalance could cause the forward tilting of the pelvis followed by hyperlordosis and compensatory kyphosis of the vertebral thoracic spine. This syndrome was termed "lower cross syndrome." In untrained boys, it was found in 50%; in the trained groups, it existed in 20 to 40% on the average.

Similar changes in the vertebral cervical spine and shoulder girdle were called the "upper cross syndrome." The shortened tonic muscles of this region are the upper part of the trapezius and the pectoralis major. The deep flexors of the neck and the lower stabilizer of the scapula are weakened. The shoulder is elevated and the head is pushed forward. This condition was found in 40% of the untrained boys. This was twice the percentage existing in boys engaged in sport training.

The next criterion in the evaluation of muscle function was the local hypermobility of the vertebral cervical spine, shoulder girdle, and lumbosacral region. A system of muscle tests was used based on the ranges of the active movement in the joints.

The lumbosacral region hypermobility was more frequent in children with greater sport activity. It was evident in 30 to 85% of this group, with the exception of the group training in swimming, where it was only 10%, the same as in untrained children (see Figure 4).

Similar findings were observed in shoulder girdle hypermobility. In trained children, this symptom was found in 20 to 45% of the members of the group. In the untrained, the swimmers and the handball players, it was present in only 10 to 15% of the group (see Figure 5).

LONGITUDINAL STUDY OF THE LOCOMOTOR SYSTEM

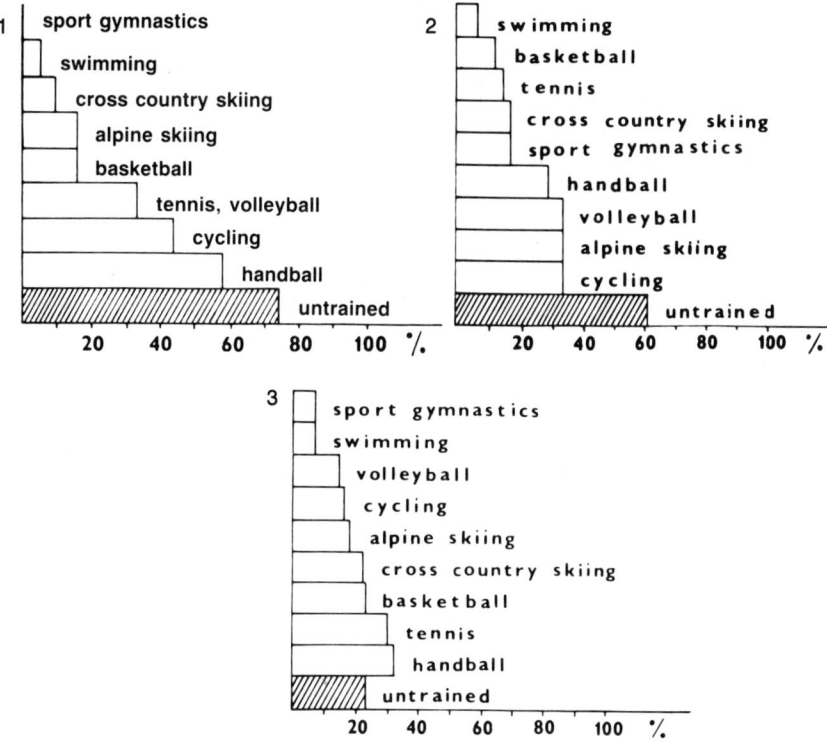

Figures 1, 2, 3—Represent the percentage of trained boys from different sports with shortened hamstrings, shortened hip flexors, and shortened trunk extensors, respectively, in comparison with untrained boys.

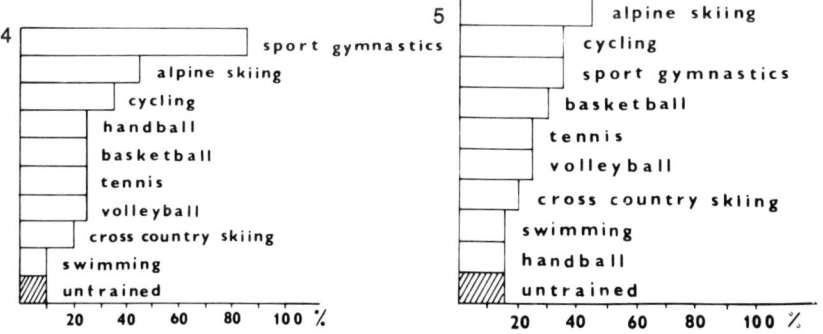

Figures 4 and 5—Represent the percentage of trained boys from different sports with hypermobility of the lumbosacral region in comparison with the untrained boys.

Discussion

According to Janda's (1978) conception of living style, industrial society lacks considerable variety of locomotor activity which supports the postural system and completely neglects the phasic one. This imbalance has serious consequences such as vertebrogenic syndrome, low back pain, spondylosis, and cervical pain. The first symptoms of the imbalances and the various troubles may be observed even in childhood. Nonadequate physical activity or one-sided overload could be the reason for these changes.

The lower incidences of shortened postural muscles and muscle imbalances in children with more sport activity could be explained by the following facts:

1. High motor activity prevents the weakening of phasic muscles.
2. The system of compensatory stretching exercises introduced prevents the shortening of the tonic muscles.
3. The selection of children for sport training possibly contributes to the better muscular function of trained boys in this study.

Because the shortening of tonic muscles is reversible and can be prevented or treated by special exercises (Spring, 1981), a more important consideration is the hypermobility in the children engaged in intensive physical activity. Hypermobility, as an irreversible prepathological condition, may cause ischemic and degenerative changes of the tendons, ligaments, and the joint capsules, which follow several years after finishing the activity. Thus, different conditions may develop after the end of a sport career when weakening muscles lose their ability to stabilize the joints.

In conclusion, the following suggestions are proposed:

1. Intensive training in children must be balanced in all muscle groups.
2. The exercise system must include stretching of the postural muscles and facilitation of the phasic muscles.
3. The local hypermobility induced by training should be avoided.
4. The physical activity after sport training should continue by performing special muscle exercises.

References

JANDA, V. (1978). Clinical aspects of moving disorders. Unpublished dissertation for professor's gradus (in Czech). Charles University, Praha.

JANDA, V. (1979) Muskelfunktionsdiagnostik (Diagnostics of muscle function). *Verlag für Medizin.* Dr. Evald Fischer, Heidelberg.

JAVUREK, J. (1982). Zkusenosti s hypermobilitou u sportovcu (The experience with hypermobility in sportsmen). *Teorie a praxe telesné výchoy,* **30**, 181-185.

SPRING, H. (1981). Muskelfunktionsdiagnostick nach Janda (Diagnostic of muscle function after Janda). *Schweizerische Zeitschrift für Sportmedizin,* **2**, 143-146.

STEINBRÜCK, K. (1980). Hypermobilität und Sport (Hypermobility and Sport). *Deutsche Zeitschrift für Sportmedizin,* **31**, 10-15.

The Composition of Muscle Fibers in a Group of Adolescents

Mornay P. du Plessis, Paul J. Smit, Louresns A.S. du Plessis, Hennie J. Geyer and Glenda Mathews
University of Pretoria

Hennie N.J. Louw
Council for Atomic Research

In sportsmen and sportswomen, the composition of muscle fiber is of the utmost importance as far as selection and achievement is concerned (Costill et al., 1976). Very little information regarding the presence of red muscle fibers (Type I), white muscle fibers (Type II), and transitional (or intermediate) fibers in growing children is available in the literature. The present study was designed to estimate the presence of these fibers in two groups of children and two groups of adults (Eriksson, Gollnick, & Saltin, 1973; Nishiyama, 1966; Sjögaard, Houston, Nygaad, & Saltin, 1978; Tunell & Hart, 1977.

Material and Methods

The first group consisted of 28 boys (ages 14 to 16 years). These boys participated in a variety of sports and super specialization was, therefore, not a factor. Similarly, the second group of 6 girls (ages 14 to 16 years) had not yet started athletic specialization. The adult group consisted of 53 white athletes (40 men and 13 women). These top track athletes were specialists in their particular events due to super specialization.

Muscle biopsies (Bergström, 1975) were performed on the vastus lateralis with a Depuy biopsy needle, 5 mm in diameter, under a local anesthetic. The sample was taken at a depth of ± 15 mm in the muscle, halfway between the trochanter of the femur and the lateral knee joint space. Tissue was frozen to -160° C by means of isopenthane in liquid nitrogen.

Frozen sections of muscle tissue 20 micron thick, were obtained by means of a cryostat microtome. The sections were subsequently stained by means of a histochemical method in order to bring out the presence of the enzyme, adenosine triphosphatase, at a pH of 4.3 (Costill et al., 1979; Dubowitz, Brooke, & Neville, 1973). This method was implemented in order to indicate the number of Type I (red or aerobic), Type II (white or anaerobic), and Type O (Type IIc) (transitional) fibers photographically. The muscle fibers were counted and the surface area of each fiber was then analyzed by means of a computer-assisted image analyzing process. (du Plessis, Louw, & Geyer, 1982). The latter method was used when it became clear that all available techniques were either too difficult or inadequate. (Edström & Nyström, 1972). A computer program was, therefore, compiled and standardized.

Results

The adolescent group consisting of 28 boys produced 2,450 fibers. The analysis showed 52.86% Type I, 34.08% Type II, as well as 13.06% fibers with a stain of intermediate hue, the so-called "transitional" fibers (Type IIc). This third group represented a relatively high percentage of intermediate fibers, 13.06% in 16 of the 28 samples (see Table 1).

In the adolescent girls' group (N = 6), 589 fibers were analyzed. The analysis in this group gave a total of 46.21% Type I fibers, 46.12% Type II fibers, and 7.65% transitional fibers. Four out of the 6 samples taken from the girls produced transitional fibers (see Table 2).

The mean surface areas of muscle fibers taken from the boys as analyzed with the texture analyzer computer technique was as follows: Type I, 1.142 micron^2, Type II, 1.352 micron^2, the difference, therefore, being 18.39%. The final analysis compares favorably with results obtained by Edström and Ekblom (1972) and Costill et al., (1976).

The mean surface areas of the muscle fibers taken from the girls were as follows: Type I, 1.168; Type II, 1.300; and transitional fibers 1.030 microns^2, respectively. The latter fibers had a mean surface area quite comparable to the 1.089 in the boys.

The difference between the surface areas of Type I and II fibers in the girls was 11.30%. Because no comparative study could be located, the results could not be compared to existing literature (see Table 4).

From the 4,443 fibers taken from the male group, the following analyses were obtained: Type I, 55.76%, Type II, 40.42%, and 3.82% transitional fibers. The latter group were found in only 16 of the 40 biopsies performed. The 529 muscle fibers taken

Table 1

Muscle Fiber Distribution and Area Estimation of 28 boys (14 to 16 Years)

	Age (years)	% Surface Type I (red) muscle fiber (Mean fiber area) (micron^2)	% Surface Type II (white) muscle fiber (Mean fiber area) (micron^2)	% Surface Type O (or C) (Mean fiber area) (micron^2)
Mean total	14.8	52.86 (1.142)	34.08 (1.352)	13.06 (1.089)
SD		15.62 (0.254)	9.62 (0.426)	14.39 (0.319)

Table 2

Muscle Fiber Distribution and Area Estimated Fiber Area of Six Girls (14 to 16 Years)

	Age (years)	% Surface Type I (red) muscle fiber (Mean fiber area) (micron^2)	% Surface Type II (white) muscle fiber (Mean fiber area) (micron^2)	% Surface Type O (or C) (Mean fiber area) (micron^2)
Mean total	14.9	46.21 (1.168)	46.12 (1.300)	7.65 (1.030)
SD		13.53 (0.244)	11.41 (0.419)	8.30 (0.310)

Table 3

Muscle Fiber Distribution (Area %)

		% Type I	% Type II	% Type O (or IIc)
Boys	N = 28			
	Mean	52.86[b]	34.08[b]	13.06[a]
	SD	15.61	1.62	11.54
Girls	N = 6			
	Mean	46.21[b]	46.12[b]	7.65[a]
	SD	13.53	11.41	8.30
Men	N = 40			
	Mean	5.76[b]	40.42[b]	3.28[a]
	SD	18.63	18.11	7.09
Women	N = 13			
	Mean	49.99[b]	50.01[b]	0.00[a]
	SD	14.69	14.69	0.00

[a]For type O (or IIc) fibers there was a statistically significant difference between boys and men and between girls and women, but no significant difference between boys and girls or between men and women ($p \leq .05$).

[b]There was no statistically significant difference Type I and II fibers of the boys and the men or between the girls and the women, but a significant difference existed between Type II fibers of boys and girls, but not between the Type I fibers ($p \leq .05$).

from the female group produced the following: Type I, 49.99%, Type II, 50.01%, with no transitional fibers (Brooke, et al., 1969; Costill, et al., 1976).

Table 4

Mean Muscle Fiber Surface Area (micron^2)

		% Type I	% Type II	% Type O (or IIc)
Boys	N = 28			
	Mean	1.142	1.352	1.089
	SD	0.254	0.426	0.319
Girls	N = 6			
	Mean	1.168	1.300	1.030
	SD	0.244	0.419	0.310
Mean		1.107	1.313	1.059
Men	N = 40			
	Mean	1.628	1.852	1.771
	SD	0.289	0.486	0.381
Women	N = 6			
	Mean	1.421	1.443	—
	SD	0.352	0.268	—
Mean		1.525	1.648	1.771

In the male group, the mean surface area of the Type I fibers was 1.628 micron^2; Type II, 1.852 micron^2; and transitional fibers, 1.771 micron^2. In the female group the Type I fibers had 1.421 micron^2 surface area, Type II, 1.443 micron^2. A difference of 13.76% and 1.55%, respectively, between male and female red and white muscle fibers was obtained in this group (Fenichel, 1963). These comparisons can be found in Tables 3 and 4.

Discussion

The staining of adenosine triphosphate (ATPase) enzyme at a pH of 4.3 indicates a strong staining tendency of the acid stable ATPase enzymes of the aerobic Type I (red) fiber. The Type II (white) fibers show no staining ability. This is due to the fact that the adenosine triphosphatase (myosine ATPase) of the anaerobic fiber is unstable at the pH of 4.3 and therefore shows no staining capacity (Costill et al., 1979).

The finding of a relatively high percentage of transitional fibers in adolescents (i.e., 13.06% in the case of the boys and 7.65% in the girls) was an interesting and a statistically meaningful finding. Some authors such as Tunell and Hart (1977), Dubowitz, Brook, and Neville (1973), and Costill et al. (1979) maintain that the fibers that remain slightly stained at certain pH values are Type IIa or IIc. Taking into consideration that there must be basic functionally developed Type I and Type II fibers at the two extreme ends of the staining abilities, one may consider the "in between fibers" as possible transitional fibers, in the sense that the functional (aerobic or anaerobic) features of the enzyme system may develop in either aerobic (Type I) or anaerobic (Type II) fibers, depending on the physical training program to which the fibers are subjected.

Theoretically, it seems logical that fibers showing intermediate staining ability contain an intermediate enzyme that seems to have the potential of changing its enzymatic characteristics to comply with the requirements of the training program to which the muscle fiber is subjected. The interchange from a fully fledged Type I to a Type II fiber in the adult athlete, depending on the demands made on the fiber, seems to be a strong possibility, if one can answer the questions of whether an enzyme can change its functional abilities. What stimulus and to what extent does it need to change (i.e., pH, lowering of PO_2, higher PO_2, or hormones)?

In light of the fact that certain researchers have reported a 50:50 distribution between red and white fibers in fetuses, newly born babies, and young infants, one wonders about the influence of puberty hormones on muscle fibers, for this age group produced a high percentage of pH 4.3 transitional fibers. (Dubowitz, 1966; Fenichel, 1963, 1966; Gollnick, et al., 1973; Johnsen, Palgar, Weightman, & Appleton, 1973).

The comparable figures between the boys and the adult men shows figures of 13.06% versus 3.28% for transitional fibers. The boys had almost four times as many of these fibers, percentagewise, as the men's group, which was a statistically significant difference (see Table 3).

In the case of girls and women, these figures were 7.65% and 0.00%, respectively, which was also meaningful. The latter figures are not representative of all groups. However, due to the fact that the presence of transitional fibers, 16 out of 28, and 4 out of 6, in the case of the boys and the girls, respectively, as against 16 out of 40, and 0 out of 13, in the case of the men and the women, respectively, were found, the deduction can be made that during periods of growth, more transitional fibers are present than in the adult athletes (Gollnick et al., 1973). An interesting fact is the presence of transitional fibers in only the top group of these adult track athletes who competed in the middle and long distance events.

It is, therefore, tempting to conclude that the adolescent transitional fibers may change to either Type I or II, and the adult fibers may change from the one type to the other by going through an intermediate phase development of the functional abilities of the enzymes (Jansson, & Kaijser, 1977).

References

BERGSTRÖM, J. (1975). Percutaneous needle biopsy of skeletal muscle in physiological and clinical research—review. *Scandinavian Journal of Clinical Laboratory Investigation,* **35,** 609-616.

BROOKE, M.H. & Engle, W.K. (1969). The histrographic analysis of human muscle biopsies with regard to fiber types. 1. Adult male and female. *Neurology,* **19,** 221-233.

COSTILL, D.L., Daniels, J., Evans, W., Fink, W., Krahenbuhl, G., & Saltin, B. (1976). Skeletal muscle enzymes and fiber composition in male and female track athletes. *Journal of Applied Physiology,* **40**(2), 149-154.

COSTILL, D.L., Fink, W.J., v. Hande, P.J., Miller, J.M., Sherman, W.M., Watson, P.A., & Witzman, F.A. (1979). *Analytical methods for the measurement of human performance.* (2nd Ed.). Muncie, IN: Ball State University.

DUBOWITZ, V. (1963). Histology—Enzymatic maturation of skeletal muscle. *Nature,* **197,** 1215-1216.

DUBOWITZ, V. (1966). Enzyme histochemistry of developing human muscle. *Nature,* **211,** 884-885.

DUBOWITZ, V., Brooke, M.H., & Neville, H.E. (1973). *Muscle biopsy: A modern approach.* Major problems in Neurology, Vol. 2. Philadelphia: W.B. Saunders Co., Ltd.

DU PLESSIS, M.P., Louw, H.N.J., & Geyer, H.J. (1982). Skeletal muscle analysis with the aid of a computer-assisted image analyzing process. *S.A. Med. J.*, **62**, 679-680.

EDSTRÖM, L., & Ekblom, B. (1972). Differences in sizes of red and white muscle fibers in vastus lateralis of musculus quadriceps femoris of normal individuals and athletes. *Scandinavian Journal of Clinical Laboratory Investigation*, **30**, 175-181.

EDSTRÖM, L., & Nyström, B. (1972). Histochemical types and sizes of fibers in normal human muscles. *Acta Neurologica Scandinavica*, **45**, 257-269.

ERIKSSON, B.O., Gollnick, P.G., & Saltin, B. (1973). Muscle metabolism and enzyme activities after training in boys 11-13 years old. *Acta Physiologica Scandinavica*, **87**, 485-497.

FENICHEL, G.M. (1963). the 'B' fiber of human fetal skeletal muscle. A study of fiber diameter size. *Neurology*, **13**, 219-226.

FENICHEL, G.M. (1963). The 'B' fiber of human fetal skeletal muscle. A study of fiber diameter size. *Neurology*, **13**, 219-226.

GOLLNICK, P.D., Armstrong, R.B., Saltin, B., Saubert, C.W., Sembrowich, W.L., & Shepherd, R.E. (1973). Effect of training on enzyme activity and fiber composition of human skeletal muscle. *Journal of Applied Physiology*, **34**, 107-111.

JANSSON, E., & Kaijser, L. (1977). Muscle adaptation to extreme endurance training in man. *Acta Physiological Scandinavica*, **100**, 315-324.

JOHNSEN, M.A., Palgar, J., Weightman, D., & Appleton, D. (1973). Data on the distribution of fiber types in 36 human muscles. An autopsy study. *Journal of Neurological Science*, **18**, 111-114.

NISHIYAMA, A. (1966). Histochemical studies on the red, white and intermediate muscle fibers of some skeletal muscles. *Acta Med. Okayama*, **20**, 137-146.

SJOGAARD, G., Houston, M.E., Nygaard, E., & Saltin, B. (1978). Subgrouping of fast twitch fibers in skeletal muscles of man. *Histochemistry*, **58**, 79-82.

TUNELL, G.L., & Hart, M.N., (1977). Simultaneous determination of skeletal muscle fiber, Types I, IIA and IIB by histochemistry. *Arch. Neurol.*, **34**, 171-173.

Passive versus Active Exposures to Dry Heat as Methods of Heat Acclimatization in Young Children

Omri Inbar, Rafi Dotan, Oded Bar-Or, and Bernard Gutin
Wingate Institute for Physical Education
and Sport, Wingate Post, Israel

Heat acclimatization is defined as an adaptive process which results in a reduction in the physiologic strain produced by the application of an environmental and metabolic stress and which, when completed, results in a remarkable increase in the capacity to function in the heat without distressing symptoms (Gisolfi, 1973; Rowell, Kraning, Kennedy, & Evans, 1967). The mechanisms responsible for the human adaptation to hot climatic conditions are not yet fully understood. However, through these mechanisms, the body is able to transport additional heat from the body core to the periphery and dissipate it to the surrounding environment. The principal element in achieving optimal level of heat acclimatization is the exposure of the body to high ambient temperature while performing a physical task. In adults, mere sitting at rest (passive exposure), even in severe heat, does not produce the physiologic responses required for full heat acclimatization (Robinson, 1967; Rowell, Kraning, Kennedy, & Evans, 1967; Shvartz, Saar, Meyerstein, & Ben-Or, 1973; Wyndham, Rogers, Senay, & Mitchell, 1976; Wyndham & Styrdom, 1969).

A possible cause for the incomplete physiological adaptation of adults following passive heat acclimatization could be the relatively low thermal strain imposed upon the organism during such heat exposures. Such low thermal stimulus may be suboptimal for the thermal and cardiovascular adjustments necessary for the complete acclimatization to work in the heat (Inbar, Bar-Or, Dotan, & Gutin, 1981; Shvartz, Saar, Meyerstein, & Ben-Or, 1973; Williams & Wyndham, 1968). In young children, however, whose geometric characteristics are conducive to greater heat influx from the surrounding environment (Bar-Or, 1980; Buskirk, Lundegren, & Magnusson, 1965; Buskirk, Bar-Or, & Kollias, 1969; Kawahata, 1960; Lofstedt, 1966), the imposed thermal load during passive exposure to heat might be sufficient to induce more complete heat acclimatization.

Therefore, this study was designed to compare the effects of passive and active heat exposures on the development of heat acclimatization in prepubertal children 8 to 10 years old.

Subjects and Methods

The overall structure of the experiment was similar to that described in two previous studies from this laboratory (Inbar, Bar-Or, Dotan, & Gutin, 1981; Inbar, Dotan, Bar-Or, & Gutin, 1983). Healthy school boys, 8 to 10 years old (n=17), were selected for participation after having their parents sign a consent form. The experiments were carried out during the winter months when all subjects were presumably unacclimatized to heat prior to the beginning of the study. The 17 prepubertal boys were randomly assigned to two groups: a passive heat acclimatization group (PHA; n=8); and an active heat acclimatization group (AHA; n=9). Their morphological and physiological characteristics are summarized in Table 1. Some data pertaining to the AHA group have been previously reported (Inbar, et al., 1981).

Both groups underwent five acclimatization sessions during a 10-day period (on alternate days), preceded by a baseline (BL) session and followed by an identical criterion (CT) session. All seven sessions for both groups were held in a climatic chamber (Hot Pack, U.S.A.) at 43° C dry bulb and 24° C wet bulb (21% relative humidity). Air velocity was less than 0.2 m·sec^{-1}.

During BL and CT, both groups performed on a cycle ergometer (Monark, Sweden) three riding bouts of 20 min each, interspersed by seven 8-min rest periods. Power was about 40 W, individually determined to elicit 85% of maximal heart rate (HR) and 40 to 45% of the previously determined maximal aerobic power. Throughout their acclimatization sessions, subjects of the PHA group sat quietly on a comfortable lounge chair, whereas the AHA subjects performed an exercise protocol identical to that described for BL and CT.

Rectal (Tre), chest, and thigh skin temperatures as well as HR were taken before entering the chamber and at 5-min intervals. Arithmetic mean of the skin temperatures (Tsk) was calculated. Body weight (Sauter, W. Germany ± 10 g) was recorded for the AHA group upon entry to the chamber and then during each rest period. The PHA subjects were weighed every 30 min. Sweating rate (SR) was taken as the net body weight loss, allowing for fluid intake and change in weight of clothing (water loss through gas exchange was not included and was assumed to be negligible under this study's conditions). The rate of metabolism ($\dot{V}O_2$) was measured halfway through the second exercise bout by collecting a 2-min expired air sample in Douglas bags. From these

Table 1

Physical and Physiological Characteristics of Subjects (M ± 1SE)

Group	Age years	Weight kg	Surface area m^2	Fat %	HRmax beats·min^{-1}	$\dot{V}O_2$max ml·kg^{1-}·min^{-1}
PHA	8.9	29.9	1.07	16.5	196.8	49.5
(n=8)	±0.2	±2.1	±0.03	±1.5	±1.4	±2.8
AHA	9.3	27.1	1.04	14.3	198.5	52.8
(n=9)	±1.3	±1.3	±0.13	±0.6	±2.7	±2.1
P	NS	NS	NS	NS	NS	NS

values, the metabolic heat production was calculated taking $\dot{V}O_2$ of 4.5 ml·kg^{-1}min^{-1} for rest and 21.1 and 23.0 ml·kg^{-1}min^{-1}, for exercise in the passive and active groups, respectively. Heat storage was calculated according to the equation: S = (0.67 Tre + 0.33 $\overline{T}$sk) x specific heat values of 0.350, 0.400 and 0.988 Kcal·kg^{-1} C^{-1}, for lean tissue, fat, and water, respectively (Bar-Or, Lundegren, Magnusson, & Buskirk, 1969). The total body water was determined according to the revised equation of Findanze (in Consolazio, Johnson & Pecora, 1963): lean body mass (% of body weight) = (1.9 x % body water) - 38.8. Radiative and convective (R+C) heat was calculated jointly from the heat balance equation: (R+C) = E + S - M, where M was taken as the net metabolic heat produced per kg of body weight (Kcal·kg^{-1}). Evaporative heat loss (E) was calculated by multiplying the total net weight loss by 0.58 Kcal (the latent heat of water vaporization). Heat activated sweat glands (HASG) were counted from five skin sites at the end of the BL session by the starch-iodine technique (Bar-Or, Lundegren, & Magnusson, 1968). Measured quantities of dilute lemonade were given upon request. However, children were encouraged to replace their fluid loss periodically.

Data treatment included descriptive analysis on each of the parameters measured. Differences between the BL and CT sessions were analyzed for each acclimatization group by paired t-tests performed on every parameter. Unpaired t-tests were done for intergroup comparisons on the differences (Δ) between BL and CT in each parameter. These Δ's were used to quantify the acclimatization effects.

Results

Table 2 depicts the metabolic, cardiovascular, and thermoregulatory responses of the two groups to their respective acclimatization procedures. As reported in a previous study (Inbar et al., 1981), the AHA group showed significant reduction in HR and Tsk, and an increase in SR per degree rise in Tre (SR↑Tre^{-1}), and HASG. In the PHA group, significant reduction was evident in HR, Tre, heat storage (S) and SR. There were no changes in $\dot{V}O_2$ or in minute ventilation as a result of either acclimatization protocol. When comparison of the changes (^{5}) between the passive and active acclimatization procedures was made (see Table 2), no significant differences in any of the parameters measured were found (P>.05).

Figures 1 and 2 illustrate the pattern of rise in Tre and HR for each group during BL and CT. A very similar pattern of Tre and HR responses in both acclimatization groups is evident. In both groups, a trend toward Tre and HR reduction during CT, compared with BL, became apparent only after some 35 to 40 min.

Illustrated in Figures 3 & 4 are the final mean values of several variables during each acclimatization exposure in the two experimental groups. In all but one parameter (Tsk), the values during each acclimatization session were significantly higher in the active than in the passive group. However, and as indicated previously, the change in all of those variables from BL to CT was not significantly dissimilar in the two groups.

Discussion

In a previous study (Inbar et al., 1981) on the effects of different heat acclimatization protocols on prepubertal boys, it was reported that, unlike in adults, mere physical

Table 2

Metabolic, Cardiovascular, and Thermoregulatory Variables at Base-Line (BL), and at the end of Acclimatization (CT), and the Changes Caused Within the Passive and Active Acclimatization Programs

Variables	Protocol	Passive BL	Passive CT	Active BL	Active CT	Δ (CT - BL) Passive	Δ (CT - BL) Active
$\dot{V}O_2$, ml•kg^{-1}•min^{-1}	M	21.1	21.7	23.0	22.9	0.60	-0.10
	SE	1.9	1.6	1.5	1.8	1.21	0.63
	P value*	NS		NS		NS	
VE, l•$^{-1}$	M	17.2	18.1	18.3	18.7	0.92	0.40
	SE	0.7	0.7	1.4	2.1	1.52	1.66
	P value	NS		NS		NS	
HR, beat•min^{-1}	M	168.9	156.7	165.4	153.2	-12.2	-11.4
	SE	5.2	3.8	6.7	4.8	4.4	2.8
	P value	<.05		<.01		NS	
Tre, °C	M	38.23	37.91	38.43	38.24	-0.32	-0.23
	SE	0.14	0.10	0.13	0.11	0.10	0.13
	P value	<.05		NS		NS	
Tsk, °C	M	37.02	36.56	37.24	36.63	-0.46	-0.64
	SE	0.20	0.15	0.15	0.24	0.17	0.15
	P value	NS		<.01		NS	
SR•SA^{-1}, g•m^{-2}•hr^{-1}	M	316.0	274.9	309.9	336.3	-41.1	26.40
	SE	29.8	15.9	31.0	23.0	20.7	23.10
	P value	<.05		NS		NS	
SR•↑Tre^{-1}, g•°C^{-1}•hr^{-1}	M	309.4	353.7	227.2	296.6	44.30	69.42
	SE	64.1	48.6	29.5	39.9	54.02	19.84
	P value	NS		<.05		NS	
Heat storage, Kcal•kg^{-1} per session	M	1.85	1.29	1.99	1.77	-0.56	-0.22
	SE	0.13	0.11	0.17	0.99	-0.10	-0.17
	P value	<.01		NS		NS	
HASG, No•cm^{-1}	M	103.1	114.3	118.1	143.4	11.2	25.2
	SE	7.2	10.4	10.7	10.4	7.0	8.3
	P value	NS		<.05		NS	

*P values are related to the differences between BL and CT within each protocol, and between the Δ's of the two protocols.

conditioning in a neutral environment by young children produces as high, if not higher, adaptive response as that caused by "classical" exercise-in-the-heat acclimatization procedure.

In the present study, an attempt was made to further investigate the child's unique heat acclimatization process, this time adding a similar group of prepubertal boys who underwent a passive heat acclimatization protocol and comparing it with the group who followed exercise-in-the-heat acclimatization program.

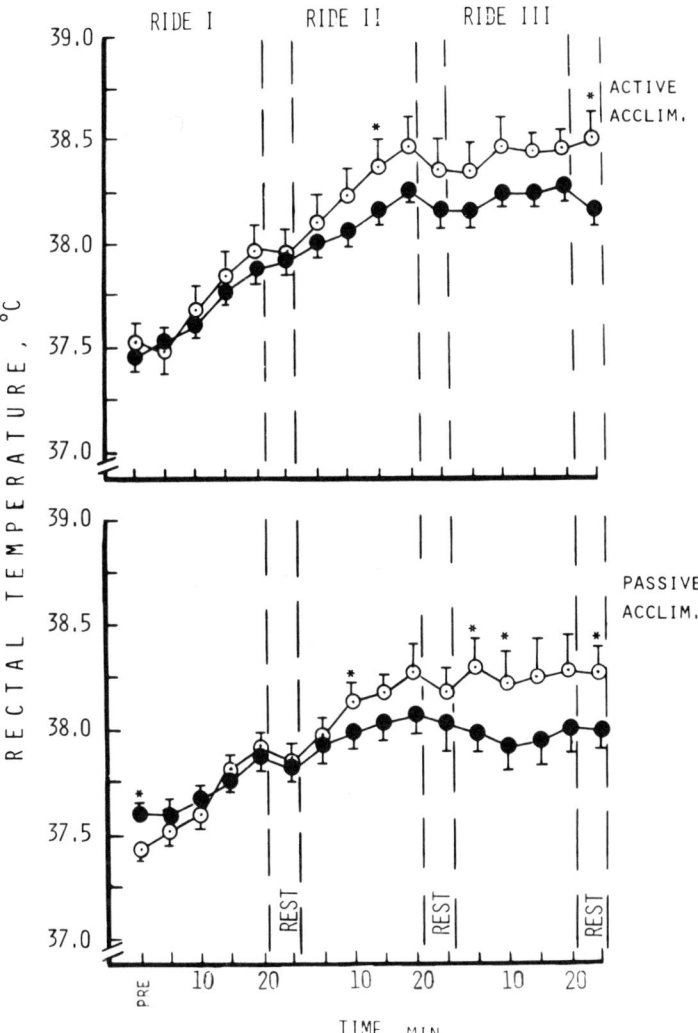

Figure 1—Rectal temperatures at 5-min intervals during BL (O) and CT (•) for the active and passive acclimatization groups. Mean ± SEM.* p<.05.

Taking differences between BL and CT (Δ) as the criteria for heat acclimatization, no statistically significant differences between the two modes could be detected in any of the measured variables (see Table 2). Furthermore, there were no clear-cut differences in the response patterns of the various parameters between the two protocols. This was true despite lower rectal temperature, heart rate, metabolic rate, and sweat loss, observed during each of the passive compared with the active acclimatization sessions.

The former observation is contrary to previous findings on adults for whom a mere passive exposure to hot environmental conditions, even when coupled with mild daily

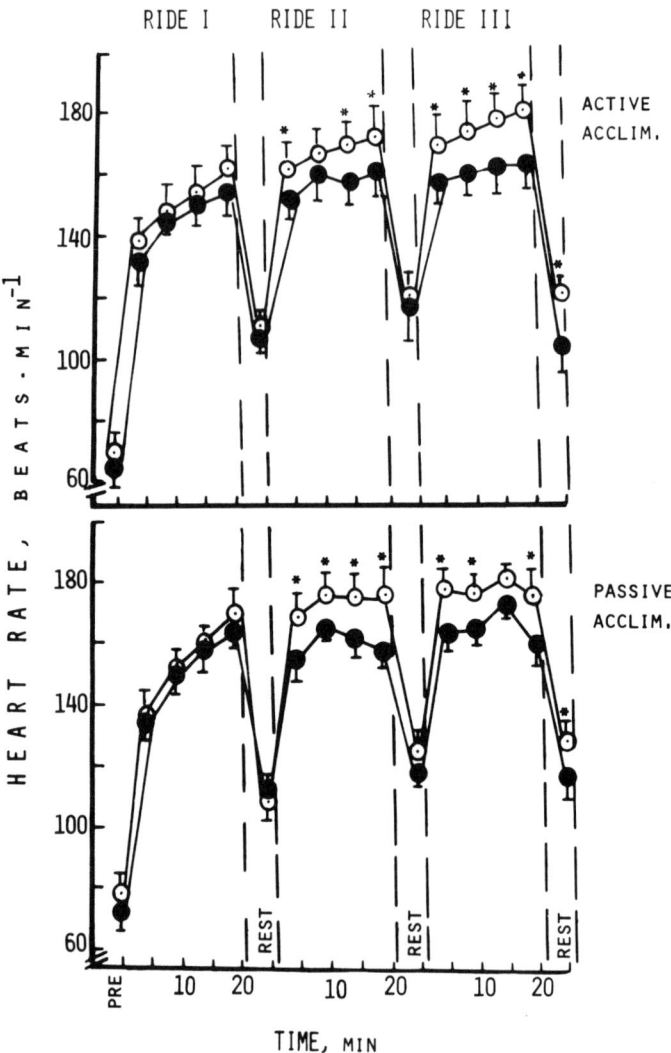

Figure 2—Heart rates at 5-min intervals during BL (O) and CT (•) for the active and passive acclimatization groups. Mean ± SEM.* $p<.05$.

activity, caused an incomplete or no acclimatization to work in the heat (Rowell, Kraning, Kennedy, & Evans, 1967; Wyndham, Rogers, Senay, & Mitchell, 1976; Wyndham, & Strydom, 1969).

Two opposing theories concerning the child's response to a passive heat protocol could be proposed based on the aforementioned considerations: (a) Unlike in adults, a combined thermal and exercise stimulus is not a prerequisite for full acclimatization in children during their first decade of life; (b) the combined thermal and exercise strain

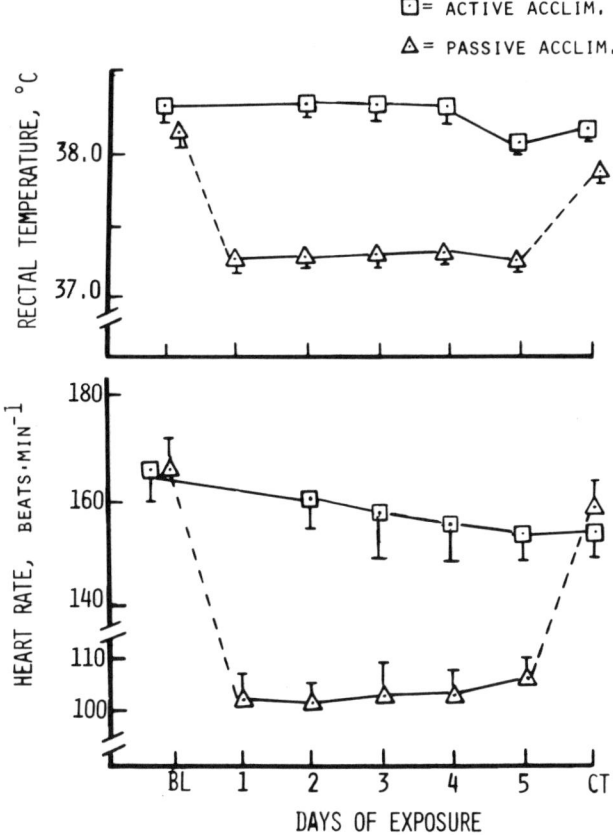

Figure 3—Changes (Δ) from BL values in rectal temperature and heart rate during each exposure. Comparison between the active (□) and passive (Δ) acclimatization protocols. Values are mean ± SEM.

imposed during the active protocol exceeded a certain optimal level for maximal heat acclimatization development.

The design of the present study could not offer a conclusive answer as to why and how, in 8- to 10-year-old boys, a response has been observed that is different from that found in adults. However, some speculations in trying to answer these intriguing questions should be attempted.

In the PHA group, the observed reduction in HR (7.2%), Tre (0.76%), Tsk (1.24%), heat storage (30%) and the increased $SR \cdot \uparrow Tre^{-1}$ (14.3%) could not be attributed to a functional improvement of the cardiovascular system because only minimal stress on that system was imposed during the passive heat acclimatization sessions (see Figures 3 & 4). An improvement in the working efficiency and consequently a reduction in metabolic heat production could not be expected either because $\dot{V}O_2$ during CT did not decrease compared to BL (see Table 2). Thus, most, if not all, of the physiologic

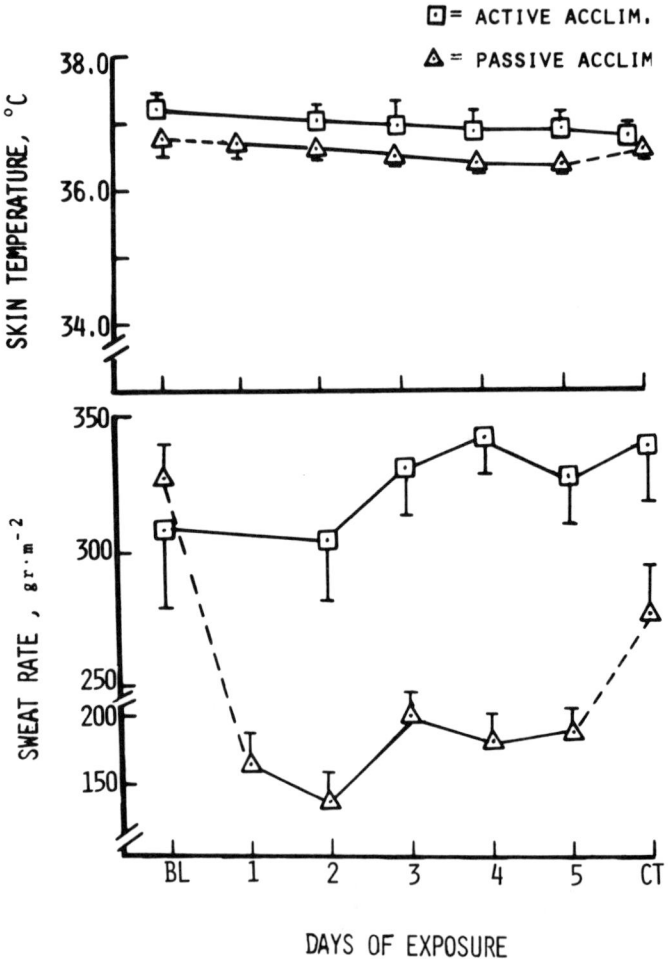

Figure 4—Changes (Δ) from BL values in skin temperature and sweat rate per body surface area. Comparison between the active (□) and passive (Δ) acclimatization protocols. Values are mean ± SEM.

adaptations caused by this procedure were the result of the mere thermal stress imposed during this acclimitization program.

Based on Table 3, most, if not all, of the reduction in body heat storage recorded for the PHA group was consequential to the significant reduction (from BL to CT) in radiative and convective heat gain. This could be brought about by a reduction in the peripheral blood flow (Bass, 1963) which in turn may result in maintaining skin temperature at relatively low levels. This possible chain of events is apt to increase the core-to-periphery temperature gradient (as the acclimatization process progresses), thereby reducing heat conductance and increasing the insulating capacity of the skin (Astrand & Rodahl, 1970). Consequently, less heat could penetrate the body shell by radiation and convection, causing R + C (and thus S) to drop.

Table 3

Heat Exchange Values (KCal·kg⁻¹·Session⁻¹) Measured Prior to (BL) and at the End (CT) of the Two Acclimatization Protocols

Group	Element	E BL	E CT	R + C BL	R + C CT	M BL	M CT	S BL	S CT
Passive	M	6.60	5.75	2.04	0.44	6.41	6.60	1.85	1.29
Group	SE	0.76	0.48	1.18	0.65	0.54	0.42	0.13	0.11
	P	N.S.		<.05		N.S.		<.01	
Active	M	6.77	7.40	1.98	1.66	7.25	7.23	1.99	1.77
Group	SE	0.65	0.54	0.85	0.85	0.42	0.50	0.17	0.09
	P	N.S.		N.S.		N.S.		N.S.	

It should be remembered that in the PHA group the fall in S was not accompanied by either an increase in evaporative cooling, nor by a reduction in metabolic heat production (see Table 3).

In contrast, the AHA group achieved its level of heat acclimatization without any meaningful drop in body heat content (see Table 3). It is likely, therefore, that its acclimatization process was developed predominantly by the marked adaptation of its sweating apparatus. Although total sweat loss did not increase significantly following either of the acclimatization procedures, sweating sensitivity, as indicated by sweat rate per °C rise in Tre above 37 °C, increased significantly (by some 30%) following the AHA protocol (see Table 2). Furthermore, the AHA protocol caused a significant increase in the population density of the active sweat glands (see Table 2), implying better wetting of the skin and possibly more efficient sweat evaporation (Inbar, Bar-Or, Dotan, & Gutin, 1981).

One possible explanation for the reported differential response of young boys compared with young men (undergoing similar passive heat acclimatization) could be sought in the different morphological characteristics of the two age groups. The large surface area to body mass ratio in the children may, under ambient temperature higher than skin temperature (the case in the present study), cause greater heat gain through radiation and convection, compared with larger individuals with small surface-to-mass ratio. In the case of passive heat acclimatization, where some minimal stress must be imposed upon the thermoregulatory system, if any adaptation of this system is to be expected, the larger SA/mass ratio of young children may be an asset in producing such stress during the heat acclimatization exposures.

One might argue that the PHA boys could become acclimatized due to habitual activities which they might have pursued on off-days when they were not in the climatic chamber. This is unlikely because none of them engaged in athletic activity during the winter when this study was performed.

The relatively high heat acclimatization induced by passive exposures among the prepubertal boys may not be explained solely by a high degree of acclimatization achieved by the PHA group, but also by a lower than optimal degree of acclimatization achieved by the AHA group. Such a possibility could be based on the theory put forward by several authors (Inbar, Bar-Or, Dotan, & Gutin, 1981; Inbar, Dotan, Bar-Or, & Gutin,

1983; Robinson, 1967; Strydom, Kotze, VanderWalt, & Rogers, 1976; Shvartz, Saar, Meyerstein, & Ben-Or, 1973; Williams, & Wyndham, 1968), who claimed that the degree of heat acclimatization is a function of the heat stored in the body during each session of a given acclimatization procedure. Moreover, Williams and Wyndham (1968) have reported that, in adults, certain combinations of thermal and exercise loads could create less than optimal development of heat acclimatization. It is possible, therefore, that the combined effects of the thermal and exercise stress imposed upon the AHA group during the acclimatization exposures was above the level needed in prepubertal children for full acclimatization to be achieved (Inbar et al., 1981; Inbar et al., 1983). The results of the present and previous investigations done in this laboratory show that the initial heat storage caused by three different acclimatization protocols (active acclimatization, exercise in neutral climate, and passive acclimatization) varied, being highest in the active procedure (1.99 Kcal·kg^{-1}·$session^{-1}$), followed by the passive (1.23 Kcal·kg^{-1}·$session^{-1}$), and then the exercise in neutral climate exposures (0.54 Kcal·kg^{-1}·$session^{-1}$) (Inbar et al., 1981), in that order (see Figure 5).

In summary, it appears that the two acclimatization protocols studied in this experiment, passive and active, produced a similar degree of acclimatization. The AHA group achieved the observed physiologic adaptations primarily by mild thermoregulatory improvement (mainly improved functioning of the sweating apparatus) caused by the continuous exposure to high thermal load, and the mild conditioning effect brought about by the relatively low power load imposed during each acclimatization session. In con-

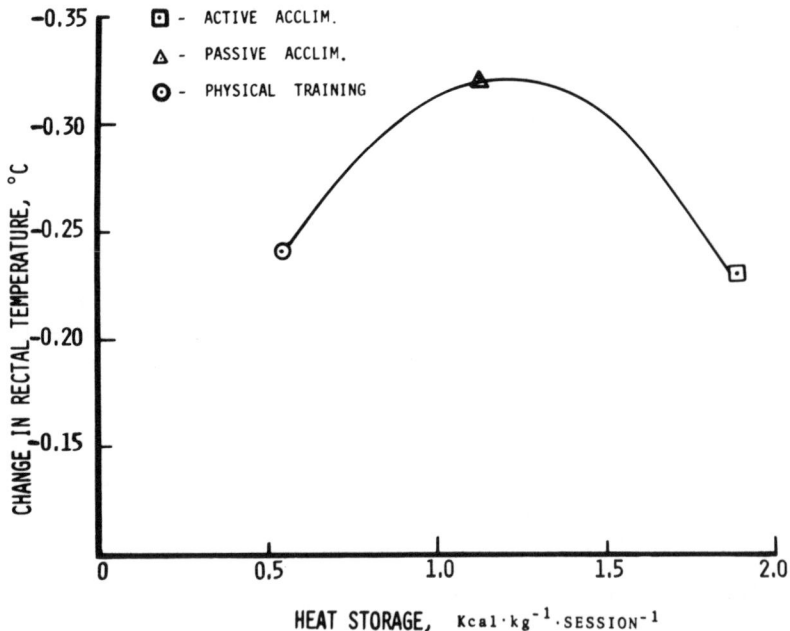

Figure 5—Relationship between change in rectal temperature (from BL to CT) and body heat storage in three different acclimatization protocols. Values for heat storage are those calculated during the first acclimatization session (following BL) for each of the respective acclimatization procedures.

trast, the PHA group achieved its degree of acclimatization by mere thermal stress which caused reduction in body heat content due to an improved insulating capacity of the body shell. The noticeable adaptation developed by the passive acclimatization group can be attributable to either the child's advantageous morphological characteristics or to the postulated theory that the thermal load encountered during the active acclimatization exposures was excessively high for an optimal rate of acclimatization to occur.

References

ÅSTRAND, P.O., & Rodahl, K. (1970). *Textbook of work physiology*. New York McGraw-Hill Book Co.

BAR-OR, O. (1980). Climate and the exercising child—A review. *International Journal of Sports Medicine,* **1**, 14-21.

BAR-OR, O., Lundegren, H.M., & Buskirk, E.R. (1968). Distribution of heat-activated sweat glands in obese and lean men and women. *Human Biology,* **2**, 235-248.

BAR-OR, O., Lundegren, H.M., Magnusson, L.I., & Buskirk, E.R. (1969). Heat tolerance of exercising obese and lean women. *Journal of Applied Physiology,* **26**, 403-409.

BASS, B.E. (1963). Thermoregulatory and circulatory adjustments during acclimatization to heat in man. In J.D. Hardy (Ed.), *Temperature: Its measurement and control in science and industry* (Vol. 3, part 3). New York: Reinhold Book Corp.

BUSKIRK, E.R., Bar-Or, & Kollias, J. (1969). Physiological effects of heat and cold. In N.L. Wilson (Ed.), *Obesity*. Philadelphia: F.A. Davis Company.

BUSKIRK, E.R., Lundegren, H.M., & Magnusson, L.I. (1965). Heat acclimatization patterns in obese and lean individuals. *Annuals of New York Academy of Science,* **131**, 637-653.

CONSOLAZIO, C.F., Johnson, R.E., & Pecora, L.J. (1963). *Physiological measurement of metabolic functions in man*. New York: McGraw-Hill.

GISOLFI, C.V., (1973). Work-heat tolerance derived from interval training. *Journal of Applied Physiology,* **35**, 349-354.

INBAR, O., Bar-Or, O., Dotan, R., & Gutin, B. (1981). Conditioning versus exercise in heat as methods for acclimatizing 8- to 10-year-old boys to dry heat. *Journal of Applied Physiology: Respiratory Environmental and Exercise Physiology,* **50**, 406-411.

INBAR, O., Dotan, R., Bar-Or, O., & Gutin, B. (1985). Heat acclimatization—A comparison between pubertal boys and young men (submitted for publication).

KAWAHATA, A. (1960). Sex differences in sweating. In H. Yoshimara, K. Ogata, & S. Itah (Eds.), *Essential problems in climatic physiology*. Kyoto, Japan: Nankodo Publishing Co.

LOFSTEDT, B. (1966). *Human heat tolerance*. Lund, Sweden: Department of Hygiene, University of Lund.

ROBINSON, S. (1967). Training, acclimatization and heat tolerance, physical activity and cardiovascular health. *Canadian Medical Association Journal,* **96**, 795-800.

ROWELL, L.B., Kraning, K.K., Kennedy, J.W., & Evans, T.P. (1967). Central circulatory responses to work in dry heat before and after acclimatization. *Journal of Applied Physiology,* **22**, 509-518.

SHVARTZ, E., Saar, E., Meyerstein, N., & Ben-Or, D. (1973). A comparison of three methods of acclimatization to dry heat. *Journal of Applied Physiology,* **34,** 214-219.

STRYDOM, N.B., Kotze, H.F., VanderWalt, W.H., & Rogers, G.G. (1976). Effect of ascorbic acid on rate of heat acclimatization. *Journal of Applied Physiology,* **41,** 202-205.

WILLIAMS, C.G., & Wyndham, C.H., (1968). The problems of "optimum" acclimatization. *Internationale Zeitschrift für Angewandte Physiologie einschliesslich Arbeitsphysiologie,* **26,** 298-308.

WYNDHAM, C.H., Rogers, G.G., Senay, L.C., & Mitchell, D. (1976). Acclimatization in hot, humid environment: Cardiovascular adjustments.

WYNDHAM, C.H., & Strydom, N.B. (1969). Acclimatization of men to heat in climatic chambers in miners. *Journal of South African Institute of Mining and Metalurgy,* **70,** 60-67.

Assessment of Biological Development by Anthropometric Variables

Mészáros Janos, Mohácsi Janos, Szabó Tamas, and Szmodis Ivan
Hungarian University of Physical Education, Budapest,
and Központi Sportiskola, Budapest, Hungary

Biological (developmental) age may differ considerably from chronological age as a result of the effects of a number of influences modifying growth and development. In the beginning of this century, Crampton (1908) described relevant observations and suggested adopting the more characteristic term, physiological age, instead of relying only on chronological age.

There are several ways to estimate the status of biological development. These were summarized by Hebbelinck (1979) as being based on (a) dentition age, (b) morphological and shape age, (c) sexual maturation age, and (d) ossification age.

In addition to these methods of estimation, Grimm (1979) considered an analysis of motor performance tests as being equally suitable in characterizing biological development. The best known methods of estimating biological age are those of Greulich and Pyle (1959), Tanner and Whitehouse (1959), and Tanner, Whitehouse, and Healey (1962). Discrepancies among the various radiological age assessment techniques have also been described (Drobná, 1979; Hebbelinck, 1979; Malina & Little, 1981; Roche, Davils, & Eyman, 1971).

While the practice of training young competitive athletes obviously requires a knowledge of developmental status, preferably expressed in years, the procedures of radiological age estimation cannot be used as extensively as might be desired because of their expensive, time-consuming, and facility-dependent nature. It was, therefore, fully justifiable to develop another method of biological age estimation that could also be utilized extensively for the study of athletic youth, without the limitations associated with radiological techniques.

Rationale and Technique for Methodology

The criteria of practical use were thought to be best met by an estimation method based on anthropometric variables. Relying on a nationwide representative study of body dimensions (N = 25,000), growth curves were constructed for the variables involved, namely, stature, body mass, and Conrad's plastic index (the sum of biacromial distance, lower arm girth, and hand circumference). The tabulated data (Mészáros & Mohácsi, 1983) include mean values for every quarter of a year, obtained by linear interpolation between the mean ages of the respective full year age groups.

Estimation of developmental age proceeds as follows:

1. Actual stature, body mass, and plastic index (Conrad, 1963) are measured and entered into the table of standards to obtain, separately for each dimension, their age equivalent to an accuracy of 0.25 year.
2. As a first approximation, developmental age is estimated by calculating the mean of chronological age and the three age equivalents of the dimensional variables.
3. When actual stature differs from the stature conforming to the subject's chronological age by more than 1 year's equivalent, the mean obtained under 2. is corrected by 5%: reducing developmental age when actual stature is taller, and vice versa. When the deviation from standard stature exceeds an equivalent of 2 years, the correction factor is 8%.

Developmental age estimated in the manner described in 195 sport school trainees, aged 11 to 13 years, was checked against their estimated ossification age obtained by the Greulick and Pyle method (1959). Correlation analysis was extended to the estimator variables as well.

Results and Discussion

The results of the correlation analyses are tabulated in Tables 1 to 3. For the 11-year-old children, bone age and the estimate of biological development correlated closely in both sexes. Estimator variables also showed a high relationship with bone age, except for chronological age (see Table 1).

Table 1

Correlation Matrix for Bone Age and Estimator Variables in 11-Year-Old Boys and Girls (25 Boys and 24 Girls)

	DA	BA	ST	BM	PI	BD
DA	—	0.64	0.62	0.49	0.50	0.70
BA	0.61	—	0.82	0.83	0.89	0.92
ST	0.57	0.82	—	0.86	0.81	0.87
BM	0.51	0.75	0.90	—	0.93	0.91
PI	0.63	0.86	0.85	0.88	—	0.93
BD	0.76	0.88	0.92	0.90	0.94	—

Abbreviations: DA = chronological age in decimal years; BA = ossification or bone age; ST = stature; BM = body mass; PI = plastic index; BD = biological development estimate. Girls are tabulated in the upper triangle, boys in the lower triangle.

Table 2

Correlation Matrix for Bone Age and Estimator Variables in 12-Year-Old Boys and Girls (30 Boys and 33 Girls)

	DA	BA	ST	BM	PI	BD
DA	—	0.34	0.32	0.13	0.22	0.31
BA	-0.16	—	0.71	0.83	0.87	0.96
ST	-0.06	0.67	—	0.79	0.79	0.80
BM	-0.06	0.80	0.91	—	0.80	0.92
PI	0.02	0.81	0.83	0.92	—	0.95
BD	0.10	0.86	0.86	0.91	0.92	—

Abbreviations as in Table 1. Top: girls; bottom: boys.

Table 3

Correlation Matrix for Bone Age and Estimator Variables in 13-Year-Old Boys and Girls (34 Boys and 49 girls)

	DA	BA	ST	BM	PI	BD
DA	—	0.24	0.12	0.16	0.08	0.32
BA	0.15	—	0.18	0.57	0.41	0.76
ST	0.03	0.79	—	0.71	0.77	0.60
BM	-0.13	0.66	0.72	—	0.85	0.89
PI	-0.15	0.68	0.74	0.96	—	0.83
BD	-0.01	0.88	0.90	0.85	0.85	—

Abbreviations as in Table 1. Top: girls; bottom: boys.

Correlations obtained in the age group of 12-year-old children were very similar to those of the 11-year-olds: High coefficients were found for biological development and low ones for decimal age (see Table 2).

In the group of 13-year-olds, there were fewer significant correlations for the girls than found either for the younger girls or for their male peers. The correlation between bone age and the estimate of biological development was only moderately high. Ossification age was unrelated to the estimator variables in this group of girls. For the 13-year-old boys, however, the obtained correlations had a pattern similar to the younger ones.

Estimates of the age of biological development obtained by the anthropometric method were numerically very close to the ones rendered by bone age assessment. Furthermore, it must be stressed that the age group in which the validity of the method was evidenced is, on the one hand, a very important one for the preparation of young athletes; on the other hand, it is regarded by other authors of estimation methods as being rather critical for an accurate estimate. Accordingly, the method appears to possess an additional advantage in that accuracy was not impaired even during the period of pubertal growth spurt which occurs in Hungary around the 12th year of age in girls, and around the 13th year of age in boys.

The time needed for taking the measurements and for obtaining the estimate is very short (2 min per subject for 1 observer), so even larger subject groups can be studied in a reasonable time.

Conclusion

Information concerning the status of biological development may be utilized not only for evaluating the motor performance of children, but also for developing training schedules, for modifying training loads when children of different ages train together, for predicting adult stature, and for analyzing child behavior under a number of practical conditions.

References

CONRAD, K. (1963). *Der Konstitutionstypus*. 2. Aufl. Berlin: Springer.

CRAMPTON, C.W. (1908). Physiological age—A fundamental principle. *American Physical Education Review*, **13**, 141-154.

DROBNÁ, M. (1979). Critical evaluation of methods of determination of skeletal age. In V.V. Novotny & Titlbachová (Eds.), *Methods of functional anthropology* (pp. 253-255). Prague: Universitas Carolina Pragensis.

GREULICH, W.W., & Pyle, S.I. (1959). *Radiographic atlas of skeletal development of the hand and wrist*. (2nd ed.). Stanford: Stanford University Press.

GRIMM, H. (1979). Criteria of biological age. In V.V. Novotny & S. Titlbachová (Eds.), *Methods of functional anthropology* (pp. 221-227). Prague: Universitas Carolina Pragensis.

HEBBELINCK, M. (1979). Methods of biological maturity assessment. In V.V. Novotny & S. Titlbachová (Eds.), *Methods of functional anthropology* (pp. 229-240). Prague: Universitas Carolina Pragensis.

MALINA, R.M., & Little, B.B. (1981). Comparison of TW-1 and TW-2 skeletal age differences in American black and white and Mexican children 6-13 years of age. *Annals of Human Biology*, **8**, 543-548.

MÉSZÁROS, J., & Mohácsi, J. (1983). *A biológiai fejlettség és a felnöt testmagasság meghatározása a városi fiatalok fejlödésmenete alapj'an (The assessment of biological development and adult stature on the basis of the growth curves of Hungarian urban youth.* In Hungarian.) Unpublished doctoral thesis, Hungarian University of Physical Education, Budapest.

ROCHE, A.F., Davils, G.H., & Eyman, S.L. (1971). A comparison between Greulich-Pyle and Tanner-Whitehouse assessments of skeletal maturity. *Radiology*, **98**, 273-290.

TANNER, J.M., & Whitehouse, R.H. (1959). *Standards for skeletal maturity. Part I*. Paris: International Children's Centre.

TANNER, J.M., Whitehouse, R.H., & Healey, M.J.R. (1962). *A new system for estimating skeletal maturity from the hand and wrist, with standards derived from a study of 2600 healthy British children. Part II: The scoring system.* Paris: International Children's Centre.

Some Notes on Physiological and Medical Considerations for Exercise and Training of Children

Oded Bar-Or
Chedoke-McMaster Hospitals
Hamilton, Ontario, Canada

With the current increase in their participation in competitive sports, children are subjected to an ever increasing physiological strain. The understanding of the physiological responses to exercise which are typical of children is therefore of relevance to coaches, physical educators, organizers of athletic events, and health professionals.

The following recommendations regarding the participation in sports of healthy and sick children are presented. These statements represent the author's biases and opinions.

Physiological Considerations

Although children can perform most sports pursued by adults, they differ from adults in various physiological capacities which may determine their level of success, or the inherent risk, in specific activities. Of special importance are the following characteristics:

1. Children's maximal aerobic power, when normalized for body weight, is similar to that of young adults (Robinson, 1938). The O_2 cost of walking (Skinner et al. 1971), of running (Åstrand, 1952) and possibly of other tasks is, however, relatively higher in children than in adults. Thus, children's "metabolic reserve" is smaller (Bar-Or, 1983a), and this limits their ability to sustain high-intensity submaximal activity. In contrast, during prolonged activities at intensities which do not exceed 60% of maximal aerobic power, cardiopulmonary responses of children are similar to those of adults (Máček, Vávra, & Novosadová, 1976).
2. Children's ability to generate power at supramaximal levels is lower than in adults (Bar-Or, 1983; di Prampero & Cerretelli, 1969; Kurowski, 1977). This is a major reason why children's performance is lower than that of adults in such activities as the 400 m run or swimming sprints.
3. Muscle strength is lower in children than in adults. It is related to body size and chronological age (Asmussen, 1973) and does not reach adult levels until some time after the growth spurt. A prepubescent cannot, therefore, be expected to perform at par with postpubescents in events which are dependent on absolute muscle strength.

4. There is a marked variability in the chronological age at which children develop and incur pubertal changes. Matching of children for competition should take this into account. An attempt should be made to consider matching by body size and sexual development.
5. Children's thermoregulatory efficiency is lower than in adults, especially when exposed to climatic extremes (Bar-Or, 1980). Due to their slower rate of acclimatization to heat (Inbar, 1978), their activities must be reduced in intensity and duration upon transition to a warm climate and then increased gradually during a 10- to 14-day period.
6. As is the case with adults, children do not voluntarily replenish all fluid losses during exercise (Bar-Or, Dotan, Inbar, Rotshtein, & Zonder, 1980). Fluid intake before and during activity must be enforced. One should teach the child to arrive fully hydrated for competition or practice sessions and to drink 100 to 150 ml every 15 to 20 min, even when not thirsty (American Academy of Pediatrics, 1982). The solute content in the fluid should not exceed 0.3 g/l NaCl, 0.35 g/l KCl and 2.0% glucose.
7. In some sports, deliberate fluid loss is a common practice. Noteworthy is adolescent wrestling (Tipton & Tcheng, 1970). New regulations should be enforced in these sports to minimize the necessity for rapid weight loss among children and adolescents.
8. In organizing an athletic event, climatic conditions must be taken into account. Health practitioners must have the authority to modify the hour of day or time of year of an athletic event, or even cancel it, if weather conditions so dictate.
9. Children lose heat in cool water faster than do adults (Sloan & Keatinge, 1973). When a swim practice takes place at water temperature less than 23° C, children—especially the lean and small—must be allowed to get out of the water every 10 to 15 min.

Medical Considerations

The health risk of participation in sports is not inherently greater in children than in adults, with the exception of greater susceptibility to injury at the epiphyseal-metaphyseal junction in long bones (Larson & McMahan, 1966). Even when some risk is involved, the physical and psychological detrimental effects of inactivity probably outweigh those of activity. All healthy children and the great majority of sick children should, therefore, be encouraged to pursue exercise and sports on a regular basis. The following diseases, discussed in alphabetical order, must be given special considerations.

Aortic Stenosis

Exercise can trigger syncope, angina pectoris, and sudden death (Doyle, Arumugham, Lara, Rutkowski, & Kiely, 1974). For children with a ventriculo-to-aortic pressure gradient of 40 mmHg or more, exertion is contraindicated. If the gradient is lower and the child is asymptomatic, mild and moderate recreational activities can be pursued. If the child is symptomatic (chest pain, syncope, but not mere "fatigue"), activity must be curtailed in coordination with a cardiologist (Bar-Or, 1983).

Bronchial Asthma

Exercise may induce bronchoconstriction. Most patients can pursue normal activity when controlled by prophylactic medication (β_2 sympathomimetic in aerosol or di-sodium cromoglycate) (Anderson, 1982). An asthmatic attack following exercise can be effectively treated by β_2 sympathomimetics (Anderson, Seale, Ferris, Schoeffel, & Lindsay, 1979). The dosage of medication may need to be increased (and activity curtailed) during cold or dry weather (Bar-Or, 1983b). Other means for reducing the effects of cold are nasal breathing (Shturman-Ellstein, Zeballos, Buckley, & Souhrada, 1978) or a face mask (Schachter, Lach, & Lee, 1981).

Swimming is the least asthmogenic activity, and some patients can benefit by switching to swimming from other sports. Asthmatic childen are trainable and they can reach top athletic levels (Fitch & Godfrey, 1976). The role of physical conditioning in improving the bronchial response to exercise is still controversial, even though some reports suggest a decrease in airway resistance following a standard task (Oseid & Haaland, 1978).

Cerebral Palsy

Patients, particularly with spasticity, tend to become overweight and hypoactive in adolescence, even if surgical and other therapies at a young age were successful in ambulating them. Sports and conditioning programs which are tailored to the residual ability of each patient are effective (Berg, 1970; Spira & Bar-Or, 1975) and are strongly recommended.

Congenital Complete Heart Block

Most patients can pursue normal activities. Exercise, however, may trigger dysrhythmia (Winkler, Freed, & Nadas, 1980) or syncope (Michaelson & Engle, 1972). Patients should therefore be exercise-tested to determine allowable levels of activity and a possible need for cardiac pacing.

Cystic Fibrosis

Recent data suggest that physical conditioning can improve bronchial clearance (Orenstein, Henks, & Cerny, 1983) and increase the endurance of the respiratory muscles (Keens et al., 1977). Children with advanced disease may respond to exercise with O_2 desaturation (Cerny, Pullano, & Cropp, 1982) Such children should refrain from intense activities.

Diabetes Mellitus

Exercise, together with diet and insulin therapy, is essential to good metabolic management in insulin-dependent diabetes mellitus (IDDM). Health practitioners, parents, and patients must learn the calorie equivalent of various activities and use this knowledge in management. An attempt must be made to spread the activities throughout the week with an equal calorie expenditure each day. Both hypoglycemia (Lawrence, 1926) and ketoacidosis (Marble & Smith, 1936) may accompany exercise in IDDM. The former can be prevented by selecting a nonexercising site for insulin injection (Koivisto & Felig, 1978), by increasing food intake prior to the activity or by reducing insulin dosage. The concept of "exercise exchanges" can be implemented in analogy to that of "food exchanges" (Bar-Or, 1983a). Ketoacidiosis can be prevented by taking insulin, as prescribed. A child should not exercise when insulin depleted or when ketoacidotic.

Epilepsy

Exercise, even when intense, does not entail a greater risk for seizures (Livingston, 1975), but seizures can occur during exercise as they do at rest (Korczyn, 1979). The risk involved in athletic participation must be weighed against the psychological trauma that results from restriction and social isolation (American Academy of Pediatrics, 1983). Patients covered by appropriate medication can be allowed to pursue all activities, excluding those which involve direct impact on the head (e.g., boxing, American football). In such activities as horseback riding, swimming, or mountain climbing, the child must be supervised. Contact sports (soccer, ice hockey, basketball) are not contraindicated, but, like any athlete, the child should be coached on the prevention of injury (American Medical Association, 1974). Patients who are not well controlled by medication should not pursue any activities which, during seizure, may cause damage to them or to others.

Hemophilia

Bleeding into joints and muscles often induces hypomobility and contractures. With the increasing availability of replacement therapy, hemophilia patients should not be restricted in their physical activity (Bar-Or, 1983). Preference should be given to noncontact sports.

Mental Retardation

Even though low maximal aerobic power (Bar-Or et al., 1971; Yoshizawa, Ishizaki, & Honda, 1975) and deficient motor skills (Kasch & Zasueta, 1971; Rarick, Widdop, & Broadhead, 1970) have been found among children with low IQ, mental retardation per se does not cause low fitness. It is the social isolation and the relative hypoactivity of many mentally retarded children that can be implicated (Bjørke, Hagen, Lie, et al., 1978; Maksud & Hamilton, 1974), in addition to a short attention span and deficient learning ability.

Both educable and trainable mentally retarded children can respond to training with improved physiological adaptation to exercise (Kasch & Zasueta, 1971; Skrobac-Kaczynski & Vavik, 1980) and some mental functions (Oliver, 1958). As stated by the American Academy of Pediatrics (1974), "Every retarded child needs a continuing program of physical maintenance with regular exercising and supervised athletic activities."

Muscular Dystrophy

Physical hypoactivity may render the child irreversibly immobile. More research is needed on the beneficial and detrimental effects of exericse. Training regimens which include strengthening of the residual muscle tissue and its endurance seem, however, to prolong the period that the child can be ambulatory, even when the disease is progressive (Vignos & Watkins, 1966).

Obesity

Obese children tend to be hypoactive due to psychosocial reasons and to detraining (Bruch, 1940; Bullen, Reed, & Mayer, 1964). Increased physical activity is of major therapeutic value for weight and fat control (Pařizková, Vaněčková, & Vamberová, 1962; Ylitalo, 1981), as well as in improving body image (Stanley, Glaser, Levin, Adams, & Coley, 1970) and instilling self-confidence in the child (Peckos, Spargo, & Heald, 1960). Optimal therapeutic regimens should combine exercise with restricted calorie intake (Bar-Or, 1983a).

References

AMERICAN Academy of Pediatrics. (1974). Joint Committee on Physical Fitness, Recreation and Sports Medicine. Athletic activities for children who are mentally retarded. *Pediatrics,* **54,** 376-377.

AMERICAN Academy of Pediatrics. (1982). Committee on Sports Medicine. Position Statement. Climatic heat stress and the exercising child. *Pediatrics,* **69,** 808-809.

AMERICAN Academy of Pediatrics. (1983). Committee on Children with Handicaps and Committee on Sports Medicine. Sports and the child with epilepsy. *Pediatrics,* **72,** 884-885.

AMERICAN Medical Association Committee on the Medical Aspects of Sports. (1974). Epileptics and contact sports. Position statement. *Journal of American Medical Association,* **229,** 820-821.

ANDERSON, S., Seale, J.P., Ferris, L., Schoeffel, R., & Lindsay, D.A. (1979). An evaluation of pharmacotherapy for exercise-induced asthma. *Journal of Allergy and Clinical Immunology,* **64,** 612-614.

ANDERSON, S.D. (1982). Exercise-induced asthma: Current views. *Patient Management,* **6,** 43-55.

ASMUSSEN, E. (1973). Growth in muscular strength and power. In L. Rarick (Ed.), *Physical activity, human growth and development.* New York: Academic Press.

ÅSTRAND, P.O. (1952). *Experimental studies of physical working capacity in relation to sex and age.* Copenhagen: Munksgaard.

BAR-OR, O. (1980). Climate and the exercising child—a review. *International Journal of Sports Medicine,* **1,** 53-65.

BAR-OR, O. (1983a). *Pediatric sports medicine for the practitioner: From physiologic principles to clinical applications.* New York: Springer-Verlag.

BAR-OR, O. (1983b). Climatic conditions and their effect on exercise-induced asthma. In S. Oseid & A.M. Edwards (Eds.), *The asthmatic child in play and sport* (pp. 61-73). London: Pitman Books Limited.

BAR-OR, O., Dotan, R., Inbar, O., Rotshtein, A., & Zonder, H. (1980). Voluntary hypohydration in 10- to 12-year-old boys. *Journal of Applied Physiology: Respiratory, Environmental, and Exercise Physiology,* **48,** 104-108.

BAR-OR, O., Skinner, J.S., Bersteinová, V., Shearburn, C., Bell, C.W., Royer, D., Haas, J., & Buskirk, E.R. (1971). Maximal aerobic capacity of 6-15 year old girls and boys with subnormal intelligence quotients. *Acta Paediatrica Scandinavica Supplement,* **217**, 108-113.

BERG, K. (1970). Effect of physical training of school children with cerebral palsy. *Acta Paediatrica Scandinavica Supplement,* **204**, 27-33.

BJØRKE, G., Hagen, R., Lie, H., et al. (1978). Physical activation of mentally retarded children. *Journal of Norwegian Medical Association,* **3**,134-136.

BRUCH, H. (1940). Obesity in childhood. IV. Energy expenditure of obese children. *American Journal of Diseases of Children,* **60**, 1082-1109.

BULLEN, B.A., Reed, R.B., & Mayer, J. (1964). Physical activity of obese and nonobese adolescent girls appraised by motion picture sampling. *American Journal of Clinical Nutrition,* **14**, 211-223.

CERNY, F.J., Pullano, T.P., & Cropp, G.J.A. (1982). Cardiorespiratory adaptations to exercise in cystic fibrosis. *American Review of Respiratory Diseases,* **126**, 217-220.

DI PRAMPERO, P.E., & Carretelli, P. (1969). Maximal muscular power (aerobic and anaerobic) in African natives. *Ergonomics,* **12**, 51-59.

DOYLE, E.F., Arumugham, P., Lara, E., Rutkowski, M.R., & Kiely, B. (1974). Sudden death in young patients with congenital aortic stenosis. *Pediatrics,* **53**, 481-489.

FITCH, K.D., & Godfrey, S. (1976). Asthma and athletic performance. *Journal of American Medical Association,* **236**, 152-157.

INBAR, O. (1978). Acclimitization to dry and hot environment in young adults and children 8-10 years old. Unpublished doctoral dissertation, Columbia University.

KASCH, F.W., & Zasueta, S.A. (1971). Physical capacities of mentally retarded children. *Acta Paediatrica Scandinavica Supplement,* **217**, 114-118.

KEENS, T.G., Krastins, I.R.B., Wannamaker, E.M., Levinson, H., Crozier, O.N., & Bryan, C. (1977). Ventilatory muscle endurance training in normal subjects and patients with cystic fibrosis. *American Review of Respiratory Diseases,* **116**, 853-860.

KOIVISTO, V.A., & Felig, P. (1978). Effects of leg exercise on insulin absorption in diabetic patients. *New England Journal of Medicine,* **298**, 79-83.

KORCZYN, A.D. (1979). Participation of epileptic patients in sports. *Journal of Sports Medicine and Physical Fitness,* **19**, 195-198.

KUROWSKI, T.T. (1977). Anaerobic power of children from ages 9 through 15 years. Unpublished Master's thesis, Florida State University.

LARSON, R.L., & McMahan, R.O. (1966). The epiphyses and the childhood athlete. *Journal of American Medical Association,* **169**, 99-104.

LAWRENCE, R.D. (1926). The effect of exercise on insulin action in diabetes. *British Medical Journal,* **1**, 648-650.

LIVINGSTON, S. (1975). Should epileptics be athletes? *Sports Medicine,* **3**, 67-72.

MÁĆEK, M., Vávra, J., & Novosadová, J. (1976). Prolonged exercise in prepubertal boys. I. Cardiovascular and metabolic adjustment. *European Journal of Applied Physiology,* **34**, 291-298.

MAKSUD, M.G., & Hamilton, L.H. (1974). *Physiological responses of EMR children to strenuous exercise. American Journal of Mental Deficiency,* **79**, 32-38.

MARBLE, A., & Smith, R.M. (1936). Exercise in diabetes mellitus. *Archives of Internal Medicine,* **58**, 577-588.

MICHAELSON, M., & Engle, M.A. (1972). Congenital complete heart block: An international study. The natural history. *Cardiovascular Clinics,* **4**, 85-101.

OLIVER, J.N. (1958). The effect of physical conditioning exercises and activities on the mental characteristics of educationally subnormal boys. *British Journal of Educational Psychology,* **28**, 155-165.

ORENSTEIN, D.M., Henks, K.G., & Cerny, F.J. (1983). Exercise and cystic fibrosis. *The Physician and Sportsmedicine,* **11**, 57-63.

OSEID, S., & Haaland, K. (1978). Exercise studies on asthmatic children before and after regular physical training. In B. Erikkson & B. Furberg (Eds.), *Swimming medicine IV* pp. (32-41). Baltimore: University Park Press.

PAŘIZKOVÁ, J., Vanecková, M., & Vamberová, M. (1962). A study of changes in some functional indicators following reduction of excessive fat in obese children. *Physiologica Bohemoslovenica,* **11**, 351-357.

PECKOS, P.S., Spargo, J.A., & Heald, F.P. (1960). Program and results of a camp for obese adolescent girls. *Postgraduate Medicine,* **27**, 527-533.

RARICK, G.L., Widdop, J.H., & Broadhead, G.D. (1970). The physical fitness and motor performance of educable mentally retarded children. *Exceptional Children,* **36**, 509-519.

ROBINSON, S. (1938). Experimental studies of physical fitness in relation to age. *Int. Z. Angew. Physiol. Einschl. Arbeitsphysiol.,* **10**, 251-323.

SCHACHTER, E.N., Lach, E., & Lee, M. (1981). The protective effect of a cold weather mask on exercise-induced asthma. *Annals of Allergy,* **46**, 12-16.

SHTURMAN-ELLSTEIN, R., Zeballos, R.J., Buckley, J.M., & Souhrada, J.F. (1978). The beneficial effect of nasal breathing on exercise-induced bronchoconstriction. *American Review of Respiratory Diseases,* **118**, 65-73.

SKINNER, J.S., Bar-Or, O., Bergsteinová, V., Bell, C.W., Royer, D., & Buskirk, E.R. (1971). Comparison of continuous and intermittent tests for determining maximal oxygen intake in children. *Acta Paediatrica Scandinavica Supplement,* **217**, 24-28.

SKROBAC-KACZYNSKI, J., & Vavik, T. (1980). Physical fitness and trainability of young male patients with Down syndrome. In K. Berg & B.O. Eriksson (Eds.), *Children and exercise IX* (pp. 300-316). Baltimore: University Park Press.

SLOAN, R.E.G., & Keatinge, W.R. (1973). Cooling rates of young people swimming in cold water. *Journal of Applied Physiology* **35**, 371-375.

SPIRA, R., & Bar-Or, O. (1975). *An investigation of the ambulation problems associated with severe motor paralysis in adolescents.* Influence of physical conditioning and adapted sports activities. Final report. Project No. 19-P-58065-F-01. Tel Aviv: U.S. Department of Health, Education and Welfare, S.R.S.

STANLEY, E.J., Glaser, H.H., Levin, D.G., Adams, P.A., & Coley, I.L. (1970). Overcoming obesity in adolescents. A description of a promising endeavour to improve management. *Clinical Pediatrics,* **9**, 29-36.

TIPTON, C.M., & Tcheng, T.-K. (1970). Iowa wrestling study. Weight loss in high school students. *Journal of American Medical Association,* **214**, 1269-1274.

VIGNOS, P.J., & Watkins, M.P. (1966). The effect of exercise in muscle dystrophy. *Journal of American Medical Association,* **197**, 843-848.

WINKLER, R.B., Freed, M.D., & Nadas, A.S. (1980). Exercise-induced ventricular ectopy in children and young adults with complete heart block. *American Heart Journal,* **99**, 87-92.

YLITALO, V. (1981). Treatment of obese schoolchildren with special reference to the mode of therapy, cardiorespiratory performance and the carbohydrate and lipid metabolism. *Acta Paediatrica Scandinavica Supplement,* **290**, 1-109.

YOSHIZAWA, S. Ishizaki, T., & Honda, H. (1975), Aerobic work capacity of mentally retarded boys and girls in junior high schools. *Journal of Human Ecology* (Tokyo), **4**, 15-26.

Long-Term Effects of Excessive Training Procedures on Young Athletes

Joseph Rutenfranz
Institut für Arbeitsphysiologie an der Universität Dortmund
Dortmund, West Germany

For most coaches, sport organizations, and doctors of all important "sport nations," epidemiology is an untried procedure. Thus, it is difficult to determine whether the usually excessive training of young athletes (children and adolescents) causes harmful effects on their psychological, social, or physical well-being. Although distinctive answers are impossible at the present time, the following indications are reasonable:

1. The extreme monotony of many training procedures should not be neglected. This is important not only for swimming, but also for several technical disciplines. Children have to learn to concentrate on sport activities as an important part of their life, for such participation may have a positive effect on their personality; however, at the same time, it may reduce nearly all other leisure time activities (Kaminski & Ruoff, 1979).

2. Another problem is the social isolation which may occur in groups of young athletes with homogeneous but reduced interests. Many curriculum vitae of athletes may be contradictory to this statement, but a lack of appropriate opportunities for different kinds of socialization processes clearly exists.

3. The improvement of physical well-being even by excessive training of young athletes seems to be evident. On the basis of our physiological knowledge, positive effects of intensive and long-lasting endurance training programs such as running, swimming, or cycling on the cardiopulmonary system are plausible and supported by many studies. However, a critical review of the literature reveals that most studies do not reflect the problems of "drop-outs," "healthy athletes-effects" and "self-selection." The results of most training studies do not support the assumption that such training programs have no adverse effects for all children who have started such training intensities early in life. Such studies may, therefore, justify only the statement that young healthy athletes are able to survive the usual heavy training programs such as 180 to 200 km of running/week (beginning at 11 to 14 years of age), 65,000 m of swimming/week (beginning at 12 to 14 years of age), or 150 to 250 km of cycling/week (beginning at 14 to 15 years of age).

However, survival without permanent physical harm is no longer undisputed for sport disciplines which require special training of muscle strength and coordination. Female gymnasts, who live in special environments as "gifted children," usually have daily training programs of about 5 to 7 hours after school. During the most important training period (6 to 16 years of age), this training may include 8,000 jumps/year or 80,000 jumps altogether (Lenhart, 1971). The jumps for high divers are more frequent: A career of a young diver may include 4,500 to 14,000 jumps/year (Groher, 1971a, b). Similar problems exist with figure skaters, trampolin jumpers, and so on (Groher, 1971a, b). Javelin throwers have to develop a special torsion or scoliosis of the vertebra for a successful throw. They need at least an 8-year training period with 6,000 throws/year, totaling 50,000 throws (Rompe, 1971).

Many of these disciplines require muscle strength, which can only be developed by conditioning and training, that is, special body-building programs. Authorities on sports medicine have on several occasions indicated that such programs are dangerous for preadolescents (Hollmann & Hettinger, 1976). However, one suspects that perhaps an unknown number of children start too early with such training procedures. It is, therefore, not surprising that the incidence of skeletal complaints, lesions, or diseases in groups of gymnasts, high divers, figure skaters, and javelin throwers who have started to train during early childhood or adolescence is higher than in control groups (Garrick & Requa, 1978; Groher, 1969, 1971a, b; Mathie, 1977; Oseid, Evjenth, Gunnart, & Meen, 1973; Refior & Zenker, 1970; Rompe, 1971; Rütt, 1971; Schwerdtner, Fohler, & Schmitt, 1976; Tütsch & Ulrich, 1973). This must be considered with respect to the fact that groups of young athletes are highly selected groups. Very little has been known until now about the incidence of such physical problems in groups of "dropouts" after a long period of hard training. It is, however, suspicious that on the average, 4 out of 10 of the best young athletes of the different sport disciplines drop out when training continues after the national junior championships. Therefore, this problem should be addressed by more effective investigations, using methods of epidemiology, particularly prospective cohort studies.

Ethical Proposals and Practical Consequences

The statements already presented may lead to the conclusion that it is unreasonable to continue to neglect such important information, or to withhold it from pediatrics, applied physiology, biomechanics, auxology, and orthopedics. In other words, pediatrics and sports medicine have the duty to protect gifted children and young athletes against coaches' training goals that may harm the integrity, the well-being, or the health of the children.

An ethical code for sports activities in childhood and early adolescence may include the following proposals and pracical consequences (Rutenfranz, 1982):

1. Use of the declarations of Helsinki and Tokyo, repsectively, in connection with human experiments on "athletic training."
2. Written consent after written explanation on forms, which must be capable of being understood regarding the special age of children and the health risks involved in specific training procedures.
3. Special health care and prophylactic measures should be performed by physicians, whose professional reputations are not dependent on the records of special young athletes.

4. Establishment of "Ethic Commissions" in the national sport organizations, that are open to questions by children and their parents. These commissions, consisting of independent people with special experience in education, pediatrics, law, and ethics, should discuss and control the risks of training methods for children.
5. Commissions or other scientific-based boards should propose or fix age limits for the participation of children at Olympic games or national and international championships. This may only be a guarantee that the ages of the athletes are adequate to participate in training procedures and particularly reduce the abnormal predominance of children at female sport games. The fascination for spectators of Olympic games of children acting as athletes does not include a responsibility for the health and safe development of these children. Therefore, it seems to be necessary to resist such illusions and fascinations in order to protect the children for themselves, their parents, their coaches, and the spectators.

References

GARRICK, J.G., & Requa, R.K. (1978). Girl's sports injuries in high school athletics. *Journal of the American Medical Association,* **239**, 2245-2248.

GROHER, W. (1969). Kreuzschmerzen und Wirbelsäulenveränderungen bei Kunst- und Trumspringern (Backaches of acrobatic and high divers). *Sportarzt und Sportmedizin,* **20**, 444-450.

GROHER, W. (1971a). Rückenschmerzen bei Kunst- und Trumspringern. (Versuch einer Analyse) (Back pains in high divers and vaulters—preliminary analysis). *Sportarzt und Sportmedizin,* **22**, 261-263.

GROHER, W. (1971b). Belastungen kindlicher und jugendlicher Lendenwirbelsäulen beim Sport (Turnen, Kunstspringen, Trampolinspringen) (Strains of the lower back in children and youth from sport: Gymnastics, skilled jumping, and trampolining). In K. Stucke (Ed.), *Deutscher Sportärztebund, Verhandlungen 24. Tagung Würzburg 14.-17.10.1971* (pp. 176-178). Gräfeling: Demeter.

HOLLMANN, W., & Hettinger, Th. (1976). *Sportmedizin—Arbeits- und Trainingsgrundlagen (Sports medicine—Work and training principles).* Stuttgart: Schattauer.

KAMINSKI, G., & Ruoff, B.A. (1979). Kinder im Hochleistungssport (Children in high performance sport). In H. Gabler, H. Eberspächer, E. Hahn, J. Kern, & G. Schilling (Eds.), *Praxis del Psychologie im Leistungssport* pp. 200-224. Berlin: Bartels & Wernitz KG.

LENHART, P. (1971). Belastungen des Bewegungsapparates beim Bodenturnen der Damen (Strains of the lower extremities in women gymnasts). In K. Stucke (Ed.), *Deutscher Sportärztebund, Verhandlungen 24. Tagung Würzburg 14.-17.10.1971* (p. 181). Gräfelfing: Demeter.

MATHIE, F. (1977). Schäden am Bewegungsapparat von Jugendlichen im alpinen Leistungssport (Injuries to the locomotor apparatus of young people in competitive alpine sports). *Zeitschrift für Orthopaedie und ihre Grenzgebiete,* **115**, 866-875.

OSEID, S., Evjenth, G., Gunnart, H., & Meen, D. (1973). Lower back trouble in young female gymnasts. Frequency, symptoms and possible causes. In O. Grupe (Ed.), *Sport in unserer Welt—Chancen und Probleme (Referate, Ergebnisse und Materialien)* pp. 564-565. Berlin: Springer.

REFIOR, H.J. (1971). Wirbelsäulenveränderungen bei Leistungsturnern—Verlaufsbeobachtungen bei Kindern und Jugendlichen (Vertebral column changes in gymnastic performers: Observations in children and youth). In K. Stucke (Ed.), *Deutscher Sportärztebund, Verhandlungen 24. Tagung Würzburg 14.-17.10.1971* (pp. 171-175). Gräfelfing: Demeter.

REFIOR, H.J., & Zenker, H. (1970). Wirbelsäule und Leistungsturnen (The vertebral column and competitive gymnastics). *Münchener medizinische Wochenschrift*, **112**, 463-467.

ROMPE, G. (1971). Wirbelsäulenschäden jugendlicher Speerwerfer (Injuries to the vertebral column in youthful javelin throwers). In K. Stucke (Ed.), *Deutscher Sportärztebund, Verhandlungen 24. Tagung Würzburg 14.-17.10.1971* (pp. 179-180). Gräfelfing: Demeter.

RUTENFRANZ, J. (1982). Ethische Probleme des Leistungsdrucks beim Kind, dargestellt am Beispiel des Hochleistungssports (Ethical problems of pressure performances of children presented for example in high performance sport). In H. Müller & H. Olbing (Eds.), *Ethische Probleme in der Pädiatrie und ihren Grenzgebieten* (pp. 279-288). München: Urban & Schwarzenberg.

RÜTT, A. (1971). Jugendsport und die Schädigungsmöglichkeiten der Wirbelsäule, insbesondere bei der Scheuermann'schen Krankheit (Youth sport and the possibilities for injury to the vertebral column especially in Scheuermann's disease). In K. Stucke (Ed.), *Deutscher Sportärztebund, Verhandlungen 24. Tagung Würzburg 14.-17.10.1971* (pp. 166-170). Gräfelfing: Demeter.

SCHWERDTNER, H.P., Fohler, N., & Schmitt, E. (1976). Vorschädigung oder Sportschäden der Wirbelsäule bei Hochleistungssportlern im Kunstturnen (Preinjury or sport injury of the vertebral column of skilled performers in gymnastics). *Sportarzt und Sportmedizin*, **27**, 155-166.

TÜTSCH, C., & Ulrich, S.P. (1973). Wirbelsäule und Hochleistungsturnen (The vertebral column and high performance gymnastics). *Schweizerische Runschau für Medizin Praxis*, **62**, 1085-1098.

DATE DUE

JUL 0 7 1999			
JUN 1 7 1980			
GAYLORD			PRINTED IN U.S.A.